Orthopaedic Care

OF THE

Geriatric Patient

Edited by

THOMAS P. SCULCO, M.D.

Clinical Associate Professor of Orthopedic Surgery,
Cornell University Medical College;
Associate Attending Orthopedic Surgeon,
The Hospital for Special Surgery;
Associate Attending Orthopedic Surgeon, New York Hospital;
Chief of Orthopedic Surgery, Bronx V.A. Hospital;
Consultant, Orthopedics, Memorial Sloan-Kettering Cancer Center;
Orthopedic Consultant, Mary Manning Walsh Nursing Home,
New York, New York

with 362 illustrations

The C. V. Mosby Company

ST. LOUIS • TORONTO • PRINCETON   1985

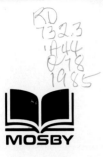

MOSBY

A TRADITION OF PUBLISHING EXCELLENCE

Editor: Eugenia A. Klein
Assistant editor: Jean F. Carey
Editing supervisor: Lin A. Dempsey
Manuscript editor: Jessica Bender
Book design: Jeanne Genz
Cover design: Kathleen A. Johnson
Production: Susan Trail

The C.V. Mosby Company
11830 Westline Industrial Drive, St. Louis, Missouri 63146

Library of Congress Cataloging in Publication Data

Main entry under title:

Orthopaedic care of the geriatric patient.

  Bibliography: p.
  Includes index.
    1. Geriatric orthopedics. I. Sculco, Thomas P.
[DNLM: 1. Orthopedics—in old age. 2. Muscular
Diseases—in old age. 3. Muscular Diseases—therapy.
4. Bone Diseases—in old age. 5. Bone Diseases—
therapy.   WE 168 07625]
RD732.3.A44078 1985   618.97'73   84-22834
ISBN 0-8016-4403-8

GW/MV/MV 9 8 7 6 5 4 3 2 1   05/C/609

CONTRIBUTORS

WALTHER H.O. BOHNE, M.D.

Clinical Associate Professor of Surgery (Orthopaedics), Cornell University Medical College; Associate Attending Orthopaedic Surgeon, Department of Orthopaedic Surgery, Assistant Attending Radiologist, Department of Radiology and Nuclear Medicine, Associate Scientist, Research Division, The Hospital for Special Surgery; Assistant Attending Surgeon, Bone Service, Department of Surgery, Memorial Sloan-Kettering Cancer Center, New York, New York

JAMES WARREN BROWN, M.D.

Clinical Associate Professor, Department of Psychiatry, Cornell University Medical College; Associate Attending Psychiatrist, New York Hospital, Payne Whitney Clinic; Associate Attending Psychiatrist, The Hospital for Special Surgery; Assistant Attending Psychiatrist, St. Vincent's Hospital, New York, New York

WILLIAM E. BURKHALTER, M.D.

Professor of Orthopaedics and Vice-Chairman, Department of Orthopaedics and Rehabilitation; Chief, Division of Hand Surgery, University of Miami, Miami, Florida

BRENDAN CLIFFORD, M.D.

Consultant, Stroke Service, Rancho Los Amigos Hospital, Downey, California

J. WILLIAM FIELDING, M.D., F.R.C.S.(C)

Director of Orthopaedic Surgery, St. Luke's–Roosevelt Hospital Center; Clinical Professor of Orthopaedic Surgery, Columbia University College of Physicians and Surgeons, New York, New York

ALEXANDER HERSH, M.D.

Emeritus Chief, Foot Service, Attending Orthopaedic Surgeon, The Hospital for Special Surgery; Consultant, Orthopedic Institute, New York, New York

RICHARD L. JACOBS, M.D.

Professor and Head, Department of Orthopaedic Surgery, Albany Medical College, Albany, New York

CHRISTOPHER JORDAN, M.D.

Clinical Associate Professor, Department of Orthopaedic Surgery, University of Southern California, Los Angeles, California; Chief, Stroke Service, Rancho Los Amigos Hospital, Downey, California

JOSEPH M. LANE, M.D.

Professor of Orthopaedic Surgery, Cornell University Medical College; Chief, Metabolic Bone Disease, The Hospital for Special Surgery; Chief, Division of Orthopaedic Surgery, Memorial Sloan-Kettering Cancer Center, New York, New York

JOHN P. LYDEN, M.D.

Clinical Associate Professor of Surgery, Department of Orthopaedics, Cornell University Medical College; Associate Attending Orthopaedic Surgeon, The Hospital for Special Surgery; Associate Attending Surgeon, Department of Orthopaedics, New York Hospital, New York, New York

RICHARD R. McCORMACK, Jr., M.D.

Assistant Attending Orthopaedic Surgeon, The Hospital for Special Surgery, New York, New York

ERIN McGURK-BURLESON, R.P.T.

Supervisor, Physical Therapy Department, Sharp Rehabilitation Center, San Diego, California

M. JOANNA MELLOR, M.S.

Assistant Program Director, Third Age Center, Fordham University; Gerontological Consultant, Network Associates, New York, New York

ROBERT L. MERKOW, M.D.

Senior Orthopaedic Resident, The Hospital for Special Surgery, New York, New York

VERNON L. NICKEL, M.D.

Professor of Surgery, Department of Orthopaedics and Rehabilitation, University of California at San Diego; Director of Rehabilitation, Sharp Rehabilitation Center, San Diego, California

EMMANUEL RUDD, M.D.

Associate Clinical Professor, Department of Medicine, Cornell University Medical College, New York, New York

KENNETH P. SCILEPPI, M.D.

Assistant Professor of Medicine, Division of Geriatrics and Gerontology, Cornell University Medical College, New York, New York

CYNTHIA D. SCULCO, R.N., Ed.D.

Associate Professor, Hunter Bellvue School of Nursing, Hunter College, New York, New York

THOMAS P. SCULCO, M.D.

Clinical Associate Professor of Orthopedic Surgery, Cornell University Medical College; Associate Attending Orthopedic Surgeon, The Hospital for Special Surgery; Associate Attending Orthopedic Surgeon, New York Hospital; Chief of Orthopedic Surgery, Bronx V.A. Hospital; Consultant, Orthopedics, Memorial Sloan-Kettering Cancer Center; Orthopedic Consultant, Mary Manning Walsh Nursing Home, New York, New York

STEVEN F. SEIDMAN, M.D.

Assistant Attending Anesthesiologist, Department of Anesthesiology, The Hospital for Special Surgery, New York, New York

EILEEN TRIOLO, R.N.

Assistant Director of Nursing, Staff Development Department, The Hospital for Special Surgery, New York, New York

PETER TSAIRIS, M.D.

Associate Professor of Clinical Neurology, Cornell University Medical College; Director of Neurology, The Hospital for Special Surgery, New York, New York

RUSSELL F. WARREN, M.D.

Associate Professor of Orthopaedic Surgery, Cornell University Medical College; Director of Sports Medicine, Arm and Shoulder Clinic, The Hospital for Special Surgery, New York, New York

ROBERT L. WATERS, M.D.

Clinical Professor, Department of Orthopaedic Surgery, University of Southern California, Los Angeles, California; Chairman, Department of Surgery, Rancho Los Amigos Hospital, Downey, California

MARC E. WEKSLER, M.D.

Wright Professor of Medicine, Department of Medicine, Cornell University Medical College, New York, New York

To
the memory of my beloved mother
Mary Rafferty Sculco

FOREWORD

Diseases and disabilities of bones, muscles, and joints are the common problems in the elderly, accounting for more than one third of significant disabilities. To give some insight to the personal and socioeconomic costs, osteoporosis has an incredible annual cost: 200,000 hip fractures that account for almost 50,000 deaths a year, millions of days spent in hospitals, and billions of dollars in cost.

Genuine progress in dealing with musculoskeletal disease will depend on basic science as well as application. We must better understand bone and cartilage cell structure and function as well as bone deposition and resorption. We must learn more about the nature of inflammatory destruction of joint cartilage.

We see that there is no shortage of research needs and opportunities for those interested in the study of the common afflictions of old age. Mechanical, degenerative, biochemical, and regenerative processes need study. Collagen appears to undergo cross-linkage with aging. Proteoglycans, compounds that account for cartilage elasticity, need to be better understood. As is so often the case, methodologic developments constitute the necessary infrastructure to uncover new findings. Sensitive radioimmunoassays and computed tomography are among such technologic steps.

The study of connective tissue cells such as fibroblasts, osteoblasts, and chondrocytes can be studied in tissue culture from young or old animals or from humans. Thus we can learn more about the synthesis of collagen, proteoglycan, and enzymes in relationship to aging. Of course, we must also study, invest, and then evaluate types of medical and surgical management of the orthopaedic and musculoskeletal problems of old age.

Fortunately, the "National Plan for Research on Aging, Toward an Independant Old Age" published in 1982 by the National Institute on Aging includes consideration of musculoskeletal aspects of aging and is a useful guide to those concerned with the discovery and application of new knowledge.

I hope and expect that this fine book edited by Thomas P. Sculco will have successive editions reflecting the continued flourishing of this important field—and so enhancing further the quality of life of older persons.

Robert N. Butler, M.D.

Brookdale Professor of Geriatric
and Adult Development; Chairman, Gerald
and May Ellen Ritter Department of
Geriatric and Adult Development,
Mount Sinai Medical Center,
New York, New York

FOREWORD

There are two common tragedies of aging that humanity presently has to live with: the aging person of sound body whose mind fails and the aging person of sound mind whose body fails. With an increasingly aging population, the incidence of each is on the rise.

Dr. Sculco and his coauthors have done a great service for our aging population by writing this book, which concerns itself with the second of these two tragedies and how to deal with it. The book brings together a team concept of how to manage musculoskeletal disability in the geriatric patient. The thrust of the text is to provide to the orthopaedist and gerontologist an overview of the spectrum of the orthopaedic problems that occur in the elderly.

The first part of the text deals with the geriatric patient in general and the changes of aging in the musculoskeletal system in particular. The second section deals with specific anatomic areas and the pathologic processes that affect these areas in the geriatric age group. The authors give details of their preferred treatment for common afflictions affecting each anatomic area. The third section deals with associated disorders of the musculoskeletal systems in the elderly and includes metabolic bone disease, fracture management (including pathologic fractures), diabetic complications, amputations, and the management of musculoskeletal complications of stroke. The fourth section deals with the nursing and physical therapy considerations in these patients, as well as long-term planning of care.

Although there have been one or two monographs on this subject, no other text exists that deals as comprehensively as this book with the musculoskeletal problems of the elderly.

Orthopaedic Care of the Geriatric Patient should be on the shelf of every physician who cares for geriatric patients, regardless of specialty, as a valuable resource of information about what to expect in the way of problems in the musculoskeletal system of the aging patient and what to do about them when they occur.

Philip D. Wilson, Jr., M.D.

Professor of Orthopedic Surgery,
Cornell University Medical College;
Surgeon-in-Chief, The Hospital
for Special Surgery,
New York, New York

PREFACE

One must wait until evening to see how splendid the day has been.
Sophocles

When sitting down to write a preface to a book dealing with the orthopaedic care of the geriatric patient, the editor is confronted with a series of questions that reflect back to the initial stimulus to organize such a book. Why collect this information at all? Who is geriatric? Should such a text be directed to orthopaedists, to gerontologists, or to all physicians (since most will deal with musculoskeletal problems in the elderly)?

Certainly the population is aging and with increasing life expectancy will continue to do so. With advancing years the musculoskeletal system is a common cause for seeking a physician's advice, and the entire spectrum of primary care providers may be approached for such advice. This text is designed to deal with the myriad disorders affecting the geriatric patient and to emphasize the overlap of disorders from other organ systems in these patients. The goal is to discuss all elements of the musculoskeletal system and conditions that affect it so that primary diagnosis and treatment can be instituted. More comprehensive consideration of the surgical treatment of these conditions is provided for the surgeon involved in their care.

Aging brings with it a subset of unique problems that are superimposed on musculoskeletal pathology. It is correct that this compendium should be available in one place, with emphasis on the pathophysiology and treatment, without subjecting the physician to multiple reference sources.

Considerable debate arises in the attempt to define what is meant by "geriatric." There is probably no absolutely correct explanation, and the societally imposed chronologic age of 65 years is inexact. In a medical sense "geriatric" refers to physiologic characteristics that may not manifest themselves until the eighth or ninth decade of life, or perhaps as early as the sixth. The intent of the text is to deal with these pathologic and age-related conditions, since often both components affect the chronologically geriatric patient.

The emphasis of this volume is on maintaining function and independence for the aged patient with a musculoskeletal disorder. Surgical treatment is feasible in these patients if careful perioperative supervision is maintained. The team approach is paramount; from the initial medical evaluation to anesthetic and surgical care to nursing, rehabilitation, and long-term care goals, all involved must develop a reasonable and coordinated plan of care if the geriatric patient is to improve his functional capabilities.

As the writer Tryon Edwards has stated, "Age does not depend upon years, but upon temperament and health." Indeed, proper care of the orthopaedic problems of the geriatric patient can improve both of these elements.

Many contributions to this text must be acknowledged, especially those of the authors who brought the idea to fruition. I would particularly like to thank Carol Tabatt and Isabel Gnau for the voluminous typing and correspondence they completed and Jean Carey of Mosby for her support and patience. Finally, I offer love and thanks to my wife and children, who persevered in my absence while this book was in progress.

Thomas P. Sculco

CONTENTS

part I
THE GERIATRIC PATIENT

chapter 1
AGING OF THE MUSCULOSKELETAL SYSTEM

Kenneth P. Scileppi

Discrimination against elderly patients as surgical candidates solely on the basis of age is a prejudice that has markedly diminished over the past several decades. Advancements in anesthetic and surgical techniques and their adaptation to suit the special problems of the elderly have reduced significantly the once prohibitive mortality of major surgery in this age group. The performance of such major feats of cardiac surgery as valve replacements and coronary artery bypasses in patients older than 75 years of age is no longer a reportable event, although not yet a routine one either. The field of orthopaedic surgery has more than shared in this process of the gradual extension of age eligibility limits for major procedures; even more impressive within the field of orthopaedics has been the development of what may be legitimately called "geriatric surgery." Techniques of joint replacement and fracture repair have been developed in the past 20 years that specifically address a spectrum of problems common only in the elderly and for whom the average patient—not the exceptional one—is in the eighth or ninth decade of life. Geriatric orthopaedics has revolutionized in such a short time the prognosis for death and disability from such conditions as arthritic and fractured hips that physicians frequently find elderly patients and their families in need of persuasive encouragement to abandon their outdated pessimistic fears of surgery.

The achievement of successful operative results in the elderly surgical patient requires not only technical skill but also an awareness of the aging changes in the human body and of the biologic variability inherent in them. Broadly stated, aging is characterized by an erosion of the physiologic reserve function existing in the organ systems of younger individuals with a consequent reduction in the older body's ability to compensate correctively for superimposed stress and to return to the original homeostatic balance. It is important to recognize, however, the tremendous variability among individuals of identical age in the degree to which such physiologic constraints of age are applicable. Superior genetic endowment at birth and a life-style of active body use can result in a fairly well defended functional reserve far into old age. Such individuals might well be superior surgical candidates compared to others a decade or two younger in whom marginal initial biologic endowment or subsequent disease, abuse, or disuse atrophy may have seriously narrowed the elastic limits of survivability. While a description of the "universal" changes of aging is important in developing an appropriate awareness of the potential problems of geriatric surgery, the application of such information to an individual patient is intelligible only as a guide to clinical evaluation of the patient; it must not become an automatic presumption because of the patient's age.

AGING OF THE NEUROMUSCULAR SYSTEM

The most conspicuous change in the human motor system with advancing old age is the decline in total body mass as a consequence of the loss in the size and/or numbers of specific types of muscle fibers.[42] Precise delineation of this effect has been made difficult by the exquisite sensitivity of muscle cells to minor fluctuations in their trophic milieu, so that the effects of "senile atrophy" are summed into other secondary effects upon muscle related to changes in the cardiovascular and endocrinologic systems. Even such psychosocial realities as the expectations of both society and the elderly themselves for participation in physical work and exercise may find their expression in reductions of muscle mass because of disuse atrophy. It appears clear, however, that independently of these other effects a significant degree of senile muscular atrophy results from the primary effect of age upon the muscle itself and/or its neural components, since some degree of atrophy with age is universal and observed even in exceptionally well conditioned individuals who remain active physical culture enthusiasts far into their senior years.

The gross pattern of senile muscle atrophy may vary somewhat between individuals inasmuch as patterns of lifelong use or disuse of particular muscle groups may have varied. In general, the muscles of the lower extremities show more significant degrees of atrophy with age than do those of the upper extremities or back.[30] Some contradictory observations have been generated regarding the effects of active muscle use in modifying the tempo of senile atrophy. Respiratory muscles kept in constant involuntary use show very little atrophy, supporting the contention that active use of a muscle perpetuates its strength.[14] Similar evidence suggests that athletic persons who remain active during their senior years maintain a differential margin of strength superiority over their peers and that their strength might be considered to be appropriate for individuals years younger.[40] In contrast, however, is the observed development of an accelerated rate of atrophy in hypertrophied muscles developed by a lifetime of occupational use in males. These individuals, who usually performed specific manual tasks during their working careers, may develop lower extremity strength performance levels in their postretirement years that ultimately fall below the age-corrected norm for the general population.

Such similarities and differences as appear in studies of senile muscle atrophy may be partly caused by the heterogenous composition of muscle itself. Individual muscle fibers are composed of variable combinations of several types of fibers whose enzymatic composition and functional properties differ.[10] Type I fibers, for example, contract slowly and with a low susceptibility to fatigue because of their enrichment with oxidative enzymes, while type II fibers, in contrast, are of the fast-twitch variety containing higher levels of adenosine triphosphatase (ATPase) than found in type I fibers. The generally lower resistance to fatigue of type II fibers varies directly with their relative levels of oxidative enzyme activity, levels that are moderate in the IIA subtype but low in the IIB. Muscle fibers appear to exist in a state of active neurotrophic determination with respect to size and functional type rather than as products of terminal pathways of cellular differentiation. Experimental studies with cross-innervation and extrinsic electrical stimulation have demonstrated the capability of one fiber type to develop some of the histochemical and functional properties of another as well as the ability to hypertrophy with continued use.[8,37]

Although individual neuromotor units are uniform with respect to fiber types, different muscles may be composed of various proportions of type I, IIA, or IIB neuromotor units, with the ultimate functional characteristics of a muscle being determined by the weighted contributions of the inherent capabilities and limitations of each fiber type. The consequent effects of exercise, disuse, and aging upon muscle can be traced in some degree to their specific effects upon the individual classes of muscle fibers. Exercise, for example, is characterized not only by the commonly recognized process of hypertrophy but also by a shift toward a greater proportion of type IIA fibers compared to type IIB.[3] Disuse atrophy is marked by a maintenance of the ratio of IIA to IIB fibers but with an overall reduction in fiber size.[16] Aging appears to result in its own differential effect upon these two fast-twitch subgroups. Type IIB fibers appear to undergo reductions in size while maintaining their numbers; type IIA fibers appear to maintain their size but undergo numerical attrition.[41] Type I fibers likewise appear to maintain their size; their numerical fate is as yet unclear. Overall there appears to be a significant reversal of the relative ratios of type II compared with type I fibers during the aging process. Cross-sectional analysis of the quadriceps muscle at the peak of adult maturity shows a 15% to 20% preponderance of type II fibers compared to type I, while by the ninth decade the summated cross-sectional area of the type I fibers at the same site is more than twice that of the type II fibers.[6]

Several ultrastructural changes within muscle fibers have been reported in aging, including patchy myofibrillar degeneration, mitochondrial enzyme depletion, and lipofuscin accumulation, but there is no evidence to date that because of these changes individual muscle fibers from elderly subjects ultimately possess any decreased capacity for the development of contractile tension compared to those of younger persons.[15,27,36] Of greater potential significance to the aging motor system than these ultrastructural changes are the observed effects of age upon the nervous system. A loss of neurons with age has been documented at various locations within the central nervous system, including the cerebellum (Purkinje's cell), brainstem (nucleus ceruleus), cortex, and hippocampus.[12] Not all areas of the brain undergo such neuronal dropouts; cell counts at a variety of other brainstem nuclear locations (e.g., the facial nucleus) reveal no appreciable changes with age. However, important age effects at other locations may nevertheless be present without an overt reduction in actual neuronal numbers; a suggestive example observed is the reduction with time of the

dopamine content of the basal ganglia.[25] This muted parallel between normal aging and similar though more severe changes characteristic of Parkinson's disease demonstrates the motor system's sensitivity not only to myopathic mechanisms of aging changes but also to the aging and disease vulnerabilities of the integrative centers of the central nervous system.

Effects of aging upon the peripheral nervous system have long been implicated as being contributory to the senile changes witnessed in the motor system. It has been proposed that with age there is a reduction either in the impulse activity level of the neuron or in its release of unidentified neurotrophic substances.[17] Certain histologic and functional characteristics of aging muscle,—for example, the tendency of muscle fiber types to be found grouped together rather than dispersed throughout the muscle, with some groups in uniform states of atrophy—are so suggestive of known cases of denervation/renervation neuropathy that some degree of "functional" denervation of muscle with age has been postulated to explain them.[4] This histologic impression is reinforced by electrophysiologic evidence to suggest that there may be a reduction in the number of functioning motor neuron units in the elderly, wherein fewer surviving motor neurons activate a larger cohort of muscle fibers brought under their influence by collateral propagation of axonal endings to recruit fibers whose original source of innervation has been lost.[9,31] Degenerative changes in peripheral nerves principally involve the loss of larger, fast-conducting alpha nerve fibers, with the relative preservation of the smaller-diameter fibers. Not coincidentally it is primarily these same large-diameter, fast-conducting nerve fibers that innervate the fast-twitch type II muscle fibers whose populations likewise show the greatest effect of senescence.

The clinical effect of these combined neural and motor senescent changes is reflected in altered strength, speed, endurance, and coordinative capabilities of the older person. Reduction in the size and/or number of muscle fibers finds direct expression in the reduction of isometric strength in the elderly. This decline in strength is proportionately greater in the proximal lower extremities than in the back or upper limbs, including hand grip.[20] Although the disuse of hypertrophied muscles may lead to their accelerated atrophy to levels below that seen in the overall population (e.g., a retired manual worker), continued vigorous exercise can probably retard muscle strength decline by the equivalent of perhaps a decade; it cannot arrest the process.[40]

Whereas the decline in muscle strength parallels the decline in bulk mass and cell numbers, the disproportionate loss of type II and the preservation of type I fibers is reflected in a reduction in the speed of contraction but with the relative enhancement of endurance (corrected for strength and the capabilities of the cardiopulmonary system). A pronounced falloff in dynamic performance at high speed in the elderly has been attributed to the preferential atrophy of type II fibers. Endurance for isotonic exercise is maintained, however, for work loads within the permissible bounds of cardiovascular function by the functional properties of type I fibers. Indeed, although endurance for isometric exercise declines in absolute terms, it may actually increase with age when corrected for the reduction in contractile muscle strength.[21,22,35] Aging athletes with good cardiopulmonary reserve are noticeably more suited for events that place a premium upon endurance (e.g., marathon running) rather then upon bursts of speed (sprinting). Likewise, reduction of the functional contribution of type II fibers to overall muscle performance may be a significant contributory cause to the slowing of movement and loss of fine motor coordination observed with age when it occurs in muscles responsible for digital dexterity and postural stability.

Although the loss of fast-conducting peripheral nerve fibers and type II muscle fibers results in a slight decrease in conduction velocity in the monosynaptic reflex time in the elderly, this reflex appears to contribute only minimally to the gross deterioration of automatic postural control seen in the elderly. Degradation of reflex postural control in the motor system appears to be more significantly linked to adverse changes in the long-latency polysynaptic reflex system that comes under brainstem and cortical influence.[45] Age-associated impairment of central nervous system processing mechanisms, possibly because of the numerical reduction of neurons in key areas (e.g., cerebellum) or a reduction of transmitter levels (basal ganglion), may produce visible degradation in the antigravitational stability of the skeletal-muscular system. Clinical experience suggests that further reductions in the quality of visual, vestibular, or proprioceptive sensory input to the elderly brain are usually the critical elements compounding existing central delays (spinal, brainstem, and cortical) that produce failures of automatic corrections in posture. Studies show that postural sway, which is very effectively suppressed in the final stages of adolescent development by cortical maturation, re-emerges in the elderly, presumably because of a loss of higher cortical control.[39] The result is a serious enhancement of the risk of falls in the elderly as a result of delayed and uncoordinated neural activation of muscle groups that have themselves suffered inherent age-associated reductions in their capacity for strong and speedy contraction.

AGING OF SKELETAL BONE

Despite its inert appearance, bone is a living organ system whose cellular elements must submit to the predictable effects of passing years as well as to the numerous daily fluctuations in their physiologic milieu. Throughout life osteoclasts and osteoblasts remain active in their respective roles—osteoclasts resorb bone matrix, which results in the release of its contained minerals and the subsequent formation by osteoblasts of new collagen-proteoglycan matrix that may become mineralized into mature bone. The linkage between these simultaneous but antagonistic metabolic activities with respect to determination of relative rates, directions, and locations is complex and only partly understood, but it includes both hormonal factors and stress-induced piezoelectric fields. More clearly understood from clinical experience, however, is the fact that bone's function as a supportive frame for the body is secondary in priority to its availability as a mineral depot for the correction of declines in the serum ionized calcium level. Differences among individuals in the bioavailability of dietary calcium to meet the primary mission of a stable serum calcium level may cause considerable variation in the degree to which skeletal calcium stores become depleted.[18]

Although the aging of any tissue may be considered to begin at birth, the practical clinical effects of age upon bone begin in young adulthood. Early childhood and adolescent years are marked by vigorous rates of osteoblast and osteoclast activity. The marked predominance of osteoblastic activity manifests itself in the growth of the skeleton during these years. Net bone formation continues for several years beyond the cessation of linear growth by epiphyseal closure but at progressively slower rates. As the metabolic activity of both osteoblasts and osteoclasts decline, they do so not only in absolute terms but also with respect to the relative difference between them. The loss of this preexisting differential advantage favoring osteoblastic bone formation brings the active process of bone remodeling into a steady-state equilibrium at approximately the fourth decade. The skeletal mass achieved at this point in life represents the peak for the individual's life span. Beyond this decade the metabolic rates of osteoblastic and osteoclastic cellular activity continue to decline further in absolute terms but with a new and reversed differential developing between them in favor of net bone resorption. The remaining decades of life are marked by a progressive and inexorable ebbing of skeletal mineral content.[13]

This loss of skeletal bone with age is marked by the appearance of several architectural variations in old bone that have important clinical consequences. Although only 20% of skeletal bone at maturity is trabecular, this compartment is the pref-

erential site of virtually all bone lost before age 50 to 55, possibly because of its disproportionately high surface:volume ratio and its good vascular accessibility.[18] The loss of trabecular bone is neither generalized nor random; rather, trabecular struts of least structural importance within a given region are preferentially resorbed, sparing as long as possible those trabeculae carrying the major compressive or tensile forces through the bone area. Beyond age 50 to 55 years the preferential site for bone resorption shifts to the cortices. Again structural considerations appear to dictate the endosteal surface to be the preferential site of bone resorption, thereby preserving the contribution to mechanical stability of the bone's normal outer diameter even though wall thickness is unavoidably sacrificed.[18]

The universality of these patterns of growth, maturation, and senile demineralization of skeletal bone argues strongly that the skeleton is "programmed" for senescence either at the level of the cellular elements themselves or by the endocrinologic systems that modulate them. Since the resistance of skeletal bone to fracture at any site is directly proportionate to its mineral density, the generalized loss of minerals with aging confers upon the elderly an overall increased risk of fracture. This risk becomes greatest for bones enriched in trabecular content, such as femoral and radial heads and thoracolumbar vertebral bodies, since these areas are disproportionately depleted of bone mineral, having been sites of preferential resorption before age 50. Modifying this universal pattern, however, are several major genetic and physiologic factors that interact with aging and materially influence the likelihood of senile skeletal failure. Conceptually, these factors may be considered to exert their effect via changes in either the peak skeletal mass at maturity and/or the relative intensity of bone resorption in later years. These determinants are considered as part of the aging of the skeletal system since they are among the normal experiences of aging and do not properly belong with the long list of identifiable diseases and disorders that can induce changes in bone mass.

Genetic factors

Men tend to attain higher peak skeletal masses at maturity than do women, an effect that significantly delays the appearance of skeletal fractures in the male senescent years. This sexual advantage is usually presumed to be due to a stronger genetic selection in males for larger body size, although to some degree the culturally influenced tendency of adolescent males to engage in greater physical activity may also contribute to the formation of denser skeletal bone at maturity.[38] Similar protective genetic differences are reported in the higher peak skeletal masses of black men and women compared to whites, while a particular susceptibility among whites to low peak adult bone masses (and fractures) has been noted in women with a light-complexioned phenotype who are of northwestern European ethnic backgrounds.[29,44]

Reproductive factors

Women who bear children generally attain 10% to 15% lower peak adult bone masses than do nonchildbearing women.[1] Presumably this difference reflects the practical difficulties in meeting the higher dietary calcium requirements for pregnant and lactating women with the consequent diversion of calcium from maternal bone into the fetal skeleton and breast milk.

Menopause

Menopause is a normal (albeit sex-specific) aging phenomenon that unlike childbearing is universal in its applicability to women. Estrogen withdrawal at menopause results in nearly a decade of accelerated bone resorption that has no physiologic equivalent in men. Although the loss of bone as a result of aging actually begins in both sexes several years before the usual age of menopause in westernized women, the rate of bone loss at menopause leaps from 0.22% of total body calcium per year premenopausally to an average of 1.5% of total body calcium per year at menopause. The bone loss rate may remain high for several years until gradually returning to a resorptive rate more nearly approximating that experienced by men throughout these years, a more modest 0.17% per year.[11]

Actual postmenopausal estrogen levels in individual women may vary over a 10-fold range depending upon differences in residual ovarian and adrenal hormonal activity, and indirect evidence suggests that the intensity of bone demineralization after menopause may directly reflect the magnitude of the drop in estrogen level.[2] Since the timing of this postmenopausal period of accelerated bone resorption places it predominantly before age 55, the trabecular compartment of the skeleton is particularly savaged. By age 80 women have lost nearly 43% of their trabecular bone compared with 27% in men, and not surprising they constitute the vast majority of patients with Colles' fractures, femoral neck fractures, and vertebral compression fractures.[28]

AGING OF ARTICULAR CARTILAGE

Like the bony skeleton, articular cartilage is a living tissue that visibly consists of a functionally important secretory product whose continued metabolic existence remains occultly dependent upon a contained cellular population. These cellular chondrocytes secrete and metabolize the essential elements of articular cartilage: type II collagen fibers, arranged in a specific spatial matrix and impregnated with a complex ground substance. Both species confer indispensible properties to the mature cartilage: collagen contributing its tensile strength and resistance to sheer; the ground substance contributing its elastic deformability. Both show identifiable physical and biochemical abnormalities in the joints of elderly patients.[32]

Articular cartilage consists of a shaped matrix of type II collagen fibers arranged in a specific functional configuration. Densely packed at the bone-cartilage interface, the collagen fibers penetrate perpendicularly into the subchondral bone, forming a secure interdigitated attachment, while those fibers at the joint surface lie in parallel along its surface. Into this collagen matrix is a ground substance composed of aggregated proteoglycan subunits bound by hyaluronic acid molecules and link proteins. The proteoglycan subunits are themselves composed of keratin and chondroitin sulfates, the latter in either the four-isomer form or a six-isomer form characteristic of mature cartilage. Rich in water content, the proteoglycan subunits reversibly release and resorb water with each successive application and release of compressive force to the cartilage. Blending their special structural strengths, the constituent elements of articular cartilage combine a high resistance to shear with the capability of effectively dissipating the force of both sudden and sustained loads to protect the bone from damage.[33]

As secretory products of the chondrocytes, both the collagen and the ground substance remain in an active state of metabolic turnover. The rate of collagen turnover is very low, while that of proteoglycans is high.[26] Attempts to identify early changes in either the cellular or the extracellular elements of articular cartilage have resulted in the observation of only minimal differences in proteoglycan aggregability and weight-bearing capability.[34,43] Biochemically and structurally significant changes have been detected only in an advanced state of articular degeneration. In such joints the earliest visible morphologic change is the focal fibrillation of the joint surface, followed by the development of small areas of ulceration and the first clear appearance of measurable biochemical abnormalities.[7] These include reductions in the proteoglycan subunit size and number and shifts in the keratin sulfate:chondroitin sulfate ratio to favor the latter, with a greater proportion of the chrondroitin sulfate appearing in its "immature" four-isomer form. The half-life of the proteoglycan subunits appears to shorten, inducing a temporary compensatory hypersecretion by the chondrocytes that ultimately exhausts itself with an eventual net loss of articular substance.[5]

The clinical effects of age upon weight-bearing joints become radiographically manifest at approximately the fourth decade of life; by the seventh decade radiographic abnormalities have become universally apparent to a variable degree[23] although only a small, unfortunate percentage of individuals ultimately develop the pain or disability that is characterized as "osteoarthritis." The distinction between the universal degenerative changes of normal aging and those of osteoarthritis exist largely as a function of the subjective perception of pain by individuals whose joint involvement lies at the severe end of a very broad spectrum. Characteristically in degeneration of articular cartilage as in other degenerative conditions, there exists no clear statistical differentiation between "normal" and "diseased."

The principal involvement of weight-bearing joints in advanced stages of degeneration suggests a primary role of repeated use or strain in the initiation of these changes—the classic "wear and tear" hypothesis. Certainly the development of these articular degenerations later in life in joints exposed to weight loading (spine, knees, first metatarsophalangeals) and strain (distal interphalangeals, first carpometacarpals) argues for this interpretation, as does the development of articular degeneration in unusual locations (e.g., shoulder) when that joint has been subjected to prolonged and unusual degrees of use (e.g., occupational). Other elements, however, remain elusive: the predisposition for women, the differing autosomal genetics for the development of painful Heberden's nodes in men[19] (recessive) and women (dominant), and the link to obesity.[24] Considerable further research remains to be done to determine the precise delineation of osteoarthritis as either an expression of or a disease of aging.

SUMMARY

The discussion in this chapter has concentrated upon the general pattern of aging changes that affect the musculoskeletal system, including those elements of the nervous system that modulate its essential vitality and confer upon it functional mobility. Although the interpretation of these changes as being the result of aging is not immune to criticism based upon the existing methodologic limitations of gerontologic research, the changes discussed appear to meet satisfactorily the twin criteria of being both universal (or nearly so) and unassociated with known patterns of disease. Whether future research validates all or some of these changes as being in fact caused solely by the effects of time upon the musculoskeletal system or whether it finds in them the footprints of a yet unappreciated disease process, the practical implications for the orthopaedic surgeon in the short term will be nearly the same. Sensitivity to their likely existence and, where possible, a determination of their quantitative significance will guide the surgeon, anesthetist, geriatrician, and physiatrist in selecting for their shared patient the most appropriate surgical and postoperative rehabilitative program for the ultimate restoration of optimal function.

References

1. Albanese, A.A.: Calcium nutrition in the elderly, Postgrad. Med. **63**:167-172, 1978.
2. Badaway, S.Z.A., Elliott, L.J., Elbadawi, A., and Marshall, L.D.: Plasma levels of oestione and oestradiol-1713 in postmenopausal women, Br. J. Obstet. Gynaecol. **86**:56-63, 1979.
3. Barnard, R.J., Edgerton, V.R., and Peter, J.B.: Effect of exercise on skeletal muscle. I. Biochemical and histochemical properties, J. Appl. Physiol. **28**(6):762-766, 1970.
4. Bass, A., Gutmann, E., and Hanzlikova, V.: Biochemical and histochemical changes in energy-supply-enzyme pattern of muscles of the rat during old age, Gerontologia **21**:31-45, 1975.
5. Bollet, A.J.: Connective tissue polysaccharide metabolism and the pathogenesis of osteoarthritis, Adv. Intern. Med. **13**:33, 1967.
6. Bowers, W.D., et al.: Effects of exercise on the ultrastructure of skeletal muscle, Am. J. Physiol. **227**(2):313-316, 1974.
7. Brandt, K.D.: Pathogenesis of osteoarthritis. In Kelly, W.N., et al., editors: Textbook of rheumatology, Philadelphia, 1981, W.B. Saunders Co.
8. Buller, A.J., Eccles, J.C., and Eccles, R.M.: Interactions between motoneurones and muscles in respect of the characteristic speeds of their responses, J. Physiol. (Lond.) **150**:417-439, 1960.
9. Campbell, M.J., McComas, A.J., and Petito, F.: Physiological changes in ageing muscles, J. Neurol. Neurosurg. Psychiatry **36**:174-182, 1973.
10. Close, R.I.: Dynamic properties of mammalian skeletal muscles, Physiol. Rev. **51**(1):129-197, 1972.
11. Cohn, S.H., et al.: Age and sex-related changes in bone mass measured by neutron activation (abstract), International Symposium on Osteoporosis, Jerusalem, 1981.
12. Curcio, C.A., Buell, S.J., and Coleman, P.D.: Morphology of the aging central nervous system: not all downhill. In Mortimer, J.A., Pirozzolo, F.J., and Maletta, G.J., editors: Advances in neurogerontology, vol. 3, New York, 1982, Praeger Publishers.
13. Gryfe, C., et al.: Pattern of development of bone in childhood and adolescence, Lancet **1**:523-526, 1971.
14. Gutmann, E., and Hanzlikova, V.: Motor unit in old age, Nature **209**:921-922, 1966.
15. Gutmann, E., and Hanzlikova, V.: Age changes in the neuromuscular system, Bristol, 1972, Scientechnica.
16. Gutmann, E., and Hanzlikova, V.: Basic mechanisms of aging in the neuromuscular system, Mech. Ageing Dev. **1**:327-349, 1972.
17. Gutmann, E., Hanzlikova, V., and Vyskocil, F. Age changes in cross striated muscle of the rat, J Physiol. **219**:331-343, 1971.
18. Jowsey, J.: Metabolic diseases of bone, Philadelphia, 1977, W.B. Saunders Co.
19. Kellgren, J.H., Lawrence, J.S., and Bier, F.: Genetic factors in generalized osteoarthrosis, Ann Rheum. Dis. **22**:237-254, 1963.
20. Larsson, L.: Aging in mammalian skeletal muscle In Mortimer, J.A., Pirozzolo, F.J., and Maletta G.J., editors: Advances in neurogerontology, vol 3, New York, 1982, Praeger Publishers.
21. Larsson, L., Grimby, G., and Karlsson, J.: Muscle strength and speed of movement in relation to age and muscle morphology, J. Appl. Physiol. **46**:451-456, 1979.
22. Larrson, L., and Karlsson, J.: Isometric and dynamic endurance as a function of age and skeletal muscle characteristics, Acta Physiol. Scand. **104**:129-136, 1978.
23. Lawrence, J.S., Bremner, J.M., and Bier, F.: Osteoarthrosis: prevalence in the population and relationship between symptoms and x-ray changes, Ann. Rheum. Dis. **25**:1-24, 1966.
24. Lee, P., et al.: The etiology and pathogenesis of osteoarthrosis: a review, Semin. Arthritis Rheum. **3**:189-218, 1974.
25. LeWitt, P.A., and Calne, D.B.: Neurochemistry and pharmacology of the aging motor system. In Mortimer, J.A., Pirozzolo, F.J., and Maletta, G.J., editors: Advances in neurogerontology, vol. 3, New York, 1982, Praeger Publishers.
26. Maroudas, A.: Transport through articular cartilage and some physiological implications. In Ali, S.Y., Elves, M.W., and Leaback, D.H., editors: Normal and osteoarthritic articular cartilage, London, 1974, Institute of Orthopaedics.
27. McCarter, R.: Aging and skeletal muscle. In Kaldor, G., and Dibattista, W.J., editors: Aging, vol. 6, New York, 1978, Raven Press.
28. Meunier, P., et al.: Physiologic senile involution and pathological rarefaction of bone, Clin. Endrocrinol. Metabol. **2**:239-256, 1973.
29. Moldower, M., Zimmerman, S.J., and Collins, L.C.: Incidence of osteoporosis in elderly whites and elderly Negroes, J.A.M.A. **194**:117-120, 1965.
30. Moore, M.J., Rebeiz, J.J., Holden, M., and Adams, R.D.: Biometric analyses of normal skeletal muscle, Acta Neuropath. (Berl.) **19**:51-69, 1971.

31. Morris, C.J.: The significance of intermediate fibres in reinnervated human skeletal muscle, J. Neurol. Sci. **11**:129-136, 1970.

32. Moskowitz, R.W.: Cartilage and osteoarthritis: current concepts, J. Rheumatol. **4**:329-331, 1977.

33. Muir, H.: Molecular approach to the understanding of osteoarthritis, Ann. Rheum. Dis. **36**:199-208, 1977.

34. Perricone, E., Palmoski, M.J., and Brandt, K.D.: Failure of proteoglycans to form aggregates in morphologically normal aged human hip cartilage, Arthritis Rheum. **20**:1372-1380, 1977.

35. Petrofsky, J.S., and Lind, A.R.: Aging, isometric strength and endurance and cardiovascular responses to static effort, J. Appl. Physiol. **38**:91-95, 1975.

36. Rubinstein, L.J.: Ageing changes in muscle. In Bourne, G.H., editor: The structure and function of the muscle, vol. 3, New York, 1960, Academic Press.

37. Salmons, S., and Vrbova, G.: The influence of activity on some contractile characteristics of mammalian fast and slow muscle, J. Physiol. (Lond.), **210**:535-549, 1969.

38. Saville, P.D.: Observations on 80 women with osteoporotic spine fracture, In Barzel, U.S., editor: Osteoporosis, New York, 1970, Grune & Stratton.

39. Sheldon, J.H.: The effect of age on the control of sway, Gerontol. Clin. **5**:129-138, 1963.

40. Spirduso, W.W.: Physical fitness in relation to motor aging. In Mortimer, J.A., Pirozzolo, F.J., and Maletta, G.J., editors: Advances in neurogerontology, vol. 3, New York, 1982, Praeger Publishers.

41. Tohgi, H., Shimizu, T., Inoue, K., and Kameyama, M.: Quantitative histochemical studies on age changes of human muscles. II. The proportion of fiber types and type grouping, Clin. Neurol. (Tokyo) **15**:798-804, 1975.

42. Tomonaga, M.: Histochemical and ultrastructual changes in senile human skeletal muscles, J. Am. Geriatr. Soc. **3**:125-31, 1977.

43. Weightman, B.: In vitro fatigue testing of articular cartilage, Ann. Rheum. Dis., **34** (Suppl. 2):108-110, 1975.

44. Whedon, G.D.: Osteoporosis, Clin. Endocrinol. **2**:349-376, 1968.

45. Woollacott, M.H., Shumway-Cook, A., Nashner, L.: Postural reflexes and aging. In Mortimer, J.A., Pirozzolo, F.J., and Maletta, G.J., editors: Advances in neurogerontology, vol. 3, New York, 1982, Praeger Publishers.

chapter 2

PSYCHOLOGIC AND SOCIAL FEATURES OF MUSCULOSKELETAL DYSFUNCTION

James Warren Brown

The purpose of this chapter is to provide the surgeon the information that may prove helpful in the care, acute and chronic, of geriatric patients. The first section will deal with acute problems that are frequently seen during hospitalization. The second section will review the more commonly used psychotropic medications. The third section will address issues that frequently arise in the treatment of chronic and/or incapacitating orthopaedic illnesses. Issues concerning the relationship between the referring physician and liaison-consulting psychiatrist will be considered in the final section.

ACUTE PROBLEMS RELATED TO SURGERY

Preoperatively there should be an evaluation of the elderly patient's mental status to ascertain signs of an organic brain syndrome, depression, and/or anxiety. A patient with a chronic organic brain syndrome is at a higher risk to develop a superimposed, acute postoperative organic brain syndrome. In the postoperative state it is often difficult to sort out what might be a delirium stemming from anesthesia and the trauma of surgery versus the sequelae of long-term organic deficits. This

differentiation is important because the prognosis of recovery from an acute delirium is usually quite favorable. With a chronic condition one can usually only hope that there will be no further deterioration. An exception to the latter generalization is a communicating hydrocephalus for which surgical intervention can often provide dramatic relief.

Patients with high levels of preoperative anxiety may also be subject to an increased incidence of postoperative delirium and their convalescence may be stormy. Serious depression can markedly disrupt the convalescent period and can adversely influence the efficacy of surgery. In my estimation, elective or semielective surgery should be postponed if the patient is significantly depressed.

The mental status evaluation of a patient with a chronic organic brain syndrome will reveal disorientation, impaired memory (recent more than remote), confabulation, lability of affect with sudden shifts in mood, irritability, and sometimes paranoid delusions. Patients who are anxious will often describe themselves as feeling frightened, worried, or apprehensive and will frequently give a history of sweating, flushing, palpitations, and tremulousness. When evaluating depression, direct observation and questioning are essential. Subjective depressive symptoms include statements about feeling blue, sad, dejected, hopeless, or despairing. Frequently patients will relate feelings of worthlessness and unfounded guilt. In every instance the patient should be questioned specifically about suicidal thoughts and inclinations. Passive suicidal thoughts (e.g., feelings that life is not worth living and/or wishing oneself dead) are not uncommon. To ascertain active suicidal inclinations, patients have to be asked whether they have seriously thought of particular ways in which to take their own life. When a patient is depressed, there is frequently impairment of sleep, which is manifested by difficulty in getting to sleep and/or early morning awakening, and of appetite and concentration. Work performance is usually impaired. Vague, nonspecific somatic complaints are often a manifestation of depression and, in some instances, they are the only manifestation. These patients will frequently deny feeling depressed despite the fact that they appear depressed and demonstrate other depressive symptoms. When physical examination and pertinent diagnostic evaluations reveal no or little organic pathology to explain these patients' symptoms and if they are told that there is nothing wrong, these patients will often react with frustrated resentment, insist upon further evaluation or treatment, and go to another doctor. Patients with this kind of depressive illness may become precipitously and seriously suicidal. They usually have gone through a number of consultations and have been told that there is no basis for their physical symptoms or they have met with mounting reactions of frustration and irritation from their doctors.

Elderly patients with depressive illnesses occasionally will demonstrate irritable paranoid behavior and on occasion may express frank paranoid delusions. It is sometimes difficult to separate an organic brain syndrome from a severe retarded depression. Indeed, some psychiatrists and neurologists believe that a severe retarded depression has, as a component, reversible dementia. It is important, however, to try to make this distinction because depression is a disease for which the prognosis is favorable with appropriate treatment. If a patient demonstrates impairment of memory and if confabulation is evident, a careful neurologic evaluation to delineate further a possible organic brain syndrome is in order.

Postoperative delirium is a frequent complication of surgery in the elderly. Alcohol abuse or inappropriate use of medications will tend to predispose patients to this condition. It is essential therefore to obtain an accurate history about the use of alcohol, drugs, and medications preoperatively. If there is even a suggestion of drug or alcohol abuse, elective or semielective surgery should be postponed. The combination of withdrawal superimposed on the trauma of anesthesia and surgery can sometimes be catastrophic.

The onset of a delirium will usually occur sometime within the second to fourth postoperative day. It is characterized by restlessness, agitation, confusion, disorientation, and clouding of consciousness. Frequently there will be hallucinations, particularly tactile. Paranoid delusions may develop, and the patient may become very frightened. Loss of reality testing and judgment in combination with impulsivity may lead to hazardous behavior. A careful medical and neurologic evaluation should be obtained to ascertain such problems as electrolyte imbalances, infections, or drug reactions. Restlessness or agitation can be symptomatically treated with tranquilizers. Except with a delirium tremens, for which detoxification with a minor tranquilizer such as diazepam would be indicated, I usually recommend a major tranquilizer such as haloperidol. In the elderly it is started with a small dose, 1 to 2 mg orally or intramuscularly every 3 to 4 hours while the patient is awake, and the dose is titrated upward according to the patient's response. Vital signs, especially blood pressure, must be carefully monitored, paying special attention to the possibility of sudden hypotension. If the medication is raised too rapidly, a confused, agitated patient may become a patient who is suddenly obfunded and unresponsive. Ancillary supportive treatment should include (1) reduction of unnecessary stimuli (if possible, the patient should be placed in a single room, and only one nurse *per* shift should be assigned to his care); (2) Subdued lighting including the use of a night light during the evening hours; and (3) limitation of visitors to the immediate family or one or two close friends.

Psychotropic Medications
Sedatives

The only sedatives I recommend for use in the elderly are chloral hydrate and flurazepam. These agents should be used as sparingly as possible.

Tranquilizers

Tranquilizers such as chlordiazepoxide or diazepam may be useful in dealing with mild to moderate *acute* anxiety states. Diazepam is useful in relieving muscle tension or spasms. For some patients, however, diazepam may precipitate and/or aggravate depression, an effect that is not characteristic of chlordiazepoxide. If these medications are used in moderately large doses, especially in conjunction with narcotic medications, the results may be oversedation, confusion, and disorientation. If symptoms of anxiety do not respond to modest doses of minor tranquilizers or if they last for extended periods of time, a psychiatric evaluation is indicated. There is usually little call for the use of major tranquilizers in the elderly except in the treatment of delirium, in maintenance therapy for chronic psychotic disorders, or to control irritability, labile affect, and impulsivity in patients with senile dementia.

Antidepressants

The major types of antidepressants are MAO inhibitors, tricyclics, and the newer "second generation" antidepressants. MAO inhibitors are used infrequently even in young or middle-aged patients because of the possibility of serious side effects and because the patient has to maintain a strict diet to avoid foods that have a high tyra-

mine content. The use of MAO inhibitors is virtually contraindicated in any patient beyond the age of 60. Tricyclic medications are used in the treatment of depression of all age groups. These medications should not be prescribed on an "as needed" basis. If indicated, they should be given in an adequate dose, every day, and for a long enough trial period to ascertain whether they will have the desired antidepressant effect.

For patients who develop an acute and relatively mild depression postoperatively, supportive care will often suffice and many of these depressions will be self-limiting. Depressions with moderate to severe symptoms or protracted depressions require treatment consisting of medication and psychotherapy. I would like to stress that a symptomatic approach with the use of medication only is often inadequate. An effort should be made to try to understand psychologic dynamics underlying the depressed state. Particular attention should be paid to how the patient is dealing with the stresses, both acute and chronic, imposed by the physical illness and its treatment. Consultations with, and involvement of, key figures in the patient's support system are essential.

Before medication is used, possible medical contraindications must be ruled out. The most important of these are cardiovascular; arrhythmias and/or conduction defects are the most serious. Orthostatic hypotension is a common side effect from these medications and it is poorly tolerated by the elderly. Clearance by an internist or cardiologist should be obtained for any patient who has significant cardiac problems. In those patients who are predisposed to closed-angle glaucoma by virtue of their family history, antidepressants may bring out the condition or aggravate it if it is already present. An ophthalmologic examination therefore should be on record either 1 to 2 years before starting medication or it should be performed 1 to 2 weeks after medication has been initiated. Urinary retention is another possible complication, especially in men with benign prostatic hypertrophy. Elderly patients usually require one third to one half the usual priming dose necessary for young adults or middle-aged patients. Medication should be started at a low dose and gradually increased over 1 to 2 weeks. The full daily dose can be given at bedtime.

Individual responses to and toleration of these medications vary widely. Before giving the medication, the patient should be informed about possible side effects such as dry mouth, constipation, sweating, signs of orthostatic hypotension, and occasionally difficulty with focusing. Many patients find these side effects, which usually appear immediately, difficult to tolerate. Unless the side effects are incapacitating, the patient will need to be encouraged to continue the medication through a trial period of 2 to 4 weeks. Once the patient experiences an antidepressant effect, the relief from the depression will usually far outweigh the irritations caused by side effects. A potentially serious complication from the use of these medications in the geriatric population is an organic brain syndrome secondary to the anticholinergic side effects. Symptoms include confusion, disorientation, and sometimes agitation. The only effective remedy is immediate discontinuance of the medication. If the patient responds to the antidepressant medication, the initial priming dose should be continued for about 6 months. At that point, if remission has persisted, a gradual reduction can be considered. If depressive symptoms recur, the dose should be raised to the level at which the patient was symptom free. Many patients will find that they can discontinue the medication; others will require further treatment at a lower maintenance dose. It should be stressed that these medications are not habit forming or addicting and that they can be taken for as long as indicated.

Sometimes compounds with stimulants such as amphetamines are used in treating the depressed elderly. In my experience I have found no use for such medication.

Lithium carbonate is used in treatment of manic-depressive affective disorders. It is particularly efficacious in the treatment of mania, and it is frequently prescribed as a prophylaxis for those patients who have a documented history of mania or hypomania.

If surgery is contemplated for patients who are taking major neuroleptics and/or antidepressant medications, the anesthesiologist should be informed in advance. The hypotensive potential of these medications, particularly in the elderly, may require that they be discontinued a day or two before surgery. The medication can usually be resumed after the patient is stable 2 to 3 days postoperatively.

CONSIDERATIONS IN THE TREATMENT OF CHRONIC AND/OR INCAPACITATING ILLNESSES

The first point to be evaluated is the effect of illness on independent functioning. It is important not only to evaluate the current impact of the illness but also to obtain a history of the level of functioning before the onset of the disorder and information on how the patient has coped during the course of the illness. This evaluation is necessary when considering major surgery, where the outcome is heavily dependent upon compliance and motivation during the convalescent period. In those situations in which the onset of the disorder has been relatively recent and the patient has demonstrated the capacity to cope in such a way so as to maximize functioning, it is reasonable to consider surgery. If, however, there is a history of resistance to programs of physical therapy or a tendency toward passive, overly dependent reliance on others, one should proceed very cautiously when considering elective surgery. The following factors should be considered in treating chronic and/or incapacitating illnesses.

Personality configuration of the patient. Passive-dependent disorders are commonly seen with long-term illnesses. Patients with these disorders are exceptionally dependent on other individuals such as the nursing staff and relatives. Frequently they will express genuine and sincere wishes for improved functioning. Their behavior, however, often reflects passive resistance to or subtle sabotaging of rehabilitative efforts. For many, chronic illness exacerbates conflicts related to dependence-independence. Often there is a history of infantile-dependent behavior and coping mechanisms before the onset of the illness. For others there may be a history of independent behavior that, on occasion, was exaggerated. With such patients reliance on others, even appropriate dependence, is associated with weakness, shame, and unacceptability. The pain of this conflict is dealt with by reaction formation, that is, an "overkill in the opposite direction." Chronic illness can then become an opportunity for the expression of *unconscious*, unacceptable infantile-regressive, dependent strivings. Consciously, such patients can only admit to the sincerely held wish to get better and function as independently as possible.

Passive-aggressive personality disorders are expressed in irritable and subtly provocative behavior. Medical and nursing staff often find themselves feeling increasingly annoyed with these patients, who steadfastly state that they only wish to be cooperative but then express one complaint or dissatisfaction after another. These patients are adept at provoking reactions of frustration and anger and then react with injured indignation. Lifelong conflicts relating to the handling of frustration and anger are often apparent. Chronic illness will inevitably provoke these emotions in anyone. Coping with these feelings, especially anger, can be difficult since there is no one to whom the anger can be reasonably directed. When the anger involves people who are important to the patient such as close relatives, doctors, and the nursing staff, there is often the fear that the emotion will be expressed and lead to swift retribution or, worse yet, to rejection and abandonment. The hostility and resentment can either be retroflexed, leading to depression, or it can be projected. The unconscious reasoning is, "It's not me who is feeling hurt and murderously angry toward you for not making me better; it's you who are being inconsiderate and mean toward me, the aggrieved victim." The subtle and almost always unconscious provocative behavior will sometimes lead to a response from the treatment staff that will serve as validation for this defense mechanism. Confrontation alone is usually ineffective and will evoke responses of rationalization or angry denial. Instead, one should attempt to address empathetically the suspected underlying conflicted emotion—that is, dependence and/or hostility—by suggesting that these feelings are to be expected with chronic illnesses and are difficult to tolerate. It is necessary to point out repeatedly that the patient should allow himself the feelings he is having and that "feeling does not equal doing." A patient may then defuse some of the affect associated with these conflicts by being able to discuss and, within reasonable limits, to express them to an understanding relative, nurse, social worker, or physician who has the time and patience to listen.

Support systems. It is extremely important to evaluate the nature and quality of the patient's relationships with the people with whom he is closely related and on whom he must depend. In some instances this may involve friends as well as relatives. For elderly patients who are still married one should ascertain the state of the spouse's health and capacity to function as part of an overall evaluation of the couple's capacity to cope with the stresses and strains of the patient's particular illness. Even in situations where the spouse's health and functioning are relatively good, the quality of the relationship should be evaluated. When there has been chronic and/or significant marital conflict, physical illness will usually intensify this conflict and, in turn, emotional problems will interfere with treatment. For those patients who have lost their spouse, it is essential to ascertain whether they have recovered from their grief or, if the death has occurred recently, how well they are dealing with the grieving process. Recently widowed patients who are depressed and without relatives or friends who can provide adequate support will find it especially difficult to deal with chronic illnesses. Elective or semielective surgery should not be considered, in most instances, until the emotional status and support systems have improved.

With all patients, but particularly the elderly, not only the patient but also the patient's relatives should understand the nature of the illness, the range of possibilities regarding the prognosis, and what will be required with respect to convalescence and maintenance care. With the elderly the effect of chronic illnesses on sexual functioning is often overlooked. Most patients will not broach this subject on their own initiative. However, if the physician tactfully raises the issue, when appropriate, and indicates a willingness to discuss it, the patient may reveal that this is an area of importance as well as concern. In many instances conjoint interviews are the most effective and efficient way of dealing with patient's relatives, especially in situations where the patient's condition and/or prognosis is grave. However, in the geriatric population an exception to this generality would be those patients whose mental or emotional status renders them incompetent to understand the nature of the problem and the prognosis (e.g., patients with senile dementia, a severe depression, or a psychotic episode). It should be kept in mind that with the geriatric population the patient and the patient's relatives will require continuing psychologic supportive care to help them cope with the consequences of a serious or protracted illness.

Evaluation of interaction between orthopaedic problems, other medical disorders, and emotional illnesses. As previously indicated, significant depression and personality disorders will usually interfere with a patient's handling of chronic orthopaedic-medical problems. The reverse is also the case; that is, chronic medical problems will often precipitate depression and aggravate personality disorders. This same generality can be applied to psychotic illnesses, but usually only if there is an interlocking between the somatic illness and the psychotic symptoms. I have seen several instances in which a patient with a documented history of a psychotic disorder, but in a state of

remission, underwent orthopaedic treatment, including surgery, without an exacerbation of the psychosis. In these situations the orthopaedic problem was relatively acute and was not incorporated into any of the patient's delusional symptoms. In each case psychiatric consultation permitted appropriate management of psychotropic medication and supportive care.

RELATIONSHIP BETWEEN REFERRING PHYSICIAN AND LIAISON-CONSULTING PSYCHIATRIST

How much a consulting psychiatrist will be able to contribute to a patient's overall care and management depends, in part, on how the patient is prepared for the consultation. If emotional problems are thought to be significant contributing factors to the patient's somatic complaints, it is important that the referring physician not convey the impression that the patient is dissimulating or fabricating. Any communication of this nature will inevitably produce a reaction of resistive resentment to the suggestion of a psychiatric evaluation. Even when patients have been reassured along these lines, they will still often express a hurt reaction of "My doctor must think it's all in my head." It is helpful to explain that emotional stress and strain, especially depression, will intensify perceived pain and diminish the capacity to cope with a physical illness. The patient should be reassured that the attending physician is not abandoning him, but rather is seeking another opinion as part of a comprehensive approach to the patient's problem. In some situations the consulting psychiatrist's services are best utilized by recommendations to treating personnel. The psychiatrist may also, of course, be of help in prescribing and managing psychotropic medications. In other situations active psychotherapeutic intervention on the part of the consulting psychiatrist is indicated. It is extremely important, however, that the patient not feel the involvement of the psychiatrist has led to a diminution of interest or concern by the attending physician.

References

1. Busse, E.W.: Stress deprivation and catastrophic illness. In Catastrophic illness in the seventies: critical issues and complex decision, New York, 1971, Cancer Care, Inc.
2. Busse, E.W.: Mental disorders in later life organic brain syndromes. In Busse, E.W., and Pfeiffer, E., editors: Mental illness in later life, Washington, D.C., 1973, American Psychiatric Association.
3. Jacobson, S.B.: Psychiatric treatment in the aged, N.Y. State J. Med. **81**(5):802-804, 1981.
4. Pfeiffer, E., and Busse, E.W.: Mental disorders in later life—affective disorders; paronoid, neurotic, and situational reactions. In Busse, E.W., and Pfeiffer, E., editors: Mental illness in later life, Washington, D.C., 1973, American Psychiatric Association.

chapter 3

EVALUATION OF THE ELDERLY PATIENT FOR SURGERY

Marc E. Weksler

The special concern about elderly candidates for surgery reflects not only their vulnerability but also the striking changes in our population with respect to age. The vulnerability of elderly surgical patients is documented by the fact that three quarters of postoperative deaths are drawn from the 30% of surgical patients who are over 60 years of age. The number of persons over 65 years of age is increasing rapidly. In 1955, 14 million Americans were over the age of 65. Now, more than 25 million Americans are over 65 years of age. Today, a disproportionately large percentage of health care is devoted to elderly persons who spend, on the average, four times more per capita on health care than persons less than 65 years of age. Although the elderly represent only 11% to 12% of the United States population, they fill more than half of doctors' ambulatory practices and occupy almost 50% of the hospital beds.

Despite this demographic imperative, medicine has been slow to respond to the changing needs of today's patients. Much of medical care remains cast in the mold established for acute, episodic diseases of the young patient. Furthermore, the data base of geriatrics is limited. Specifically, the natural history of many diseases in the elderly is not known in sufficient detail to permit in many cases a rational decision between the risks of medical and surgical therapy. Nevertheless, medical experience

has defined at least some of the special considerations required in evaluating the elderly for surgery.

EVALUATING THE ELDERLY PATIENT FOR SURGERY

This chapter will describe the role of the geriatric consultant in evaluating the elderly patient for surgery. The consultation has several goals. The first goal is to review the need for surgery because the indications for surgery in the elderly are not always clear and at times a second surgical opinion may be helpful. Surgical second opinion programs have revealed that certain operations are more frequently associated with conflicting recommendations.[3] Prostatectomy and cataract extraction, which are operations frequently recommended to elderly patients, are not recommended by the second surgeon in 20% to 40% of the cases. The second goal of the consultation is to identify risk factors that increase the morbidity and mortality of surgery. Many risk factors can be ameliorated, thus increasing the patient's chance for uncomplicated surgery. The third goal is to provide the patient and family with a description of what can be expected before, during, and following surgery.

Homeostatic reserves are progressively narrowed with age. This age-associated process I have termed "homeostenosis." The

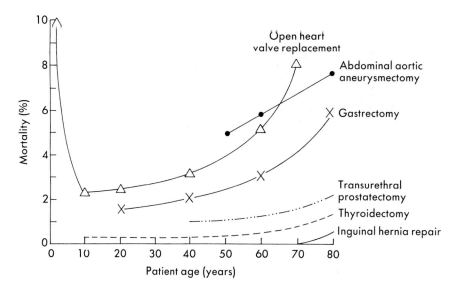

FIG. 3-1. Percentage of postsurgical mortality according to patient age (From Polk, H.C.: In Gardner, B., Polk, H.C., Stone, H.H., and Sugg, W.L., editors: Basic surgery, New York, 1978, Appleton-Century-Crofts.)

limitation in physiologic reserves described by this term suggests that "fine tuning" of the physiologic systems before surgery will maximize the capacity of the elderly patient to sustain the stresses of surgery. The goal is to bring into balance the decompensated physiologic systems that would otherwise complicate surgery. This can best be achieved if a geriatric evaluation is arranged 4 to 6 weeks before elective surgery. Obviously, this is not possible when emergency surgery is necessary. Nonetheless, the preoperative evaluation of the elderly patient who requires emergency surgery should consider the same risk factors within the time available.

Many authorities believe that morbidity and mortality following surgery increase (Fig. 3-1) with age.[14] Some believe that surgical risk increases only in patients over the age of 70.[4] Others believe that age is not an independent risk factor but rather that it reflects the physiologic limitations and diseases that accompany aging.[2] This may be a semantic point because it is usually difficult to distinguish clearly between aging and the pathologic processes that accompany aging.

The reported surgical morbidity and mortality vary with the operative procedure, the ratio of elective-to-emergency surgery, and the population of patients. It is generally acknowledged that older patients are particularly vulnerable to emergency surgery. The varied conclusions drawn from studies in which the distribution of these factors differed would be expected. Recently, the results of surgery in 500 patients over the age of 80 were reported.[2] Mortality approached 20% for exploratory laparotomy, usually performed on an emergency basis, whereas it was 12% for colectomy, 5% for open reduction and fixation of hip fractures, and less than 2% for transurethral prostatectomy.

DISCUSSING THE OPERATION WITH PATIENT AND FAMILY

An acute decline in physical and intellectual functions frequently follows surgery in the elderly. The family frequently believes that the patient is worse off after surgery than before. A surgical success may be viewed by the patient or, more frequently, by the patient's family as a therapeutic failure, at least in the postoperative period. The patient who may have been leaving his bed at home only with difficulty may become bedridden, or even worse incontinent, following surgery. For this reason, the examination of the elderly patient before surgery should include an assessment of mental and physical functions. A formal "mini-mental status" examination should be administered to document the level of intellectual function. Similarly, if possible, the ability of the patient to get out of bed and walk should be tested. Intellectual and physical activity are critical determinants of independence and must be known in order to plan for convalescent care.

In part, the acute deterioration that occurs after surgery in the elderly represents the stresses of hospitalization and surgery that fall disproportionately upon the elderly. In part, however, these changes may be only apparent and reflect denial by the patient and family of intellectual and physical impairments that the patient had before surgery. Disorientation and sundowning may become obvious for the first time following admission to the hospital when the patient is in an unfamiliar environment. Confusion and delirium during the postoperative period are more frequent than commonly realized in all age groups. This is particularly true with older patients. Acute psychiatric disturbances are particularly common in intensive care units and when contact with the environment is compromised, as for example when visual or auditory function is lost. In careful studies, approximately 25% of postoperative patients have been found to suffer mental aberrations following surgery.[8] It is helpful to warn the elderly patient that visual and/or auditory aberrations may occur postoperatively. This information allays the anxiety that these psychologic disturbances may otherwise provoke. Reorientation by the health care team is very helpful in the days following surgery and is far better than sedatives in quieting the agitated postoperative patient.

Fortunately, the mental and physical deterioration that follows surgery is usually reversed with time although this may take as long as 6 to 8 weeks. The use of a convalescent or intermediate care facility is of great benefit to the elderly patient following surgery. If the possibility of temporary deterioration of an elderly patient following surgery is anticipated and discussed with the patient and family before surgery, premature and inappropriate institutionalization of the elderly patient may be avoided.[9]

THE MEDICAL HISTORY

Most of the relevant information concerning the elderly patient's risks from surgery will be derived from the history. The patient's history should be reviewed with special emphasis on chronic diseases and impairments, current medications, and past hospitalizations and operations, particularly including information on complications and unexpected problems that developed in the past and might occur again. For example, postoperative deep venous thrombosis, wound infection, or hemorrhage frequently recurs. In medical history as in political history the past is often prelude to the future.

A most important part of the history relates to medication. A knowledge of the drugs and anesthetics taken in the past and those being taken before surgery is crucial to the preoperative evaluation. For example, reexposure to halothane may produce chills and fever and less frequently hepatic damage 7 to 14 days after surgery. Medications that have caused allergic or other untoward effects should be identified in order to prevent their use. Patients who have received corticosteroids for 10 to 14 days or more during the year before surgery should receive parenteral hydrocortisone preoperatively and for 5 to 7 days after surgery to prevent acute adrenal insufficiency.

Some drugs, such as levodopa and oral hypoglycemic agents, cannot be given parenterally. It must be decided whether these drugs can be discontinued during surgery and during the immediate postoperative period or whether alternative preparations that can be given parenterally should be substituted. For example, some patients with Parkinson's disease controlled with levodopa may deteriorate if the drug is withdrawn. To prevent this, drugs such as benztropine (Cogentin), which can be administered parenterally, may be used. Finally, some drugs should be discontinued before surgery. For example, aspirin, which inhibits the hemostatic function of platelets, should be discontinued at least 1 week before surgery. Clonidine and MAO inhibitors, which potentiate the response to pressor agents, should also be discontinued at least 1 week before surgery. Beta-adrenergic blockers need not be discontinued. These drugs, frequently used to treat angina, may protect cardiac patients from arrhythmias or reinfarction. Elderly patients with head trauma, infections, and shock are at great risk for stress ulcers and may benefit from prophylactic antacids or cimetidine.

NUTRITION AND SURGERY

A dietary history, including the use of alcohol, is important. Signs and symptoms of alcohol withdrawal including tremor, confusion, delirium, and convulsions may occur in the postoperative period, and if not recognized, they present a complex diagnostic problem.

Overnutrition and undernutrition are recognized to be risk factors for surgery. Obese patients are at greater risk of deep venous thrombosis, pulmonary emboli, atelectasis, and pneumonia. Unfortunately, it is rare that significant weight reduction can be achieved before surgery. Weight loss may reflect a catabolic state or malnutrition. Malnutrition associated with a serum albumin concentration of less than 3.4 mg/ml, lymphopenia less than 1500 cells/mm^3, and anergy compromises wound healing and increases susceptibility to infection. Very thin elderly patients had significantly higher morbidity following hip fractures than did well-nourished patients who were otherwise well matched.[1] There is increasing evidence that enteral or parenteral nutrition with vitamin and mineral supplements can replete nutritional deficits and decrease the complications following surgery. Thus, patients given a short course of parenteral nutrition before surgery for gastrointestinal carcinoma had decreased postoperative morbidity and mortality.[13]

Many elderly patients without cancer who deny weight loss may be malnour-

ished. Many elderly exist on a "tea and toast" diet. A well-balanced diet is expensive, and its ingredients are heavy to carry home from the store. Furthermore, cooking is an effort, especially if the socialization that normally occurs at meal time is lacking. Not surprisingly, vitamin and mineral deficiencies are common in these patients. Since wound healing depends to a considerable extent upon adequate nutritional reserves of protein, vitamins, particularly vitamin C, and minerals, particularly zinc, it is reasonable to provide supplemental protein, vitamins, and minerals when the nutritional state of a patient before surgery might be compromised.

RESPIRATORY DISEASE AND SURGERY

Pulmonary function shows the most rapid age-associated decline of any organ system. Lung volumes and flow rates at 65 years of age are only 60% of their values at 20 years of age. These changes increase the susceptibility of elderly patients to postoperative pulmonary complications. A history of obesity, obstructive pulmonary disease, cardiac disease, deep venous thrombosis, pulmonary emboli, and smoking all increase the risk of postoperative pulmonary disease. Spirometry should be performed if there is significant exercise intolerance or a significant medical history.

Arterial blood gas measurements should be obtained in patients with a significantly impaired FEV_1 before surgery. A raised PCO_2 is associated with increased postoperative pulmonary complications. Similarly a PO_2 below 55 mm Hg on room air places the patient at high risk. With significantly impaired pulmonary function, local or spinal anesthesia should be considered to avoid the 30% to 50% fall in tidal volumes that routinely occur following general anesthesia.

While many of the functional abnormalities are fixed in pulmonary disease, there is considerable evidence that discontinuing smoking for as little as 1 to 4 weeks significantly improves pulmonary function, decreases bronchial secretions, and improves bronchial ciliary function.

All patients should be urged to discontinue cigarette smoking before surgery. The benefit of prophylactic bronchodilators or antibiotics is debated.

An increased respiratory rate may be a clue to lung disease. Elderly patients who are obese or are cigarette smokers must be suspected of having obstructive pulmonary disease. The physical examination of the lungs and pulmonary function tests should be used to measure respiratory function in the elderly patient. If respiratory function is severely compromised, the stress of the operative procedure must be weighed against the degree of pulmonary insufficiency. Patients with chronic obstructive pulmonary disease should have preoperative postural drainage with chest percussion. This has been shown to decrease pulmonary complications following surgery.[7]

THROMBOEMBOLIC DISEASE
AFTER SURGERY

Thromboembolic complications of surgery are very common. Patients with a history of deep venous thrombosis or pulmonary emboli are at very high risk of thromboembolic disease following surgery. The elderly patient is at particular risk because postoperative thromboembolic disease increases with age.[12] The chance of deep venous thrombosis and pulmonary emboli is increased following surgery not only because bed rest increases venous stasis but also because the operative procedure may obstruct blood flow or traumatize vessels. Furthermore, the fibrinolytic activity of the blood is reduced following surgery. Certain operations frequently performed on elderly patients, for example, hip surgery and prostatectomy, are associated with a particularly high rate of deep venous thrombosis and pulmonary emboli. Radioisotope scanning or venography documents deep venous thrombosis in 70% of elderly patients operated on for hip fractures, in 50% of elderly patients after prostatectomy, and in 35% of all surgical patients over the age of 40.[11]

It appears therefore that all elderly patients, especially those for whom hip or prostate surgery is planned, should have prophylaxis for deep venous thrombosis and pulmonary emboli. What type of prophylaxis should be chosen? Early ambulation, physical therapy, and pneumatic boots that compress calf muscles carry little risk and should be employed. Drugs used in the prophylaxis of deep venous thrombosis and pulmonary emboli include low-dose heparin, aspirin, and dextran. Patients to be considered for such therapy must have normal coagulation studies and not be taking oral anticoagulants or aspirin.

Low-dose heparin therapy (5000 units 2 hours before surgery and 5000 units two or three times per day for 1 week) prevents the activation of the clotting cascade and has been shown to decrease deep venous thrombosis and pulmonary emboli in patients undergoing major elective surgery.[10] However, such therapy is not effective in decreasing deep venous thrombosis and pulmonary emboli after prostatectomy or hip surgery, and low-dose heparin is inadequate for patients with an active thrombotic process. Heparin therapy should not be used before neurologic or ophthalmic surgery. Aspirin (300 mg twice a day) has been shown to reduce deep venous thrombosis in men but not in women following hip surgery, while dextran has been reported to decrease both deep venous thrombosis and pulmonary emboli.[11] Dextran produced a reduction in thromboembolic disease similar to that of low-dose heparin. Although blood losses at surgery were not significantly different and transfusion requirements were the same, heparin therapy was associated with more wound hematomas.

CARDIAC DISEASE AND SURGERY

A history of cardiac disease is important in assessing the risks of surgery for the elderly patient. A history of angina or a previous myocardial infarction increases the risk of reinfarction in the postoperative period. The degree of risk is related to the interval between the myocardial infarction and the surgery. Thus, 37% of patients who had a myocardial infarction in the 6-week-period before surgery and 16% of patients who had a myocardial infarction between

TABLE 3-1
Cardiac risk in noncardiac surgery

Criteria	Points
History	
Age over 70 years	5
Myocardial infarction previous 6 months (potentially reversible)	10
Physical examination	
S₃ gallop, jugular venous distension (potentially reversible)	11
Significant aortic valvular stenosis	3
Laboratory examination	
EKG	
Premature atrial contractions or rhythm other than sinus	7
More than 5 premature ventricular contractions/minute	7
General status (potentially reversible)	3
Abnormal blood gases	
Electrolyte abnormalities	
Abnormal renal function	
Liver disease, bedridden	
Operation	
Emergency (potentially reversible)	4
Intraperitoneal, intrathoracic, aortic	3
TOTAL POSSIBLE	53
TOTAL POTENTIALLY REVERSIBLE	28

Modified from Goldman, L., et al: N. Engl. J. Med. **297:**845, 1977. Reprinted by permission of the New England Journal of Medicine.

TABLE 3-2
Correlation of cardiac risk points and postoperative cardiac problems

Point total	Life-threatening complications (%)	Cardiac deaths (%)
0-5	0.7	0.2
6-12	5.0	2.0
13-25	11.0	2.0
>26	22.0	56.0

Modified from Goldman, L., et al.: N. Engl. J. Med. **297:**845, 1977. Reprinted by permission of the New England Journal of Medicine.

6 weeks and 6 months before surgery had a postoperative myocardial infarction.[10] Most investigators believe that delaying surgery more than 6 months after a myocardial infarction does not further reduce the risk of postoperative reinfarction. Postoperative myocardial infarction, which occurs most frequently 4 to 7 days after surgery, has a high (50%) mortality rate.[5] For this reason surgery should, if at all possible, be delayed until at least 6 weeks and preferably 6 months after a myocardial infarction. One half of postoperative myocardial infarctions in elderly patients are not associated with chest pain. These "silent" myocardial infarctions may be manifested only by increasing congestive heart failure, by a fall in blood pressure, or less frequently by a cardiac arrhythmia. Confusion or other mental aberrations, sometimes the result of reduced cerebral circulation, may be the only clue to a silent myocardial infarction.

Cardiac complications are a leading cause of postoperative morbidity and mortality in elderly patients.[2] A multifactorial analysis of cardiac risks in over 1000 patients who had noncardiac surgery found that one third of the postoperative death rate (the total death rate was 6%) was attributed to cardiac disease and 4% of the patients who survived had life-threatening but nonfatal cardiac complications following surgery.[4] A point system has been devised to quantitate significant risk factors for postoperative cardiac complications (Table 3-1). Risks are detected through the history and by physical and laboratory examinations of the surgical candidate. Two historical risk factors, an age over 70 and a history of myocardial infarction less than 6 months before surgery, are highly significant risk factors. Other risk factors are detected by physical or laboratory examinations.

The point system for cardiac risk provides a means to divide patients into four groups according to the degree of risk with respect to mortality and life-threatening but nonfatal complications (Table 3-2). Goldman et al.[4] recommended that "only truly life-saving procedures be performed on patients with risk index scores of 26 or more points." Fortunately, 28 of the 53 points are reversible to some degree, and the geriatric evaluation should offer a therapeutic plan to lower these risks.

The pulse, taken for at least 30 seconds, may offer a clue to cardiac arrhythmias. All abnormal rhythms increase the risk of surgery. Premature atrial contractions add less to the risk of surgery than do premature ventricular contractions. Multifocal premature ventricular contractions, more than 5 premature ventricular contractions per minute, and premature ventricular contractions exhibiting the "R-on-T" phenomenon are of particular concern. If abnormal rhythms are suggested by the history or by the physical or laboratory examination, a 24-hour Holter monitor recording should be obtained. Patients with serious arrhythmias may benefit from the insertion of a temporary pacemaker.

Many elderly patients have implanted cardiac pacemakers. Some operate only "on demand." Since electrical interference from equipment in the operating room can disturb the operation of a demand pacemaker, fixed-mode pacing should be instituted during surgery to prevent malfunctioning of the pacemaker during surgery.

As many as 50% of elderly patients have blood pressures above 160/90. Although hypertension in the elderly is a significant risk factor for cardiovascular disease, it is not a risk factor with regard to cardiovascular morbidity and mortality following surgery.[4] If the diastolic blood pressure is less than 110, bed rest alone usually lowers the blood pressure so that antihypertensive therapy is not necessary before surgery. If hypertension contributes to congestive heart failure, antihypertensive therapy should be instituted to improve cardiac function.

Auscultation of the carotid vessels is another important aspect of the preoperative evaluation. If a bruit is discovered, symptoms of transient neurologic deficits should be sought. If a history of a transient ischemic attack is obtained, Doppler studies and angiography should be used to evaluate carotid blood flow. Since the risk of cerebrovascular accidents during or following surgery is very high in patients with symptomatic carotid artery disease, vascular repair should be carried out before all except emergency surgery is performed. On the other hand, if no symptoms of neurologic disease are elicited, the course of action is less clear. Since 15% of patients over 65 have bruits, it is not reasonable to subject all patients to angiographic studies. Perhaps candidates for coronary bypass surgery who are at particular risk of cerebrovascular accidents should have Doppler studies. Patients with carotid bruits without any history or signs of neurologic deficit appear to be at no greater risk of cerebrovascular accidents following surgery than are patients without carotid bruits. Thus, in a study of 700 patients examined before surgery, the frequency of cerebrovascular accidents was comparable in patients with and without carotid bruits.[15]

Cardiac disease in general and congestive heart failure in particular contribute much to the morbidity and mortality following surgery. Therefore, careful assessment of cardiac function is a crucial part of the preoperative assessment. Cardiomegaly, jugular venous distension, and hepatomegaly are important signs of congestive heart failure. Peripheral edema in the elderly is a less useful sign of congestive heart failure. Venous disease is a common cause of swelling of the lower extremities. Patients in heart failure or patients who have been in heart failure in the past are at greater risk of developing postoperative pulmonary edema. Therapy with digitalis, diuretics, and/or agents that reduce cardiac afterload improves cardiac compensation and reduces the risk of acute postoperative heart failure. Venous disease increases the risk of thromboembolic disease and may suggest the need for anticoagulant therapy. Finally, cardiac auscultation may reveal abnormalities in cardiac rhythm or valvular heart disease.

Patients who have had valvular heart disease and/or a prosthetic valve implanted require special care before surgery. Many of these patients are receiving oral anticoagulant therapy. It is therefore necessary to provide a period of hemostatic competence during the surgical procedure without exposing the patient to undue risk of thromboembolic disease. This can be achieved by stopping the coumarin drug 24 hours before surgery and giving 50 mg of vitamin K_1 intravenously. Intravenous heparin (1000 units/hour) is begun 12 hours after surgery if there is no postoperative bleeding and is continued until the effect of oral anticoagulants, begun usually on the third postoperative day, is established.

INFECTIONS AFTER SURGERY

Increasing data suggest that patients given antimicrobial prophylaxis before certain operations have a lower incidence of sepsis and wound infection (Table 3-3). Patients with valvular heart disease, prosthetic heart valves, or prosthetic joints are at particular risk from infections. These patients are at risk not only from sepsis but also from bacteremia, which can result in bacterial colonization of the prosthesis. Prophylactic antibiotics are given to such pa-

TABLE 3-3
Antibiotic prophylaxis for surgery

Operation	Antibiotic
Clean	
Cardiovascular: prosthetic valve insertions, vascular reconstruction, coronary bypass	Cefazolin
Orthopaedic: joint replacement, Internal fixation of fracture	Penicillinase-resistant penicillin
Clean-contaminated	
Entry into upper respiratory tract	Penicillin
Gastric surgery with obstruction or hemorrhage	Cefoxitin
Biliary surgery with jaundice, with cholecystitis, age 70 or older	Cefoxitin
Hysterectomy	Cefoxitin
Urologic surgery with infected urine	Antibiotic appropriate to bacteria
Colorectal	Cefoxitin plus oral erythomycin and neomycin
Dirty	
Ruptured viscus	Clindamycin
	Gentamicin
	Penicillin
Traumatic fracture	Cefazolin
Amputation with ulcer or compromised blood flow	Cefazolin
Patients with prosthetic valves or prosthetic joints: as above with these additions:	
Upper respiratory tract procedures: intubation, bronchoscopy	Penicillin
Urinary tract procedures: cystoscopy	Penicillin and gentamicin
Gastrointestinal tract procedures: enema, barium enema, colonoscopy	
Podiatry: callus	Penicillinase-resistant penicillin

Modified from Med. Lett. **25**:113, 1983.

tients to prevent sepsis, bacteremia, and wound infection. Patients with prosthetic valves or prosthetic joints require prophylactic antibiotics for surgical procedures involving the upper respiratory tract (e.g., penicillin for bronchoscopy), procedures involving the urinary tract (e.g., penicillin and streptomycin for cystoscopy), and procedures involving the lower gastrointestinal tract (e.g., penicillin and streptomycin for proctoscopy and barium enema). Even foot care is a potential risk in patients with prosthetic implants because an infected callus may be silent. A single dose of 500 mg of an oral penicillinase-resistant penicillin should be given before podiatric surgery. If an infected area is uncovered, the antibiotic therapy should be continued for 2 days.

For most patients the advantages of antibiotic therapy before surgery outweigh the risk of untoward reactions (in the absence of known allergy) to these drugs. A concern in the use of prophylactic antibiotics is infection with drug-resistant microorganisms. For this reason, antibiotics with a narrow spectrum that covers the most likely organisms should be chosen. Prophylactic antibiotics should be given for surgery in which foreign bodies, such as prosthetic valves or joints, are implanted. Drugs are given by the parenteral route immediately before surgery and continued for 24 hours after surgery, the period when bacteria are most likely to enter the bloodstream. Surgical entry into the gastroduodenal tract or biliary system requires prophylactic antibiotics only under special circumstances (Table 3-3). On the other hand, surgical procedures involving the upper respiratory tract, colon, or an infected wound are always an indication for antibiotics. Cefazolin is frequently the drug of choice because it has a longer half-life than other cephalosporins and injection is less painful. Cefoxitin is chosen when infections with anaerobic bacteria are likely. Urologic surgery in the absence of urinary tract infection does not require prophylactic antibiotics. If the urine is infected, appropriate antibiotics should be chosen based on the urine culture and sensitivity results. Gramnegative sepsis may follow instrumentation of the urinary tract if the urine is infected.

HEMATOLOGIC DISEASE AND SURGERY

Polycythemia vera, multiple myeloma, and chronic lymphocytic leukemia occur most frequently in the elderly. These diseases may be associated with impaired hemostasis. Patients with polycythemia vera are at risk both from hemorrhage, because of platelet dysfunction, and from thrombosis caused by increased blood viscosity. Increased blood viscosity results primarily from the increased erythrocyte count. These complications are minimized if the red blood cell and platelet counts are in the normal range. Phlebotomy is the safest method for reducing the red cell mass but it may stimulate thrombocytosis. Patients with platelet counts above $800,000/mm^3$ should be treated with cytostatic drugs.

Patients with multiple myeloma may have impaired platelet function, resulting either from thrombocytopenia or from the effects of myeloma proteins on the platelets or on fibrin clot formation. Patients with multiple myeloma should be tested for platelet function as well as for platelet number. Patients with chronic lymphocytic leukemia are at increased risk of pyogenic infection because of hypogammaglobulinemia. Parenteral gamma globulin should be given to enhance the opsonization of bacteria.

ENDOCRINE DISEASE AND SURGERY

Diabetes mellitus is a very common disease among the elderly. Many patients with diabetes mellitus are treated with oral hypoglycemic agents. These agents cannot be used during the period when surgical patients are denied oral feeding. A decision must be made as to whether therapy for diabetes can be discontinued for a short time or whether insulin therapy is required to prevent hyperglycemia. Careful attention to blood glucose homeostasis is particularly important because elderly patients are particularly sensitive to the effects of both hypoglycemia and hyperglycemia. Most elderly patients have impaired renal function. Such patients are at particular risk from hyperglycemia, which because of peripheral resistance to insulin and a decreased capacity to clear glucose from the blood into the urine may lead to hyperosmolar, nonketotic coma. It is usually reasonable to manage glucose metabolism during surgery and the immediate postoperative period with intravenous glucose and insulin. The dose is established by frequent blood glucose determinations.

Thyroid disease is frequently difficult to recognize in the elderly. The signs and symptoms of hypothyroidism may be attributed to "slowing down" with age. The signs of hyperthyroidism may be masked. Eye signs, tremors, sweating, and heat insensitivity frequently observed in the young usually are not seen in the elderly hyperthyroid patient. One third of elderly hyperthyroid patients do not have an enlarged thyroid. Atrial fibrillation may be the only clue to hyperthyroidism in the elderly. The danger of thyroid storm following surgery, however, is not any less in masked hyperthyroidism in the elderly patient. Despite greater awareness of apathetic hyperthyroidism, 10% to 30% of thyroid storm is still precipitated by surgery.

THERMOREGULATION AND SURGERY

Temperature regulation is known to be impaired in the elderly. Exposure of many elderly patients to cool temperatures fails to elicit the normal physiologic responses to conserve heat, such as vasoconstriction or generation of body heat by shivering. Body temperature therefore may fall. Rectal temperatures should be obtained on all elderly patients. Rectal temperatures below 37° C may be of minor concern in the young patient but may be a clue to impaired thermoregulation in the elderly. Patients with low body temperatures have a higher risk of morbid and fatal events following surgery.[1] Surgery stresses the thermoregula-

tory capacity of the patient. The operating room is cool; intravenous fluids are at room temperature; peritoneal surfaces are exposed to ambient temperature; and drapes conserve little body heat. Warming blankets may be used during surgery to compensate for heat loss, but nothing is more important than measuring body temperature during and after surgery. Hypothermia depresses cardiac and respiratory function and may lead to hypotension, impaired ventilation, and cardiac arrhythmias. Such complications, which are frequently noted in the recovery room, may be the results of hypothermia.

UROLOGIC ABNORMALITIES AND SURGERY

Rectal examinations should be performed on all elderly patients not only to obtain a stool specimen to be tested for occult blood but also to detect rectal masses and an enlarged prostate. Rectal masses or prostatic hypertrophy may be the cause of a newly discovered hernia. An enlarged prostate also presents a risk factor for urinary retention following surgery. In older men with prostatic hypertrophy, overhydration during or following surgery, anticholinergic drugs, and bed rest may precipitate acute urinary retention. If the patient has prostatic hypertrophy or a history of urinary infection or if a urologic procedure will be performed, a urine culture should be obtained to rule out bacteriuria. Appropriate treatment for bacteriuria should be given before surgery. Renal function may be estimated by blood urea nitrogen (BUN) and creatinine concentrations. However, in the elderly "normal values" do not ensure normal renal function because 50% of renal function can be lost before either BUN or creatinine rises above the normal range. Furthermore, in elderly patients with low protein intake and/or low muscle mass, even more renal function can be lost before BUN or creatinine levels become abnormal. If renal function may have been compromised by infection, prostate enlargement, hypertension, or prior renal disease, creatinin clearance should be tested. The glomerular filtration rate not only documents the level of renal impairment but also serves as a guide to the proper dose of many drugs excreted by the kidney. Impaired renal function does not become a significant risk to surgery until renal perfusion falls below 45 to 50 ml/minute. Below this level of kidney function, wound healing is compromised.

LABORATORY TESTS BEFORE SURGERY

A number of routine laboratory tests should be obtained before surgery. Elderly patients should have a urinalysis, complete blood count, serum chemistries (BUN, creatinine, alkaline phosphatase, SGOT, SGPT, and electrolytes), a chest x-ray examination, and an electrocardiogram before surgery. The integrity of the coagulation system should be tested by platelet count, prothrombin time, and partial thromboplastin time. If there is any suggestion of a hemorrhagic diathesis or ingestion of drugs that inhibit platelet function, the bleeding time should be tested. Finally, blood for typing and crossmatching should be obtained.

Acknowledgment

I wish to thank Dr. Kenneth P. Scileppi and Dr. Anita Herdan for reviewing the original manuscript. The information in this chapter is derived from my contribution to Practical Geriatric Medicine.

References

1. Bastow, M.D., Rawlings, J., and Allison, S.P.: Undernutrition, hypothermia and injury in elderly women with fractured femur: an injury response to altered metabolism, Lancet 1:143, 1983.
2. Djokovic, J.L., and Headley-Whyle, J.: Prediction of outcome of surgery and anesthesia in patients over 80, J.A.M.A. 242:2301, 1979.
3. Finkel, M.L., McCarthy, E.G., and Ruchlin, H.S.: The current status of surgical second opinion programs, Surg. Clin. North Am. 62:705, 1982.
4. Goldman, L., et al.: Multifactorial index of cardiac risk in non-cardiac surgical procedures, N. Engl. J. Med. 297:845, 1977.
5. Goldman, L., et al.: Cardiac risk factors and complications in non-cardiac surgery; Medicine 57:357, 1978.
6. Gruber, U.F., et al.: Incidence of fatal post operative pulmonary embolism after prophylaxis with dextran 70 and low dose heparin: an internal and multicare study, Br. Med. J. 280:69, 1980.
7. Harman, E., and Lillington, G.: Pulmonary risk factors in surgery, Med. Clin. North Am. 63:1289, 1979.
8. Heller, S.S., et al.: Psychiatric complication of open heart surgery. N. Engl. J. Med. 283:1015, 1970.
9. Levilan, S.J., and Kornfeld, D.S.: Clinical and cost benefits of liaison psychiatry, Am. J. Psychiatry 138:790, 1981.
10. Low dose heparin prophylaxis and pulmonary embolism, Med. Lett. 19:71, 1977.
11. Mitchell, R.A.: Can we really prevent postoperative pulmonary emboli? Br. Med. J. 1:1523, 1979.
12. Morrell, M.T., Truelove, S.C., and Barr, A.: Pulmonary embolism, Br. Med. J. 2:830, 1963.
13. Muller, J.M., Brenner, U., Dienst, C., and Pilchmaier, H.: Preoperative parenteral feeding in patients with gastrointestinal carcinoma. Lancet 1:68, 1982.
14. Polk, H.C.: The mathematics of clinical judgement. In Gardner, B., Polk, H.C., Stone, H.H., and Sugg, W.L., editors: Basic surgery, New York, 1978, Appleton-Century-Crofts.
15. Ropper, A.H., Wechsler, L.R., and Wilson, L.S.: Carotid bruits and the risk of stroke in elective surgery, N. Engl. J. Med. 307:1388, 1982.
16. Tarhan, S., Moffitt, E.A., Taylor, W.F., and Ginliani, E.R.: Myocardial infarction after general anesthesia, J.A.M.A. 220:1451, 1972.

chapter 4

ANESTHESIA FOR GERIATRIC ORTHOPAEDIC SURGERY

Steven F. Seidman

As life expectancy has increased and surgical technology has progressed, anesthesiologists have been presented with increasing frequency with the perioperative management of geriatric patients. Early studies indicated that the overall operative mortality in patients over age 70 was in the range of 16% to 20%. The higher mortality rates were associated with thoracic, abdominal, and major vascular procedures. Operations performed on an emergency basis had the poorest outcome. These figures have improved with time so that more recent work indicates that for elective procedures the overall mortality rate is less than 5% in the geriatric population.[3]

More specifically, with regard to orthopaedic procedures performed on the geriatric patient, Ziffren and Hartford[18] in 1972 reported on mortality rates for amputations both below and above the knee and for the closed reduction and internal fixation of hip fractures. Mortality figures in their series were in the range of 2% to 17%. Most certainly, mortality statistics in geriatric orthopaedics have improved significantly since their work was first reported.

Although mortality statistics for operative procedures on the elderly have improved, the geriatric population still remains at higher risk for mortality associated with anesthesia and surgery than its younger counterpart. The explanation for this fact lies in the older patient's diminished capacity to withstand physiologic insults. As a patient ages he becomes pro-

gressively less able to compensate for derangements in homeostasis. Surgery and anesthesia may challenge physiologic reserves to the point of decompensation. To understand why the anesthetic management of the geriatric patient requiring orthopaedic intervention often proves hazardous, it is necessary to focus on some of the physiologic changes associated with aging. It must be emphasized that there is a distinction between the general reduction in organ reserves associated with aging as opposed to the deterioration of specific organ systems as a result of disease. We may have some ability to limit or reverse changes associated with disease, but we have no control over the natural diminution in organ function secondary to aging.

PHYSIOLOGIC CHANGES
Cardiovascular changes

Overall cardiovascular reserves diminish with age. Cardiac output is noted to decrease as a result of the reduction in both heart rate and stroke volume. There is an increase in circulation time of 33% at age 80 compared with that at age 30 years. Atherosclerotic changes result in narrowing of the vascular lumen, causing increased vascular resistance and decreased tissue perfusion. Vascular changes associated with aging are associated with increased systolic pressures, while the diastolic pressures may increase somewhat or remain unaffected. Upper limits of normal blood pressure in the older patient range up to 160 torr systolic and 100 torr diastolic.[17] Alterations in heart size and morphologic changes in the conduction system, both associated with the aging process, help to explain, in part, the increased incidence of arrhythmias seen in these patients. Aging also results in a diminution of function of the medullary cardiovascular control centers. The resultant decrease in sympathetic nervous system activity is associated with an impairment in cardiovascular compensatory responses. This loss of sympathetic function in addition to the decreased cardiac contractility and heart rate causes a reduction in cardiac reserve. This reduction in reserve may not be apparent during normal activity, but under the stress of anesthesia and surgery (e.g., blood loss, hypotension, cardiac depressant anesthetic agents), cardiac failure may ensue.[17]

The cardiovascular changes listed above are normally associated with the aging process. It should be appreciated that superimposed cardiovascular disease (e.g., valvular disease, cardiomyopathy, coronary artery disease) serves to accentuate the changes associated with aging, resulting in an increased likelihood for decompensation during anesthesia and surgery.

What effects might these changes in cardiovascular function with aging have on anesthetic management? Geriatric patients are quite sensitive to the cardiac depressant effects of various anesthetic agents. Their limited cardiac reserves may well result in marked decreases in cardiac output and blood pressure after exposure to such cardiac depressants. Doses must therefore be altered and anesthetic agents chosen with the potential for decompensation always kept in mind. Volume depletion is not well tolerated by the geriatric patient. Blood loss, insufficient volume replacement, or preoperative hypovolemia all might result in insufficient cardiac function especially after the introduction of anesthetic agents. Geriatric patients are often incapable of handling extremes of blood pressure. Those with preexistent disease (e.g., myocardial infarctions or cerebrovascular accidents)

are severely stressed by hypotensive states. Similarly, patients with myocardial disease may develop cardiac decompensation in the face of severe hypertension. It is imperative in these geriatric patients with narrowed coronary arteries that, with regard to the heart, favorable ratios of oxygen supply versus oxygen demand be maintained. Otherwise myocardial ischemia may result that could progress to a fulminant infarction.

Pulmonary changes

The aging process causes changes in lung function and structure that impair the ability of the lung to serve its function in gas exchange and as a conduit for the uptake and elimination of anesthetic gases. With aging the thoracic wall becomes stiffer, there is degeneration of pulmonary parenchymal tissue, and the ventilatory muscles weaken. There is an increase in the dead space, closing volume, and residual volume with aging, but vital capacity and forced expiratory volume in 1 second (FEV_1) diminish. These changes result in increased ventilation-perfusion mismatching with a resultant decrease in the efficiency of gas exchange. The normal reduction in arterial oxygen tension (PaO_2) is progressive with age. These degenerative changes occur normally with aging and are only accelerated with conditions such as emphysema, restrictive lung disease, and pulmonary emboli. Anesthetic agents in and of themselves cause changes in pulmonary mechanics, volumes, and ventilation-perfusion balance that result in impaired gas exchange and resultant hypoxemia. Therefore, the geriatric patient who is to undergo surgery and anesthesia is at risk from the changes induced by aging, by prior pulmonary disease, and by perioperative impairments of pulmonary function (e.g., anesthetic agents, postoperative pulmonary emboli, atelectasis). These factors act synergistically to place the geriatric patient at increased risk for ventilation-perfusion imbalance, hypoxemia, and atelectasis. As a result, anesthetic regimens that produce minimal derangements in pulmonary function are to be selected in caring for the geriatric patient. Proper anesthetic management includes a careful preoperative evaluation to minimize risk factors such as bronchospasm and infection and, if necessary, the use of pulmonary function testing and preoperative arterial blood gas determinations to evaluate further those patients thought to be at high risk. Attention must also be directed preoperatively to adequate pulmonary toilet. Intraoperatively it is best to avoid those anesthetic regimens that cause progressive pulmonary impairments. From this standpoint, the use of spinal or epidural anesthesia and peripheral nerve blocks is suggested over general anesthesia. Intraoperatively and postoperatively care must be taken to avoid aspiration, ensure adequate pulmonary toilet, and, if respiration is impaired, to use proper ventilatory support. If appropriate attention is not paid to these matters, respiratory failure with consequent hypoxemia and respiratory acidosis may easily occur in the geriatric patient undergoing anesthesia and surgery.[17]

Central nervous system changes

In the geriatric patient, age-related changes in the central nervous system affect anesthetic management. The overall reduction in the activity of the central nervous system results in a corresponding decrease in the dose of anesthetic drugs and analgesics necessary for the geriatric patient. The progressive loss of the integrity of protective airway reflexes with aging makes the patient more susceptible to aspiration. Because of the increased sensitivity to analgesics, the geriatric patient is more likely to experience respiratory depression and airway obstruction after exposure to analgesics. Prior central nervous system disease (e.g., stroke) and/or concurrent conditions such as weakness or tremors require consideration before using anesthetic regiments such as spinal or epidural anesthesia or peripheral nerve blocks. The possibility of confusion and impaired communication must be considered before determining which anesthetic technique should be chosen.

Renal changes

Age-related changes in both renal function and structure are also noted in the geriatric patient population. Total renal blood flow, glomerular filtration rate, and creatinine clearance all decrease with age. Tubular function is also impaired in the geriatric population, resulting in impaired concentrating ability and a decline in the excretory and resorptive capacity of the renal tubules. These changes occur normally with aging, but superimposed renal disease can augment these changes. A further deterioration in renal function may be caused by extrarenal factors such as cardiac failure, intravascular volume depletion, and the use of diuretics.

These changes in renal function have important implications toward anesthetic management. The geriatric patient will normally have impaired renal excretion of drugs. The addition of general anesthesia into this situation further reduces renal blood flow and glomerular filtration and thereby further impairs the renal excretion of drugs. Hypotension and a decrease in cardiac output, both of which may well accompany general, spinal, or epidural anesthesia, can augment the decline in renal function. Finally, some anesthetic agents (e.g., methoxyflurane, enflurane) may under some circumstances have nephrotoxic effects through the production of inorganic fluoride. Since geriatric patients are already known to have some decline in renal function, the preoperative evaluation should point out those patients with superimposed renal disease and those with extrarenal pathology (e.g., cardiac failure) who are at risk for developing renal decompensation. The anesthetic management of such patients includes the avoidance of potential nephrotoxic agents and hypotension, appropriate intravascular volume repletion, and attention to the maintenance of an adequate urine output.

Hepatic changes

Changes in hepatic function associated with aging center around reduced hepatic perfusion, decreased hepatic enzymatic activity, and lower levels of serum albumin.[3] These changes result in delayed metabolism of drugs and increased plasma levels of unbound, free drug. As a result, drugs used during anesthesia may have both prolonged and excessive effects. Drug doses must be reduced accordingly in the geriatric patient. In patients with concurrent hepatic disease, agents such as halothane that are potentially hepatotoxic are best avoided.

The combination of the decrease in metabolic function of the liver along with the decreased excretory capacity and glomerular filtration of the kidney acts synergistically to prolong and accentuate the effect of drugs given to the geriatric patient. The induction and maintenance of the anesthetic state must be titrated against these changes to avoid an excessively deep or prolonged state of anesthesia. Furthermore, not only is the geriatric patient at risk from the standpoint of decreased metabolism and excretion of drugs but also they are placed at risk from the standpoint of drug interactions and untoward side effects because elderly patients often receive multiple prescription drugs.

Concurrent diseases

Aging involves not only changes in cardiovascular, pulmonary, central nervous system, renal, and hepatic physiology, but also changes in all other organ systems. The systems that have been discussed here are of primary importance to the anesthesiologist with regard to the maintenance of bodily homeostasis intraoperatively and in making the choice as to which anesthetic modality to utilize. As mentioned before, a distinction must be made between the reduction in organ reserves associated with aging as opposed to the deterioration of specific organ systems caused by disease. The geriatric patient is faced with diminished physiologic function as a result of both these phenomena. Obviously older patients are much more likely than their younger counterparts to have developed some form of disease that has added a superimposed diminution in organ function (e.g., congestive heart failure, emphysema, nephritis,

cirrhosis). These facts must be considered before anesthetizing the geriatric patient for orthopaedic surgery.

ANESTHETIC PROBLEMS ASSOCIATED WITH ORTHOPAEDIC SURGERY
Tourniquet use

Let us now direct our attention to those phenomena that are of singular importance to orthopaedic anesthesia. Because of its involvement with the extremities, orthopaedics provides a broad range of anesthetic choices including general, spinal, or epidural anesthesia, peripheral nerve blocks, and intravenous regional anesthesia. To provide for a dry surgical field and to minimize blood loss, tourniquets are often used in orthopaedic surgery. Tourniquet inflation may well result in hypertension and tachycardia. Kaufman and Walts[4] reported on tourniquet-induced hypertension in patients undergoing leg surgery. They reported an overall 11% incidence of hypertension after tourniquet inflation. It was noted that the incidence of hypertension was significantly higher in the geriatric population, reaching as high as 67% of those patients over 80 years of age in whom narcotic nitrous oxide anesthesia was used. The incidence of hypertension in those patients over 80 years old was 12% if regional anesthesia was used. Furthermore, the incidence of tourniquet-induced hypertension was noted to be higher in those patients with cardiac enlargement and in those receiving general anesthesia utilizing narcotics and nitrous oxide. Tachycardia and hypertension represent cardiovascular stresses to which the geriatric myocardium may not respond well. Myocardial work and hence myocardial oxygen demands increase, putting the geriatric patient at risk of developing cardiac ischemia. If severe enough such an ischemic state can progress to frank infarction.

Methylmethacrylate

The use of methylmethacrylate potentially poses many problems regarding anesthetic management. Charnley[2] first reported transient decreases in blood pressure 1 to 2 minutes after the insertion of the acrylic cement into the femur. Peebles et al.[9] believed that the mechanism responsible for this hypotensive effect was peripheral vasodilation, whereas others suggested pulmonary fat and bone marrow emboli as the possible causes of the hypotension.[1] Wong et al.[16] reported that methylmethacrylate induced mild cardiovascular depression in patients undergoing total hip replacements, but that these changes were not statistically significant. However, currently most authors agree that hypotension occurs frequently after the placement of acrylic cement and that the mechanism is the monomer-induced vasodilation. As pointed out by Charnley,[2] the greatest drops in blood pressure resulting from methylmethacrylate placement occurred when the blood pressure was already high as opposed to those patients receiving hypotensive anesthesia in whom there was a minimal reduction in blood pressure after the insertion of the cement.

An additional physiologic derangement follows the use of methylmethacrylate. Following PaO$_2$ levels during total hip replacement, Park et al.[8] noted a sharp but transient decrease in PaO$_2$ after the placement of acrylic bone cement. This change in PaO$_2$ occurred without any concurrent change in either the pulse rate or systemic blood pressure. Hence, Park et al. concluded that the etiologic cause was most likely not pulmonary emboli. Rather, they concluded that the drop in PaO$_2$ was related to the amount of acrylic polymer absorbed into the circulation.

These physiologic changes induced by methylmethacrylate, hypotension and decreased PaO$_2$, place the already high-risk geriatric patient in further jeopardy. Hypotension can result in decreased perfusion of the coronary, cerebral, and renal circulations, which could result in coronary and cerebral ischemia and renal failure. Aging itself is associated with atherosclerotic changes resulting in decreased coronary, cerebral, and renal perfusion even without concurrent hypotension. In some patients, hypotension induces a compensatory tachycardia that may further aggravate cardiac ischemia by decreasing the diastolic filling time of the coronary arteries. Patients who cannot respond to this decrease in blood pressure by increasing cardiac output (i.e., those patients with valvular heart disease, with fixed heart rates, with cardiomyopathy, or taking propranolol [Inderal]) are at risk for insufficient systemic perfusion. The decreased cardiac reserves associated with the aging process and the cardiovascular changes induced by anesthesia (e.g., decreased cardiac output, vasodilatation) further aggravate the methylmethacrylate-induced hypotension.

As for the methylmethacrylate-induced decrease in PaO$_2$, it too is adversely affected by the aging process and anesthesia. PaO$_2$ normally decreases with age and may well be reduced by anesthesia because of factors such as ventilation-perfusion mismatching and atelectasis. Therefore, the anesthetized geriatric patient in whom acrylic bone cement has been applied must be considered at risk for developing hypoxemia.

Aspiration pneumonitis risks

Orthopaedic procedures in the geriatric population may be performed on an emergency basis on patients who have recently eaten or patients with delayed gastric emptying. This fact, coupled with the age-related decrease in the integrity of the protective laryngeal reflexes, places the geriatric patient at risk for aspiration pneumonitis during anesthesia. For this reason, it is suggested that for such orthopaedic procedures performed on an emergency basis the patient should either receive general endotracheal anesthesia with a rapid sequence induction, or if spinal or epidural anesthesia or peripheral nerve block is chosen, the patient should receive only light sedation.

Fat emboli

Additional problems experienced by the geriatric patient undergoing orthopaedic procedures include the risk of fat emboli. The risk of fat emboli seems highest in orthopaedic procedures such as intramedullary nailings and joint replacements. The use of a tourniquet seems to decrease the incidence of fat emboli.[14] The clinical signs associated with fat embolization include pulmonary dysfunction causing hypoxemia and central nervous system derangements such as alterations in consciousness, restlessness, and delirium. Those pathologic changes induced by fat emboli serve to aggravate the pulmonary and central nervous system alterations that are already noted in the geriatric patient undergoing anesthesia.

ANESTHETIC MODALITIES

Let us now shift our attention to the specific anesthetic modalities and see how they interact with the changes induced by the aging process and with orthopaedic operative procedures. Anesthesia for such procedures may be accomplished with general anesthesia, spinal or epidural anesthesia, peripheral nerve block, or intravenous regional anesthesia.

General anesthesia

The popularity of general anesthesia rests, in large part, in its virtually guaranteed analgesia and amnesia, its controllability, and its ease of administration. There are few, if any, absolute contraindications to its use, but under certain circumstances alternate forms of anesthesia are preferable. Major drawbacks to its use include alterations of cardiovascular, pulmonary, and renal function and the risk of aspiration pneumonia. General anesthesia results in cardiac depression (e.g., decreased myocardial contractility and decreased cardiac output) that is additive to the degenerative changes associated with aging. This cardiac depression is especially noted with the use of the halogenated hydrocarbons (halothane, enflurane [Ethrane], and isoflurane [Forane]) and may well cause hypotension and decreased systemic perfusion; in the case of halothane, it may predispose the patient to ventricular arrhythmias. General anesthesia is also associated with changes in pulmonary volumes, mechanisms, and ventilation-perfusion matching, all resulting in potential hypoxemia and atelectasis. The changes induced by general anesthesia, as with aging, are associated with diminished pulmonary function. For this reason, general anesthesia is often avoided in geriatric patients with preexistent pulmonary disease if alternative anesthetic modalities are available. As for the effects on the kidneys and liver, general anesthesia is known to decrease renal blood flow (especially with concurrent hypotension) and glomerular filtration as well as to diminish hepatic perfusion. These facts together with the potential nephrotoxicity of enflurane, and methoxyflurane (Penthrane) and the hepatotoxicity of halothane force the anesthesiologist to reconsider the use of general anesthesia and/or certain anesthetic agents in the geriatric population with preexistent renal or hepatic dysfunction. Since the geriatric patient already has some age-related impairments of cardiovascular, pulmonary, hepatic, and renal function, the use of general anesthesia, which can further impair the function of these organ systems, is not always physiologically sound.

Aside from its negative effects on various organ systems, general anesthesia is not very protective against the hypertension and tachycardia that can accompany tourniquet inflation. The study by Kaufman and Walts[4] points out that general anesthesia is poorly protective regarding tourniquet-induced hypertension in the geriatric population. Regional anesthesia (i.e., spinal anesthesia, peripheral nerve block) was found to be more protective. This fact is of importance to the patient with coronary artery disease, congestive heart failure, or valvular heart disease in whom a significant increase in blood pressure and/or pulse rate may result in cardiac decompensation or ischemia.

Spinal and epidural anesthesia

Spinal and epidural anesthesia represent anesthetic possibilities for patients undergoing lower extremity surgery. Both yield adequate analgesia and muscle relaxation if appropriate concentrations of local anesthetics are used. Although neither spinal nor epidural anesthesia results in a loss of consciousness, both techniques may be supplemented with sedatives to provide intraoperative amnesia. As pointed out by Murphy,[7] the use of a thigh tourniquet requires that the spinal or epidural anesthetic reaches a level cephalad of at least T10. Apparently afferents that travel along with the sympathetic nerves enter the neuraxis at this level and they must be blocked if tourniquet inflation is to be carried out painlessly. In the study by Kaufman and Walts[4] regarding tourniquet-induced hypertension, spinal anesthesia was found to be quite protective in preventing the onset of hypertension after tourniquet inflation. Furthermore, if the spinal anesthetic travels no farther cephalad than T10, then usually only mild changes in cardiovascular and virtually no changes in respiratory function occur. The usual cardiovascular sequela of a spinal or epidural block is hypotension, the drop in blood pressure being more abrupt after spinal anesthesia than epidural. The more cephalad the block travels, the more profound the blood pressure drop. Bradycardia may result after a spinal block extending to high thoracic levels since the cardiac accelerator nerves emerge from the T1 to T4 levels. Furthermore, as a spinal or epidural block extends cephalad there is progressive weakness and possibly paralysis of the respiratory intercostal muscles. Even with total intercostal paralysis, however, the phrenic input to the diaphragm is sufficient to maintain respiratory homeostasis. Usually respiratory failure after a spinal block is caused by hypotension with resultant ischemia of the medullary respiratory centers.[7] Because of the inherent cardiovascular changes that occur with aging, the geriatric patient is at particular risk of developing circulatory insufficiency after spinal or epidural blocks that inadvertently ascend to high thoracic levels. As stated previously, however, if the block extends no higher than T10, circulatory and respiratory changes are minimal, and surgery can safely proceed on the lower extremity even with a tourniquet.

Peripheral nerve blocks

Peripheral nerve blocks for extremity surgery are most useful in the geriatric population. Under most circumstances such nerve blocks are performed without any untoward effects on the cardiovascular, respiratory, or central nervous systems. Also the commonly used local anesthetics have no renal or hepatic toxicity. A well-administered nerve block allows one to anesthetize an extremity selectively and, if indicated, the addition of adequate sedatives brings about intraoperative amnesia.

The drawbacks regarding peripheral nerve blocks center about the intravascular injection of local anesthetics and the possibility of complications such as pneumothorax, recurrent laryngeal nerve paralysis, or subarachnoid needle placement. The inadvertent injection of excessive local anesthetic into a vascular channel is associated first with the central nervous system manifestations of excitation and seizures. Cardiac depression in terms of both depressed rhythmicity and contractility may also accompany the intravascular injection of an excessive dose of local anesthetic. Certain peripheral nerve blocks (i.e., axillary blocks) are contraindicated in the presence of infection or malignancy in the involved extremity.[15] In the presence of a coexistent neuropathy in the involved extremity, the performance of a peripheral nerve block is not suggested. Obesity makes the performance of a peripheral nerve block technically quite difficult. Another major drawback of such blocks lies in their possibility of failure. Analgesia is not always guaranteed with a nerve block, and this possibility of failure has diminished their popularity with many anesthesiologists and surgeons. In spite of these drawbacks, peripheral nerve blocks are usually excellent choices for the geriatric patient undergoing extremity surgery since they involve the most minimal physiologic derangements of all the anesthetic modalities.

In geriatric patients with compromised pulmonary function who are to undergo upper extremity surgery, there seems little indication for the use of a supraclavicular block since the incidence of pneumothorax as reported by Moore[6] is 0.5% to 4%. In such patients axillary blocks or interscalene approaches to the brachial plexus are both excellent alternatives to the supraclavicular route and do not carry the high risk of pneumothorax. It should also be mentioned that peripheral nerve blocks protect against tourniquet-induced hypertension. In the upper extremity such protection requires the blocking of the intercostobrachial nerve on the medial aspect of the arm in addition to the performance of the axillary, supraclavicular, or interscalene block. If the intercostobrachial nerve is not blocked, the patient will experience discomfort along the upper, inner aspect of the arm after tourniquet inflation, and hypertension and/or tachycardia may ensue.

Intravenous regional anesthesia

Intravenous regional anesthesia, the so-called Bier block, is similar to the peripheral nerve block in that the involved extremity alone can be anesthetized. This technique is usually performed for upper rather than lower extremity surgery because of the large dose of local anesthetic that would be required to anesthetize the leg properly. The major advantages of this technique revolve around its ease of performance and virtually guaranteed success, unlike the situation with peripheral nerve blocks. However, the possibility of tourniquet failure makes this technique fraught with a danger of local anesthetic overdose with the resultant sequelae of seizures and cardiac decompensation.

Anesthesia for arthroplasty

With total joint replacements being performed so commonly, the issue of anesthetic techniques has been addressed more frequently. Total hip replacements are now performed using general, spinal, and epidural anesthesia. Thompson et al.[13] compared patients undergoing total hip arthroplasty under both general anesthesia and hypotensive general anesthesa utilizing either high-dose halothane or nitroprusside to induce hypotension. It was found that none of these methods affected the results

of postoperative cerebral, hepatic, or renal function or myocardial status. Intraoperative blood losses decreased from 1183 ± 172 ml in the group with normal pressure to 406 ± 102 ml and 326 ± 41 ml in the groups with halothane and nitroprusside hypotension, respectively. The conclusions drawn by Thompson et al.[13] were that deliberate hypotension added no morbidity and significantly shortened operating time, decreased blood losses, and minimized the number of blood transfusions needed. This finding of reduced blood loss under hypotensive anesthesia was also noted by Rosberg et al.[10,11] in Sweden. In a study performed by Sculco and Ranawat[12] comparing spinal anesthesia to general anesthesia in patients undergoing total hip arthroplasty, it was noted that the patients under spinal anesthesia had reduced blood losses (the average reduction being 600 ml), less postoperative suction drainage, and required fewer transfusions. The postoperative complications were fewer in the spinal anesthesia group. Studying 60 patients undergoing total hip arthroplasty, Modig[5] demonstrated a significantly lower incidence of deep vein thrombosis and pulmonary emboli with epidural anesthesia compared to general anesthesia. Modig attributed the differences in thromboembolic phenomena to increased blood flow and better fibrinolytic function with epidural anesthesia.

Total knee replacements are performed using general, spinal, or epidural anesthesia. The use of a thigh tourniquet minimizes the importance of anesthetic technique and blood loss during this procedure. Of great importance in knee replacement surgery is the issue of tourniquet-induced hypertension and/or tachycardia that often results. As mentioned before, spinal anesthesia appears more protective regarding tourniquet-induced hypertension than does general anesthesia.

In joint replacement surgery the effects of methylmethacrylate must always be considered. As noted previously, the effects of methylmethacrylate include hypotension and hypoxemia. Hypotension may result in inadequate coronary or cerebral perfusion in the patient with severe atherosclerosis. Hypoxemia can pose a problem in the patient with concurrent pulmonary disease who is receiving a general anesthesic. These factors must be kept in mind when choosing the anesthetic modality for arthroplasty.

References

1. Bernstein, R.: Anesthesia for total hip replacement. In Zauder, H., editor: Anesthesia for orthopedic surgery, Philadelphia, 1980, F.A. Davis Co.
2. Charnley, J.: Acrylic cement in orthopaedic surgery, Baltimore, 1970, The Williams & Wilkins Co.
3. Janis, K.M.: Anesthesia for the geriatric patient. A.S.A. refresher course, Anesthesiology, **7**:143, 1979.
4. Kaufman, R.D., and Walts, L.F.: Tourniquet induced hypertension, Br. J. Anaesth. **54**:334, 1982.
5. Modig, J.: Thrombosis risk less with epidural block, Anesthesiol. News **8**(11):1-11, 1982.
6. Moore, D.: Regional block, Springfield, Ill., 1978, Charles C Thomas, Publisher.
7. Murphy, T.: Spinal, epidural and caudal anesthesia. In Miller, R.D., editor: Anesthesia, New York, 1981, Churchill Livingstone.
8. Park, W., et al.: Changes in arterial oxygen tension during total hip replacement, Anesthesiology **39**:642, 1973.
9. Peebles, D., et al.: Cardiovascular effects of methylmethacrylate cement, Br. Med. J. **1**:349, 1972.
10. Rosberg, B., et al.: Blood loss reduced during hip arthroplasty, Anesthesiol. News **8**(10):120, 1982.
11. Rosberg, B., et al.: Blood loss reduced during hip arthroplasty, Acta Anaesthesiol. Scand. **26**:189, 1982.
12. Sculco, T., and Ranawat, C.: The use of spinal anesthesia for total hip replacement arthroplasty, J. Bone Joint Surg **57A**(2):173, 1975.
13. Thompson, G.E., et al.: Hypotensive anesthesia for total hip arthroplasty, Anesthesiology **48**:91, 1978.
14. Wilkins, K.: Fat embolism. In Zauder, H., editor: Anesthesia for orthopedic surgery, Philadelphia, 1980, F.A. Davis Co.
15. Winnie, A.: Regional anesthesia of the upper and lower extremities. In Zauder, H., editor: Anesthesia for orthopedic surgery, Philadelphia, 1980, F.A. Davis Co.
16. Wong, K.C., et al.: Cardiovascular effects of total hip replacement in man, Clin. Pharmacol. Ther. **21**(6):709, 1977.
17. Zamost, B., and Benomof, J.: Anesthesia in the geriatric patient. In Katz, J., et al., editor: Anesthesia and uncommon disease, Philadelphia, 1981, W.B. Saunders Co.
18. Ziffren, S., and Hartford, C.E.: Comparative mortality for various surgical operations in older versus younger age groups, J. Am. Geriatr. Soc. **20**(10):487, 1977.

chapter 5

RHEUMATIC DISEASE IN THE ELDERLY

Emmanuel Rudd

DEFINITION

The elderly may be arbitrarily defined as persons having reached the age of 60. The average span of life in the Western World is now between the ages of 70 and 80. For 10 to 15 years the majority of the elderly will remain independent for self care and household work; many will continue in the work force and will participate in recreational activities. Some will retire earlier than others by choice, because of various circumstances or for health reasons. Diseases of the joints in the elderly will affect each person with a different speed and an individual pattern. The condition of the locomotor system plays a particularly important role in modulating the ability of the elderly to function at home and in the community.

Until 50 years ago it was commonly accepted that aging was accompanied by constant or recurrent aches in the back and limbs. The words "rheumatism" and "arthritis" were used indiscriminately to label joint pain, stiffness, and limitation of mobility. It is still common for lay people, and unfortunately for some health professionals, to equate joint pain with old age.

Advances of contemporary rheumatology allow us to distinguish between the aging process and pathologic states, to recognize various diseases of the joints, and to formulate hypotheses of the cause and pathogenesis. We still have only a tentative classification of the more than 100 clinical entities considered rheumatic diseases, but we have some insight about their natural history[34] The epidemiologic studies have provided information on sex and age distribution and the relative frequency of rheumatic diseases in the general population.[22,40] Of some 30 million people in the United States reported to be suffering from "arthritis and rheumatism" two-thirds have been diagnosed as having osteoarthritis.[24,25] Among the elderly this is the most frequent diagnosis.

Rheumatoid arthritis, which afflicts about 6 million people, can start at any age and not infrequently after the fifth decade. It is a chronic illness, and many elderly have long-standing disease. One million gout patients are better managed because of our present understanding of this metabolic disease and its control. However, some cases of gout become chronic, and one sees this condition in the elderly. Pseudo-gout, or chondrocalcinosis, is a disease of the elderly discovered and investigated only in the last 20 years. Septic arthritis, when recognized and treated early and adequately, is curable. However, in the elderly, its presentation is often atypical and masked by other diseases.

Many elderly have complaints of pain and decreased mobility in joints, which are attributed to "soft tissue rheumatism." Polymyalgia rheumatica is one of the more characteristic soft tissue diseases of the older person.

DIAGNOSIS AND PATIENT CARE

A general internist sees in order of decreasing frequency, patients with osteoarthritis, rheumatoid arthritis, soft tissue rheumatism, gout, pseudogout, and septic arthritis. Patients with musculoskeletal complaints of pain, stiffness, and limited mobility make up 10% of an average general practice. For an internist specializing in geriatrics, this number goes up to approximately 30%.[38,39]

In the United States the referral pattern has been changing in the past 15 years because of access to a larger number of clinical rheumatologists and the rapid increase in joint replacement skills of the orthopaedic surgeons. Traditionally, the rheumatologist consults or manages patients with inflammatory spondylarthropathies, rheumatoid arthritis and other diffuse connective tissue diseases, gout, and pseudogout. Regional problems of the spine and limbs caused by osteoarthritis or soft tissue rheumatism are seen in consultation and are often managed by the orthopaedic surgeon.

The clinician should be aware of pitfalls in the diagnostic approach and assessment. Pain in the limbs and spine can be caused by cardiovascular disorders and neoplastic diseases, which like the rheumatic disorders increase in frequency with advancing age. The elderly are prone to have several diseases concomitantly. An exhaustive history and a comprehensive examination are mandatory. Clinical judgment should place in perspective the abnormal findings from the laboratory and roentgenograms and their relevance to the patients' symptoms and signs. The significance of the rheumatic disease component should be judged within the overall health status of the individual. The patient may minimize complaints or concerns about aching joints or spine. In fact, he might fear a disabling or potentially fatal illness.

After evaluation by the physician, the elderly patient is in need of reassurance. He may be told of the lack of evidence for any cancer and given advice about his cardiovascular system. However, it is undesirable to tell the patient that he is in good health and that he has only "arthritis." In simple terms he should be given an explanation of the type of suspected or diagnosed rheumatic disease. The patient should also be told of the chronic nature of his affliction, its usual course, and how it may or may not affect him in his later years. Older persons tend to accept arthritis as a normal part of the aging process and they have a low expectation of help from the physician. They are not aware of new knowledge and skills that health professionals can offer.

An early and accurate diagnosis can lead to the cure of septic arthritis and to the control of polymyalgia rheumatica and gouty arthritis. The majority of patients with severe rheumatoid arthritis will benefit from a comprehensive program of a multidisciplinary team. Continuity of care should be assured by the patient's personal physician who knows his health needs, environment, and available resources.

This chapter gives an overview of rheumatic disease of the elderly as seen by a clinical rheumatologist. The focus is on the individualized treatment and continuity of care in chronic illness. The patient is informed and guided by his personal physician. Gerontologists, orthopaedic surgeons, and allied health professionals often participate in patient care and support.

OSTEOARTHRITIS
Definition and pathology

Osteoarthritis is a disease of one, a pair, or a small number of joints. Most frequently involved are the terminal and proximal finger joints, the first carpometacarpal and the first metatarsophalangeal joints, the knees, the hips, and the apophyseal joints of the lumbar and cervical spine. Osteoarthritis, also called degenerative joint disease and osteoarthrosis, has no systemic or constitutional features (Fig. 5-1). The disease is characterized by degeneration of the articular cartilage and remodeling of the subchondral bone with proliferative spur or osteophyte formation. Concomitant manifestations include a variable amount of low grade synovial inflammation and capsular thickening. When the inflammatory component is significant and persistent, causing extensive structural damage, the disease is described as an erosive form of osteoarthritis.

Radiologic changes of osteoarthritis are found in most persons after age 60[23] though often they are not accompanied by any symptoms. Primary generalized osteoarthritis[18,19] is seen mostly in postmenopausal women. It involves symmetrically multiple joints, particularly in the hands. Secondary osteoarthritis predominates over the idiopathic primary form. It is the final common path that arises from different causes: long-standing inflammatory arthropathies, metabolic and endocrine diseases, congenital and developmental abnormalities. Study of biomechanical dysfunction of joints has greatly expanded the list of causes leading to osteoarthritis of the hips and of the knees. Detailed information on pathology, pathogenesis, and experimental models of osteoarthritis has appeared in recent literature.[12,29,36]

Clinical features

The chief complaint in osteoarthritis is pain in one or several joints. The other complaint is gradual loss of mobility. The onset of pain is insidious and at first the discomfort occurs only with motion. As the disease advances pain becomes present at rest and can interfere with sleep. Pain in osteoarthritis comes from periosteal elevation associated with spur formation, pressure on exposed subchondral bone, trabecular microfractures, and periarticular muscle spasm. Acute joint pain is brought on by trauma and repetitive motion. It is associated with low grade synovitis and capsulitis. Acute flare may be induced by crystal shedding in patients with calcium pyrophosphate and calcium hydroxyapatite tissue deposits.[6] Pain has often been present intermittently for years. Its level and impact on the individual's comfort and activities have been tolerable. What brings the elderly to consult is the worsening of the pain, the resulting restriction of mobility,

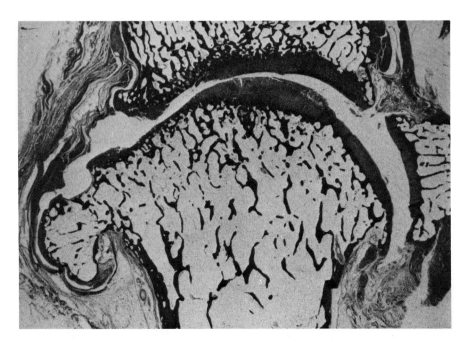

Fig. 5-1. Osteoarthritis of first metatarsophalangeal joint with partial erosion on both surfaces of articular cartilage and condensation of subchondral bone. Osteophyte extends above dorsal margin of metatarsal head. (From the Arthritis Foundation Clinical Slide Collection on the Rheumatoid Diseases. Copyright 1972. Used by permission of the Arithritis Foundation.)

and fear of loss of independence. Although the common complaint is pain in large weight-bearing joints, history will often bring out the existence of recurring spells of neck and lower back pain.

Examination may reveal the presence of painless deformity of finger joints. A common presentation is the middle aged or elderly woman with osteoarthritis limited to distal interphalangeal joints (Heberden's nodes) or proximal interphalangeal joints (Bouchard' nodes). A frequent associated deformity is of the first carpometacarpal with squaring of the joint, adduction, and internal rotation of the thumb. The patient has had pain and paresthesias in the hands early in the disease. She is now relatively pain-free but is concerned about possible future disability and the cosmetic appearance of her fingers (Fig. 5-2). The involved joints may be moderately tender. There may be crepitus or grating on moving the joint passively.

In hip disease the first motion to be lost is internal rotation. In the knee the earliest change is usually in the patellofemoral joint, manifested by the difficulty the elderly person experiences on stairs and on getting on and off buses. Eventually the knee shows deformity related to tibiofemoral disease; it is more often a varus than a valgus deformity.

The diagnosis of osteoarthritis is made clinically and confirmed by roentgenograms. There are no abnormal findings in the blood tests that are valuable to rule out other diseases. Synovial joint aspiration shows a normal fluid with a low cell count and a normal viscosity.

Regardless of whether the symptoms are in the large weight-bearing joints or the hands, the elderly have a fear of developing a crippling disorder that might interfere with independent living. Arthritis in the elderly is often associated with disabilities such as decreased vision and impaired hearing. Multiple illnesses lead to inactivity and depression. Involvement of hips and knees intensifies the problem by limiting ambulation and self care.

The course of osteoarthritis is slowly progressive with flares of pain and increas-

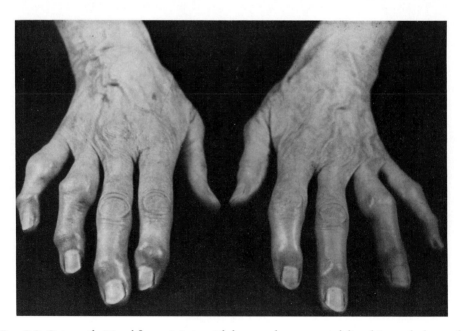

FIG. 5-2. Osteoarthritis of finger joints with bony enlargement of distal interphalangeal joints (Heberden's nodes) and proximal interphalangeal joints (Bouchard's nodes). (From the Arthritis Foundation Clinical Slide Collection on the Rheumatoid Diseases.) Copyright 1972. Used by permission of the Arthritis Foundation.

ing disability. The site of joint disease, the degree of anatomic changes, functional limitations, and the elderly person's overall health condition will determine the prognosis and the strategy for management.

Management

Physical measurers. For osteoarthritis of hips and knees, relief or pain should be attempted first by reducing the level of physical activity and by balancing rest and non–weight-bearing exercises. The patient may assume that more walking will improve the joints. Pain can be reduced by changing this behavior. Rest should be prescribed and the patient instructed to lie down for 1 to 2 hours during the day and 8 hours at night. A pillow should not be placed under the knees to reduce pain. A walking cane should be prescribed after instruction for its proper use. Bilateral canes or a walker are preferred for bilateral severe hip and knee disease. It should not come as a surprise that the majority of the elderly and women in particular are resistant in accepting the use of a cane. A raised toilet seat, a higher chair with arms, a reacher, and a long-handled shoe horn can be of great help for the elderly with hip and knee disability.

The painful low back and neck of an older person are often the result of apophyseal joint osteoarthritis combined with degenerative disc disease and paraspinal muscle spasm. Pain can be relieved by the use of local heat and intermittently wearing a lumbosacral corset and a neck collar. Excessive loading of the back and weight-bearing joints should be reduced by a sensible weight loss.

To maintain and improve range of motion and to strengthen muscles, the patient is given an exercise program. Advanced age is not a contraindication for exercises but compliance is not always satisfactory. Exercise programs need to be simple, beginning after the pain has been somewhat relieved. The patient is instructed in two or three exercises to be done once or twice daily at home. If the patient is forgetful, a family member should be responsible for supervision. The basic exercises are the quadriceps and glutei setting, the straight leg raising, and the pelvic tilt. Heat application before exercises can be helpful. A hot bath or shower is the best modality for home use. Proper railings and appliances need to be provided for safety.

For osteoarthritis of the hands, warm soaks or melted parafin dips provide relief from pain and stiffness. A thumb splint is useful for a painful osteoarthritis of the first carpometacarpal joint.

Drug therapy. The patient does expect help from medication. Pain relieving medicines are prescribed with a definite schedule. Some elderly people may be forgetful, and to help them remember, it is best to prescribe medication to be taken twice daily—with breakfast and with dinner, or on arising and on retiring. A third dose can be added at lunchtime as needed.

An analgesic dose of aspirin, 600 mg morning and night, is often sufficient for pain relief. In case of gastrointestinal intolerance, it can be replaced by a buffered or a coated preparation of aspirin, well tolerated by a majority of patients.

Although the role of inflammation in producing the symptoms of osteoarthritis is not well established, it is generally accepted that some of the pain and stiffness is related to inflammatory changes in and around the joints. An antiinflammatory dose of aspirin, 4 gm, is rarely well tolerated or accepted by the elderly. When the need arises, it is preferable to prescribe a nonsteroidal antiinflammatory medication such as naproxen (250 mg or 375 mg) or sulindac (150 mg or 200 mg) twice daily. Either medication should be taken at the end of a meal, breakfast and dinner, or on arising and on retiring, accompanied by a glass of milk. Another antiinflammatory medication, piroxicam (20 mg), has a long half-life and can be given once daily. The patient should be alerted to the possibility of side effects such as nausea, vomiting, and occasional diarrhea. Any of these drugs should be given a trial of 2 weeks, if tolerated, to determine the possible beneficial effect on pain. If the medication is indeed helpful, it can be continued for several additional weeks. The patient should be told that the medication is given for a limited time for a specific purpose of relieving pain related to inflammation and to facilitate the use of physical measures.

Other antiinflammatory agents, taken three to four times daily, can be tried: indomethacin, tolmetin, ibuprofen, mefenamic acid. Compliance is more difficult to obtain when medication has to be taken more than once or twice a day, and the possibility of side effects is always present.

Systemic corticosteroids should not be used in the treatment of osteoarthritis in the elderly. Intraarticular steroids can be helpful but should be given selectively. An inflamed osteoarthritic knee that did not respond to rest and antiinflammatory medication for 2 weeks could be helped by an intraarticular injection of a long-acting steroid such as methylprednisolone (40 mg). If the pain is relieved for a month or more, the injection could be repeated. If relief is fleeting and if a second injection is not followed by similar or longer relief of pain and inflammation, some other mode of treatment should be sought. Osteoarthritic finger joints rarely require intraarticular steroid injections except for the first carpometacarpal joint.

Surgery. Most patients with osteoarthritis are treated conservatively. They are prescribed medication for spells of pain and given advice to retard or prevent disability by monitoring and adjusting their activities at home and in the community. Psychologic support and patient compliance with behavior modification are part of the treatment. The patient with osteoarthritis of the hip and the knee, unilateral or bilateral, should be told of the possibility of joint replacement if pain or disability becomes unacceptable. Options between continuation of conservative measures and surgical intervention should be discussed, and the patient should make the decision for elective surgery. Advanced age is not a contraindication for joint replacement, but an assessment of the patient's overall health and psychologic status must be made. Any infection, particularly in the genitourinary tract, should be evaluated, and whenever possible, eliminated. Relative indications for

joint replacement in osteoarthritis of the hip or knee include the following:
1. Pain interfering with sleep
2. Difficulty or inability to perform activities of daily living
3. Unacceptable limitation in walking ability and the use of stairs
4. Inability to use public transportation and to work

Joint replacement has been a breakthrough in the management of osteoarthritis when it reaches the disabling stage. Details of hip and knee replacement are found elsewhere in this book.

Conclusion

Osteoarthritis remains a disease of unknown cause. Trials of medicinal agents designed to prevent or reverse degenerative lesions have been carried out on an investigational basis. Degradation of cartilage results from release of enzymes from chondrocytes and leukocytes. Agents that inhibit the degradative process or can stimulate cartilage repair may be beneficial. No such agent has yet been proved to be clinically acceptable.

In the elderly, the problem of osteoarthritis is complicated by the psychologic and socioeconomic impact, multiple disabilities, and progressive isolation of the individual. Each patient requires repeated intervention with an assessment of pain, physical and psychologic consequences of disease, and the patient's understanding and goals.

RHEUMATOID ARTHRITIS
Definition and clinical features

Rheumatoid arthritis is a diffuse connective tissue disease characterized by a polyarticular involvement, which is usually symmetric. It is a systemic disease with constitutional symptoms of weakness, generalized stiffness, and at times, weight loss and fever. About 15% of the patients have nonarticular manifestations involving the eyes, heart, and lungs.[3] Such symptoms justify the name rheumatoid disease rather than rheumatoid arthritis. It predominately affects women with a 3:1 female to male ratio. The cause of rheumatoid disease is unknown, and there is no specific treatment. It has a wide spectrum from mild limited involvement of a few joints to very severe generalized and disabling forms. The course is unpredictable and functional prognosis is guarded.

In the elderly, there are essentially two clinical presentations:

1. Onset of rheumatoid arthritis after age 60, which is uncommon
2. Rheumatoid arthritis that has started many years before, frequently in the fourth and fifth decade, and that has evolved to a late stage disease either through a continuously progressive course or through a succession of remissions and relapses

The onset is insidious with fleeting pain in multiple joints, particularly in hands and feet, progressive weakness, and easy fatigability. Generalized stiffness comes on during the night and is particularly troublesome on arising and for several hours thereafter. The patient feels better in the afternoon but becomes fatigued and has more pain and stiffness in the early evening.

Less frequently, the onset is abrupt, with fever, malaise, loss of appetite, and weight loss.

The characteristic sign is joint synovitis with capsular distention and effusion. The first joints involved are often the wrists and the joints of the fingers, particularly the metacarpophalangeal joints and the proximal interphalangeal joints. Metatarsophalangeal joints can be involved early in some 25% of cases. Although the larger, more proximal joints are usually affected later in the course of the disease, it is not uncommon, particularly in the elderly, to have the onset with knee or shoulder disease, and only later does the disease spread to the more peripheral joints.[9]

Symmetric synovitis of multiple joints is characteristic of, but not specific or limited to, rheumatoid arthritis. One extraarticular manifestation, which is quite specific but found in only approximately one third of cases, is the rheumatoid nodule. It is most frequently found on the extensor surface of the forearms but also over the fingers, toes, and ischial tuberosities (Fig. 5-3).

Laboratory investigations show an ele-

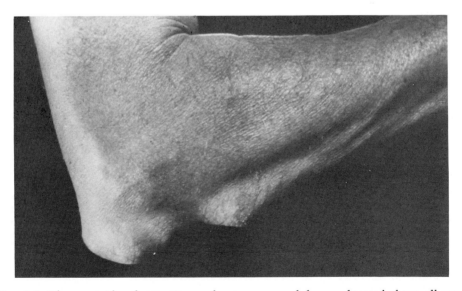

FIG. 5-3. Rheumatoid arthritis. Two subcutaneous nodules are located about elbow: one is in olecranon bursa and the other on extensor surface of forearm. (From the Arthritis Foundation Clinical Slide Collection on the Rheumatoid Diseases. Copyright 1972. Used by permission of the Arthritis Foundation.)

vated sedimentation rate, best measured by the Westergren method, in which the normal reading is 20 mm in 1 hour. Readings of 80 to 100 mm are common in patients with active rheumatoid arthritis. Although a high sedimentation rate has no specificity and is an acute phase reaction of an inflammatory process, it is a useful test for following the disease course and the effect of antiinflammatory measures used to control the symptoms.

The blood count is also not specific. Usually a hypochromic microcytic anemia parallels disease activity and improves when the inflammatory phase decreases but does not respond to iron therapy. The white blood cell count can be normal or can show relative leukopenia or leukocytosis. The platelet count is high when the disease is particularly active.

The most characteristic laboratory finding is the presence in the serum of proteins known as the rheumatoid factor or factors, which are antibodies to patients' own altered gamma globulins.[7] Rheumatoid factor is detected by an agglutination test known as latex fixation for rheumatoid arthritis factor. Inert particles of latex are coated with gamma globulin. An agglutination takes place when these particles are mixed with the patient's serum, and the degree of agglutination can be quantitated and reported with a titer. It is important to have the test quantified particularly when it is performed with the serum of an elderly individual since a high proportion of normal individuals agglutinate the latex particles at a low titer of 1:40 and 1:80. A titer of 1:160 should be the lowest considered clinically significant. The titer can go quite high with the upper limit in most laboratories reported as 1:5120.

Seventy-five percent of patients with rheumatoid arthritis will have a positive latex fixation with an appreciable titer, but about 25% are so-called seronegative rheumatoid arthritis patients. Another diagnostic pitfall is the possible presence of a positive latex fixation test in other diffuse connective tissue diseases, chronic infections, and liver disease. The exact significance of the rheumatoid factor and its role in the pathogenesis of the disease are unknown.

In the early stages of rheumatoid arthritis and sometimes for many months or years, roentgenograms do not show any abnormalities other than regional osteoporosis of involved joints without cartilage thinning or bony changes.

The diagnosis of rheumatoid arthritis is thus difficult and remains a clinical judgment diagnosis with limited help from laboratory and roentgenograms. In the elderly it is particularly important to consider the possibility of neoplastic disease, which can have the same type of onset with consitutional symptoms and ill-defined limb pain. It is not unusual to question the diagnosis for several months while observing the patient's clinical course and offering symptomatic care.

Management of early disease

It is helpful to have the patient hospitalized for 1 to 2 weeks to complete the examinations, to start on a program of comprehensive management, and to educate the patient about the disease and involvement in the treatment. In the early phase of a chronic illness, it is essential to establish communication between the patient and the health professionals. The patient should learn about the unpredictable course and the ups and downs of the disease manifestations. With the guidance of a personal physician, helped by advice from consultants and allied health professionals, the patient should return home from the hospital with clear instructions about activities and the necessary rest. The person with rheumatoid arthritis should be taught joint positioning and a program of simple exercises, which should include range of motion of the involved joints, particularly the shoulders, and strengthening exercises for the knees.

The patient should learn the difference between analgesic medications such as acetaminophen or aspirin in small doses of 2 to 4 tablets per day and antiinflammatory medication, which relieves pain by decreasing the inflammatory process in and around the painful joints. Aspirin when given in sufficient amount has antiinflammatory activity. To achieve it, the patient will have to accept and tolerate 4 gm of aspirin divided in four daily doses, usually given at meals and at bedtime. The majority of patients actually tolerate this dosage quite well, particularly if aspirin is given in a buffered form or in coated tablets. It is, however, difficult to take the large number of pills for long periods. Rheumatoid arthritis, unlike osteoarthritis, is characterized by inflammation. Unless the disease goes into remission, antiinflammatory medication has to be given as long as the inflammation persists, which may mean many months or years.

As an alternative to aspirin, various nonsteroidal antiinflammatory medications have been developed in the past 20 years. Indomethacin, one of the early ones, still remains much in use. It is given in a dose of 25 to 50 mg three to four times daily. Side effects may include gastrointestinal distress, headaches, and dizziness, particularly in the elderly individual. It is advisable to test for tolerance by starting with a trial dose of 25 mg twice daily before increasing the dose. The newer medications are ibuprofen, tolmetin, naproxen, fenoprofen, sulinadac, mefenamic acid, and piroxicam. Their tolerance and effects on inflammation are variable. The present trend is to use one at a time for approximately 2 weeks to test both tolerance and beneficial effect before switching to the next. This is all confusing to the patient who often gets discouraged and does not give the new drug a fair trial if immediate relief does not occur within days. The principle of this approach to symptomatic relief of pain needs to be explained and the patient encouraged to observe and report his reaction at regular intervals.[15,16]

Systemic corticosteroids have potent antiinflammatory effects. The one most often used is prednisone. Side effects are dose related and increase with the length of time the medication is given. After 30 years of experience with the administration of corticosteroids to patients with rheumatoid ar-

thritis, most authorities conclude that steroids should be given selectively and sparingly. The original concept of giving a substantial dose to "suppress" inflammation and then maintain the suppression with a small dose has not lived up to expectations, yet this practice is common.

In a patient who has a rapidly progressive disease, who is becoming incapacitated and has not obtained relief from simple analgesics and nonsteroidal antiinflammatory medication, particularly in the elderly, it is justifiable to give a small amount of prednisone, such as 5 to 7.5 mg daily. It is best to take this dose on retiring, so that there is less morning stiffness and easier function on arising. Some patients, however, prefer to have a small dose given to them the first thing in the morning. The alternate day steroid administration is not very effective in patients with rheumatoid disease since symptoms worsen on days when the drug is not taken.[15,16]

Although no specific treatment for rheumatoid arthritis exists, practitioners can offer the patient "remittive agents," which have a more sustained effect on inflammation and may actually slow down and possibly stop disease progression. Remittive agents are parenteral gold, an antimalarial medication, penicillamine, and azathioprine. These agents have in common slow action on the inflammatory process. Relief of symptoms does not occur before 2 to 4 months, sometimes longer. Their beneficial effects are unpredictable: 30% to 70% of subjects respond favorably. These remittive agents have potential toxicity.[15,16]

The antimalarial hydroxychloroquine is not used much at present, mostly because of occasional toxicity to the eyes and irreversible retinal changes. Parenteral gold has been used for some 40 years and has survived a great deal of criticism and skepticism. It has the disadvantage of intramuscular administration. However, an oral gold preparation is currently under investigation and might become available in the near future. Weekly injection of one of the two available gold preparations (gold sodium thiomalate, aurothioglucose) is given intramuscularly weekly in 50 mg doses. The beneficial effect usually results after a total of 500 mg has been given. After a total of 1000 mg, the dose of 50 mg is continued at 2-week intervals for an additional 500 mg, and thereafter a maintenance therapy of 50 mg once a month is given to prevent recurrence of the disease process. Gold must be monitored both for its beneficial effect and for possible side effects. Because the most common intolerance is manifested by skin and mucous membrane lesions, the patients should be told of that possibility, which can occur in approximately 25% of cases. About 5% of the patients develop proteinuria, and a urinalysis should be done before each injection. Bone marrow suppression is a rare but dreaded complication, seen in less than 1% of gold-treated patients. It is mandatory to have a blood count including a platelet count after every third or fourth injection, even more often at the beginning of therapy.

Those patients who improve with gold go into a remission that is manifested by disappearance of constitutional symptoms of weakness and stiffness and a slow decrease of joint inflammation and pain. [5]

Penicillamine is given orally in a dose of 125 to 250 mg per day for the first 2 months with close clinical monitoring and biweekly urinalysis and blood count. If no benefit occurs after 2 months, the dose is doubled, and the monitoring continues. At 4 months, if there is enough improvement, the same dose is continued; otherwise the dose is increased from 500 to 750 mg per day. At 6 months the patient is assessed and a decision is made about whether the medication should be continued in case of good tolerance and beneficial effect on pain and inflammation. Long-term use of penicillamine is not well defined and should be determined by clinical parameters.[17]

Azathioprine is an immunosuppressive agent with potential carcinogenic effect. It can be tried when other remittive agents have failed.

A quick acting antiinflammatory medication and a slow acting remittive agent can be used in combination. The former gives the necessary rapid relief, and the latter is used to slow down and possibly arrest the disease process. Because of potential side effects of the remittive agents, and because of the need for long and tedious treatment, it is obvious that patients need to understand and cooperate in the program.

Late stage of rheumatoid arthritis

A more common presentation in the elderly is rheumatoid disease that has started earlier in life. What one sees 15 or 20 years after the onset was appropriately called by Dr. Harold Robinson "the consequences of age and disease."[32]

At this late stage the diagnosis is obvious. What is needed is an assessment of past events and present status. A review might reveal that in all the years that the patient had rheumatoid disease, hospitalization or confinement at home was never required and the person was able to carry on gainful employment with little or no loss of time from work or usual activities. Some 50% of patients with rheumatoid arthritis are fortunate to have a mild course with no significant disability from their disease. Eventually, some 25% to 35% develop moderate disability from rheumatoid arthritis. Eventually, some of the joints will show disease sequelae, such as mild flexion deformities of elbows, wrists, and fingers or deformed toes. Nevertheless, they are independent for self care and not necessarily a burden to their families and to the community. They do periodically require, when the disease flares, pain-relieving medication usually for a limited time. They do require periodic evaluation and adjustment of treatment.

The other 50% of the elderly with long-standing rheumatoid disease do not fare as well. History will reveal that they had several hospital admissions, some of them in recent years for surgical procedures including joint replacements. This group includes a subset of about 15% for whom the disease has been relentlessly progressing in spite of all therapeutic efforts. Years ago, these patients had to give up their jobs and rely on the family and hired help for household chores. The severely afflicted patients can do little more than eat independently. They have to depend on others for assistance in most activities of daily living. They are usually confined to their homes, with limited ambulation, in wheelchairs, or bedbound.

The review of past events leads to the assessment of the patient's present status, his disease, his reaction and understanding of what can and cannot be done, the environment in which he lives and functions, and his goals and expectations.

An assessment of the patient with rheumatoid arthritis should take into account:

1. Complaints: pain, stiffness, fatigue
2. Course and disease activity since the onset: remissions, relapses, treatments
3. Anatomic changes
4. Functional disability
5. Psychosocial overview

In late disease, one has to recognize irreversible changes of the joints with deformities and subluxations and limited mobility. Pain can be secondary to degenerative changes and bone-to-bone contact. There might still be disease activity as manifested by constitutional symptoms of morning stiffness, fatigability, and inflamed joints.

The assessment of the past and the present leads to a formulation of a comprehensive program of management. More than ever, at this stage the patient has to be involved and made to understand that his frustrations are shared by the health professionals. However, with their help his existence can become more acceptable and the outlook more hopeful.

If pain results from active disease and the inflammatory process, one should administer antiinflammatory medication and consider remittive agents after explanation to the patient of not only their potential value but also their drawbacks. More often, pain is secondary to structural changes and one has to rely on analgesics but not resort to narcotics whenever possible.

Use of a cane, crutches, or a walker can sometimes make a big difference in the patient's ability to function independently. The same can be said for assistive devices, especially toilet activities and dressing.

The elderly individual, handicapped by rheumatoid arthritis, should be evaluated with regard to his overall medical condition, and some projection made about his life span. The person should be told of the options available. He might be satisfied with a program stressing pain relief with medication and accept sheltered existence at home or in an institution. He should also be told of the possibility of improving function by joint replacement. The patient's goals should be specific and his expectations realistic. His personal physician and the consultants should understand them and offer an acceptable program. Rheumatoid arthritis is a chronic and progressive disease. The treatment that can be offered is symptomatic and supportive.

Although much less frequent than osteoarthritis, rheumatoid arthritis is a greater challenge because of its systemic nature, its unpredictable course, and its impact on the individual.

DIFFUSE CONNECTIVE TISSUE DISEASES

Besides rheumatoid arthritis there are diffuse connective tissue diseases much less frequent and generally not thought of as diseases of the elderly.[25]

Systemic lupus erythematosus (SLE)

Older patients account for about 10% of the total SLE cases,[8] with a high female preponderance. The disease has an insidious onset with fatigue, fever, weight loss, arthralgia, and low grade arthritis particularly of finger joints. The course is progressive with frequent appearance of nonspecific rashes and spells of chest pains brought on by pleurisy or pericarditis. Kidney disease is manifested by proteinuria and microscopic hematuria. Blood studies show an elevated erythrocyte sedimentation rate and a low white blood cell count. In the majority of cases immunofluorescence detects the presence of antinuclear antibodies (ANA). The test is not specific and can be positive in patients with other diseases and in normal individuals. A test showing the presence of antibodies to native DNA is, however, highly specific for SLE. It can be quantitated and when the titer is high and this finding is associated with a low complement level the disease is present and active.[21]

Other blood abnormalities suggesting the diagnosis of lupus are a false positive test for syphilis and a circulating anticoagulant. The prognosis of lupus in the elderly is relatively favorable with limited kidney disease and rare central nervous system involvement. Most patients respond to treatment with aspirin and nonsteroidal antiinflammatory medication. For acute crises of visceral disease prednisone (60 mg a day) is given and the dose is decreased gradually based on clinical parameters.

A lupus-like syndrome can develop in patients taking procainamide or hydralazine for cardiovascular disease. Other drugs can cause a lupus-like disease with presence of ANA in the blood, but an absence of antibodies to native DNA and a normal level of complement. Discontinuation of the offending drug results in disappearance of symptoms.

Progressive systemic sclerosis (PSS)

PSS causes diffuse connective tissue fibrosis with skin changes known as scleroderma and a multisystem disease involving the gastrointestinal tract, heart, lung, and kidney.[33] Women are affected three to four times as often as men.

Initial symptoms of Raynaud's phenomenon and puffiness of hands usually occur in middle life. The disease evolves slowly and is found in the elderly as a widespread thickening of the skin and progressive visceral involvement. One-third of patients experience arthralgia and joint stiffness but few have true polyarthritis. As the disease progresses the skin becomes taut with a loss of normal wrinkles and folds particularly over the hands, feet, and face. Subcutaneous calcifications appear frequently over the joints and in the fingertips. There are fibrous deposits on the surfaces of the joints, the tendon sheaths, and overlying fascia. Many patients develop flexion contractures of the fingers. Visceral involvement is generally less severe in the elderly and occurs several years after the skin changes. Gastrointestinal symptoms result from loss of peristalsis and from fibrosis resulting in dysphagia, abdominal fullness, and constipation. Most patients develop pulmonary fibrosis with exertional dyspnea but many remain asymptomatic. Cardiomyopathy and renal disease with severe hypertension are major causes of death in patients with PSS.

No effective treatment is available for this disorder. However, for patients with Raynaud's phenomenon, supportive measures such as avoidance of smoking and exposure to cold are helpful. Newer antihypertensive drugs have been used to control blood pressure and stabilize kidney function in some patients with progressive systemic sclerosis.[34]

Polymyositis and dermatomyositis

These are diffuse inflammatory muscle diseases that can occur at any age and commonly in the sixth and seventh decade and are twice as frequent in women than in men.[30] Muscular weakness of the limb girdles and neck is present in nearly all patients. The course is one of spontaneous remissions and relapses. In some cases the weakness develops slowly and first affects the lower extremities, causing difficulty in getting up from a low chair and going on stairs. Progression of weakness of shoulder girdles interferes with dressing activities. Arthralgia and low-grade polyarthritis are usually short lasting. Periorbital edema may occur.

The rash of dermatomyositis occurs in about 40% of patients with inflammatory myopathy. It is a red patchy and scaly eruption found over the elbows, the dorsum of the finger joints, the knees, and the ankles. A heliotrope rash may appear on the upper eyelids. Visceral involvement is manifested by esophageal and bowel disturbances secondary to hypomotility. A clinical diagnosis is confirmed by laboratory findings of elevated serum creatine phosphokinase, aldolase, and transaminases and by a muscle biopsy showing primary degeneration of muscle fibers, infiltrates of inflammatory cells, and interstitial fibrosis.[36]

A majority of patients respond to corticosteroid treatment. Prednisone (60 to 80 mg) is given daily in divided doses and continued for 3 to 6 months or longer in decreasing doses guided by clinical response and lowering of serum enzymes. About 15% of the elderly with polymyositis have an underlying malignancy.[2] In some cases resection of the primary tumor has resulted in an improvement. Prognosis of polymyositis of the elderly is guarded and the mortality rate is higher in older persons.

Soft Tissue Rheumatism
Polymyalgia rheumatica

Soft tissue rheumatism, also known as nonarticular rheumatism, can be secondary to osteoarthritis, rheumatoid arthritis, and other inflammatory arthropathies. It is then also called secondary fibrositis or fibromyositis.

Primary soft tissue rheumatism is localized or generalized. Some of the local conditions are common in the elderly, particularly tendinitis of the shoulder and stenosing tenosynovitis of the fingers. These entities are described in other chapters of this book. A primary generalized form, polymyalgia rheumatica, has been known under this name in the United States for the past 25 years.

Polymyalgia rheumatica is a clinical syndrome that occurs in persons over the age of 60, twice as frequently in women as in men. It is characterized by pain and stiffness in the shoulders and upper arms and by bilateral stiffness of the pelvic girdle, which can actually predominate in about 10% of this group of patients. The stiffness is worse in the morning and can last for several hours. Systemic symptoms include malaise, low grade fever, and weight loss. The most consistent objective findings are tenderness on palpation of the shoulder and arm muscles and restriction of motion of shoulders and hips, particularly in the morning. One-third of all patients with polymyalgia develop sysptoms of temporal arteritis. Careful examination may reveal tenderness of the temporal artery on one side or bilaterally.

The most consistent laboratory abnormality is the finding of a markedly elevated erythrocyte sedimentation rate, often higher than 100 mm in 1 hour (Westergren). A mild anemia is common, and there may be modest elevation in white blood cell and platelet counts. The serum enzymes and electromyography are normal and help to rule out polymyositis. An association between polymyalgia rheumatica and temporal arteritis, also known as giant cell arteritis, has been recognized for many years, but the nature of this relationship is still not fully understood. In giant cell arteritis the branches of the arteries originating from the arch of the aorta are involved.[41] The onset of the arteritis may be sudden, but in many instances, symptoms are present for months before the diagnosis is established. Patients have headaches, often localized to the regions of the temporal or occipital arteries with tenderness of the involved portions of the head. Sudden loss of vision is a potential complication of this disease. Once established, a visual deficit is permanent.

Polymyalgia rheumatica occurs in 50% of patients with giant cell arteritis and may appear in any phase of the disease. The cause of giant cell arteritis and polymyalgia rheumatica is unknown. It has been suggested that patients with polymyalgia have arteritis and that the musculoskeletal symptoms result from vasculitis. The internal elastic membrane of the artery is the focus of the inflammatory reaction in giant cell arteritis, and the presence of an antigen in this structure has been considered. This would support the concept that immunologic mechanism is involved in the pathogenesis of the disorder.[13]

Polymyalgia and temporal arteritis respond dramatically to treatment with corticosteroids. Prednisone is a drug most commonly used, and the dose varies according to the clinical presentation. For polymyalgia alone, 10 to 15 mg per day is given. In patients with temporal arteritis without visual symptoms, the dose is increased to 20 mg daily, and in those with visual symptoms, 40 to 60 mg daily. Patients require prolonged steroid therapy to control pain and stiffness and to guard against development of visual changes. The dose of medication can be cautiously reduced in stepwise fashion based on clinical findings. Pain and stiffness are usually controlled within 2 or 3 weeks, and the sedimentation rate falls below 30 mm in 1 hour after 2 to 3 months of treatment. A maintenance dose of prednisone, 10 mg daily, is given for approximately 6 months. Further reduction, 1 mg every month, is then attempted unless symptoms recur. An abrupt withdrawal of steroid treatment could be followed by severe recurrence of both polymyalgia rheumatica and temporal arteritis. This disorder tends to run a self-limited course, but it can last from several months to several years.

Polymyalgia rheumatica is a clinical diagnosis. Rheumatoid arthritis ultimately develops in 5% of a large series of cases. The neoplastic diseases mimic some features of polymyalgia, and a screening evaluation is indicated. Prominent muscular symptoms often suggest the diagnosis of polymyositis; however, in this disease the muscle tenderness and weakness are more marked, and the diagnosis can be confirmed by elevated serum enzymes and biopsy findings.

CRYSTAL DEPOSITION DISEASES
Gout

Clinical features. Gout appears in adult males and lasts a lifetime with some 40% of cases seen in men aged 55 years and over. In females gout does not appear until after menopause with an overall male to female ratio of about 6:1.[11]

Patients with gouty arthritis show symptoms and signs that should facilitate an early diagnosis. An acute attack is an intensely inflammatory arthritis often with tenosynovitis. The episode may appear and resolve spontaneously within 3 to 7 days and may be followed by an asymptomatic period which lasts days, months, or years. Factors that frequently precipitate an acute attack include local trauma, surgical procedures, infections, and excessive intake of alcoholic beverages. The common sites are the first metatarsophalangeal joint, the ankle, the knee, and the wrist. Gouty tenosynovitis is often on the dorsum of the foot and the dorsum of the wrist. A family history of gout, a record of renal stones, and hyperuricemia strengthen the likelihood of diagnosis although none of these findings is pathognomonic of gout.

Gouty arthritis in an older person, particularly a woman, sometimes poses a difficult challenge of differential diagnosis. Elevation of serum uric acid is not sufficient to establish a diagnosis of gouty arthritis. The laboratory procedure of choice is an aspiration of joint fluid and demonstration of intracellular needle-shaped crystals of monosodium urate by polarizing light microscopy.[42] Many months or years may intervene between recurrent attacks of gouty arthritis.

Ten to 20 years after the initial attack of arthritis and without effective treatment, chronic tophaceous gout may develop. This is a common clinical presentation in an elderly person.[4] The patient gives a history of progressive disease with attacks of gouty arthritis appearing more frequently, lasting longer, and with an increasing number of large and small joints becoming permanently involved. Characteristic findings are the presence of tophi, which are deposits of monosodium urate. They are subcutaneous nodules, firm and nontender, which are found on the extensor surfaces of the forearm and hand, the olecranon bursa, next to the finger joints, anterior tibial surface, and Achilles tendon. Tophi may occur anywhere in the body—classically in the helix of the ear, but most often next to bones and articular cartilage where they cause destruction recognized on roentgenograms as "punched out" areas. The clinical picture sometimes resembles nodular rheumatoid arthritis. A definitive diagnosis of tophaceous gout can be made by needle aspiration of a nodule and demonstration of needle shaped crystals of monosodium urate.

Fifteen to 30% of patients with chronic tophaceous gout demonstrate evidence of renal insufficiency. This is the result of depositions of monosodium urate in the kidneys in association with variable degrees of pyelonephritis and nephrosclerosis.[43]

Treatment. The management of gout should be considered for the control of an acute attack of arthritis or tenosynovitis, for the intercritical period to prevent recurrence of attacks, and for the prevention of the progression of the disease and deposition of crystals.

In the treatment of an acute attack of gout, phenylbutazone and indomethacin are equally effective. The optimal dose of phenylbutazone is 100 mg given 4 times a day for 3 to 5 days. In the treatment of such short duration serious toxic manifestations are rare. One occasionally sees the worsening of an existing peptic ulcer, phenylbutazone can also cause water retention and congestive heart failure.

Indomethacin given at a dose of 50 mg 3 times a day for 5 days is effective but can produce dizziness, headaches, and gastrointestinal side effects. The newer nonsteroidal antiinflammatory agents have been used with a good clinical response.

Colchicine has been the only drug available for the treatment of acute gout until the past 25 years. A dose of 0.5 mg of colchicine was given hourly for a total of 8 to 10 mg. Administered to patients suspected of having an acute gouty attack, it had diagnostic value because it resulted in a rapid objective response to the treatment. Eighty percent of patients receiving a full therapeutic dose of colchicine by mouth have significant gastrointestinal side effects, particularly diarrhea. For this reason its use in control of acute gout has been replaced by the nonsteroidal antiinflammatory medications. In selected cases a single intravenous dose of 2 mg of colchicine is an effective treatment but with potential side effects.

For long-term care colchicine by mouth, 0.5 to 1 mg daily, is gievn to prevent recurrences of gouty attack while the patient is started on a treatment to control his hyperuricemia.

Dietary therapy with a decreased purine intake is mostly ineffective and rarely used.

Reduction of serum uric acid is achieved by increasing the renal excretion of uric acid or by decreasing its formation. The aim is to reduce the serum uric acid level to below 6.0 mg/dl. The drug administered to increase uric acid excretion is probenecid. It is administered in a dosage of 0.5 to 2.0 gm per day in divided doses and is indicated for the gouty patient with normal renal function, no renal calculi, and normal excretion of uric acid. The treatment is started with a low dose, maintenance of a large fluid intake, and alkalization of the urine with oral sodium bicarbonate. Allopurinal, 200 to 400 mg per day, reduces the serum and urine uric acid by decreasing uric acid synthesis. It is particularly indicated in the elderly with gout complicated by renal insufficiency and the presence of tophi.[20]

Hypouricemic drugs are not given during an acute attack of gout. They are started after acute symptoms have subsided. Prophylactic treatment with colchicine is given concomitantly for several months until the serum uric acid reaches an optimal level.

Many patients are needlessly placed on hypouricemic drugs as a result of the finding of an elevated serum uric acid. In the older age group hyperuricemia can occur from the use of diuretics and from polycythemia, leukemia, and myeloproliferative disorders. Secondary gout may result from the induced high uric acid level. However, asymptomatic hyperuricemia should be treated only when it is persistent and severe and not related to some readily preventable factor.

Pseudogout

The technique of polarized light microscopy, which identified microcrystals of sodium monourate in gouty joint fluid, led to the discovery of crystals of calcium pyrophosphate dihydrate (CPPD). Arthritis associated with CPPD deposition is described as pseudogout and is characterized by acute joint inflammation.

The prevalence of CPPD arthritis does rise sharply with age.[28] From autopsy findings it has been observed that about 5% of the adult population has knee joint CPPD deposits at the time of death. The average age of patients with pseudogout is about 70 years, but many patients have symptoms beginning in the sixth and seventh decades. Several clinical patterns of inflammatory and degenerative CPPD arthropathies have been noted. About one-fourth of all patients with CPPD disease have pseudogout characterized by synovitis with an effusion. An acute attack involves one or a few joints and lasts from one day to several weeks. An attack may be triggered by surgery, an infection, or trauma. It is not unusual to have episodes of gout and pseudogout in the same individual. The knee joint is most frequently involved in pseudogout. Between attacks the patient is asymptomatic although roentgenograms of the knees and other joints often show calcium deposits described as chondrocalcinosis.

Examination of the joint fluid using polarized light microscopy will show weakly positive birefringent 3 to 5 mm rhomboid or rod-like crystals of CPPD.

About half of all the patients with CPPD crystal deposition disease show progressive degenerative changes in multiple joints. The most commonly involved are the knees, followed by the wrists, metacarpophalangeal joints, and hips. Involvement is generally bilateral. Only half of these patients have acute episodic attacks. Many joints with CPPD deposits visible on roentgenogram remain asymptomatic. In rare cases there is a destructive neurotrophic-like arthritis in a patient with CPPD disease.[27]

An elderly individual may show one pattern of arthritis early in the course of the disease and a different pattern later in life.

The treatment of CPPD crystal deposition disease is symptomatic. There is no known prevention or reversal of progressive deposition of crystals, unlike the situation in urate gout.

An acute crystal-induced synovitis is best treated by a joint aspiration and an intraarticular injection of a corticosteroid preparation. CPPD induced joint inflammation does respond to colchicine but to a lesser degree than gouty arthritis. Nonsteroidal antiinflammatory agents are effective during the subacute stage.

Treatment of clinically symptomatic weight-bearing joints associated with CPPD deposition consists of analgesic medication, muscle strengthening exercises, weight reduction when indicated, and the use of crutches or canes. In advanced cases of degeneration of the knees or hips, joint replacement needs to be considered.

SEPTIC ARTHRITIS
Diagnosis

Septic arthritis is rare in the healthy adult. The elderly with long-standing rheumatoid arthritis, individuals with chronic illness such as diabetes mellitus, cirrhosis of the liver, or a malignancy are at risk to develop infected joints. Many of these debilitated patients have an infection of more than one joint, which can confound the diagnosis and delay appropriate treatment.[10]

The high morbidity and mortality of joint sepsis warrants a high index of suspicion. Septic arthritis must be considered when rheumatoid patients develop a sudden exacerbation of pain and swelling in one or several joints. Patients treated with corticosteroids or immunosuppressive agents who have skin infections and urinary tract disease are the most susceptible. The knee is most commonly involved but any joint can be the site of infection. Signs of sepsis, such as fever and leukocytosis, can be absent. Roentgenograms of the affected joints are not always helpful in the early diagnosis.

Whenever infection is suspected, the joint must be aspirated and the joint fluid examined and cultured. A cell count of 100,000 or more white cells per mm^3 with predominance of polynuclear cells points toward the diagnosis of an infection. A low synovial fluid glucose level is not always helpful. It can be low in a noninfected rheumatoid joint.

A Gram stain can give a presumptive diagnosis. Septic arthritis can be definitely diagnosed by a positive joint fluid culture. Culture of blood and of possible sources of infection, especially ulcerated skin and genitourinary tract, should be performed simultaneously. Ninety percent of septic arthritis in the rheumatoid population results from positive organisms, 80% of these from *Staphylococcus aureus.*[35]

Most cases of septic arthritis caused by gram-negative bacilli occur in individuals with chronic disease, particularly cancer and impaired immune function.

Management

Gram-positive cocci are treated with a penicillinase resistant semisynthetic penicillin, effective against the staphylococcal organisms. In septic arthritis resulting from pneumococcal pneumonia, penicillin is the drug of choice. Gentamycin is used against the gram-negative bacilli.

Parenteral therapy is preferred, particularly for initiation of therapy. Because synovial fluid antibiotic levels are directly related to blood levels, it is important to achieve effective blood levels. The use of intraarticular antibiotics is not recommended since all the antibiotics commonly used in the treatment of septic arthritis achieve adequate synovial fluid levels. Parenteral antibiotic therapy also offers the advantage of treating the concurrent systemic infection.

Duration of treatment must be assessed for each patient. Various host factors, allergic reactions, and toxic reactions should always be considered.

Pus is destructive to joint tissue and interferes with the effectiveness of most antibiotics. The infected joint should be aspirated frequently, daily if necessary to keep it dry. If the fluid is difficult to remove percutaneously, surgical drainage should be used.

An infected joint should be placed in the position of least tension. A light splint could be used during the active stage of infection. Passive range of motion should be started as soon as pain permits. Active exercise with gentle stretching is added progressively when inflammation and pain subside. Efforts are made to reduce contractures and increase mobility and muscle strength so that maximum function is obtained.

Joint infection can follow joint replacement surgery. Roughly 100,000 total hip replacements and an equal number of other joint replacements are performed each year in the United States, the majority in the elderly; an infected prosthesis is a significant category of septic arthritis.

Factors predisposing to postoperative infection are previous operations on the same joint, use of corticosteroids, and immunodeficient states.

Patients with an infected prosthesis generally have pain, often in the absence of systemic illness. The problem is to differentiate prosthetic loosening caused by infection from sterile loosening. Roentgenograms and joint scanning are helpful but a definitive diagnosis is established by joint aspiration and fluid culture. In spite of the most vigorous antibiotic treatment with or without surgical drainage, fewer than one third of infected prostheses can be saved. Eradication of sepsis requires removal of prosthetic components. In the hip this results in several inches of shortening and limited functional ability. When the prosthesis is removed from the knee there is an option to carry out arthrodesis or to preserve a gap between the bone ends for an eventual prosthetic replacement. Salvage of an infected prosthetic joint may require repeated operations and prolonged parenteral antibiotic treatments. It requires close cooperation between the orthopaedic surgeon, the rheumatologist, and the infectious disease specialist.

References

1. Alarcon Segovia, D.: Drug-induced ANA and lupus syndrome, Drugs **12**:69-77, 1976.
2. Barwick, D.D., and Walton, J.N.: Polymyositis, Am. J. Med. **35**:646-660, 1963.
3. Bluestone, R., and Bacon, P.A., editors: Extraarticular manifestations of rheumatoid arthritis, Clin. Rheum. Dis. **3**(3), 1977.
4. Boss, G.R., and Seymiller, J.E.: Hyperuricemia and gout: classification, complications and management, N. Engl. J. Med. **300**:1459-1468, 1979.
5. Cooperating Clinics Committee of the American Rheumatism Association: A controlled trial of gold salt therapy in rheumatoid arthritis, Arthritis Rheum. **16**:353, 1973.
6. Dieppe, P.A., et al.: Mixed crystal deposition disease in osteoarthritis, Br. Med. J. **1**:150, 1978.
7. Egeland, T., and Munthe, E.: Rheumatoid factors, Clin. Rheum. Dis. **9**(1), 1983.
8. Estes, D., and Christian, C.L.: The natural history of SLE by prospective analysis, Medicine **50**:85-95, 1971.

9. Fleming, A., Benn, P.T., Corbett, M., and Wood, P.H.N.: Early rheumatoid disease: patterns of joint involvement, Ann. Rheum. Dis. **35**:361, 1976.

10. Goldenberg, D.L., and Cohen, A.S.: Acute infectious arthritis: a review of patients with non-gonococcal joint infection, Am. J. Med. **60**:369-376, 1976.

11. Grahame, R., and Scott, J.T.: Clinical survey of 354 patients with gout. Ann. Rheum. Dis. **20**:895-900, 1977.

12. Howell, D.S., and Talbott, J.M.: Osteoarthritis symposium, Semin. Arthr. Rheum. **2**(suppl. 1): 111, 1981.

13. Hunder, G.G., and Allen, G.L.: Giant cell arteritis: a review, Bull. Rheum. Dis. **29**:980-987, 1978.

14. Hunder, G.G., Disney, T.F., and Ward, L.E.: Polymyalgia rheumatica, Mayo Clin. Proc. **44**:849-875, 1969.

15. Huskisson, E.C., editor: Anti-rheumatic drugs, Clin. Rheum. Dis. **5**(2), 1979.

16. Huskisson, E.C., editor: Anti-rheumatic drugs, Clin. Rheum. Dis. **6**(3), 1980.

17. Jaffe, D.A.: D-penicillamine, Bull. Rheum. Dis. **28**:948, 1978.

18. Kellgren, J.H., Lawrence, J.S., and Bier, G.: Genetic factors in generalized arthritis, Ann. Rheum. Dis. **22**:237, 1963.

19. Kellgren, J.H., and Moore, R.: Generalized osteoarthritis and Heberden's nodes, Br. Medical Journal **1**:181, 1952.

20. Klinenberg, J.R.: Current concepts of hyperuricemia and gout, Calif. Med. **110**:231-243, 1969.

21. Koffler, D., Agnello, V., and Kunkel, H.G.: Polynucleotide immune complexes in serum and glomeruli of patients with SLE, Am. J. Pathol. **74**:109-122, 1974.

22. Lawrence, J.S.: Rheumatism in populations, London, 1977, William Heinemann Medical Books.

23. Lawrence, F.S., Brenner, J.M., and Bier, G.: Osteoarthrosis, Ann. Rheum. Dis. **25**:1-24, 1966.

24. Lawrence, R.C., and Shulman, L.E., editors: Epidemiology of the rheumatic diseases: proceedings of the Fourth International Conference, National Institutes of Health, New York, 1984, Gower Medical Publishing, Ltd.

25. Madison, P.J., Michael, F.R., and Scott, D.G.: Other connective tissue disorders. In Wright, V., editor: Bone and joint disease in the elderly, New York, 1982, Churchill Livingstone.

26. Masi, A.T., and Medsger, T.A., Jr.: Epidemiology of the rheumatic diseases. In McCarthy, D.C., editor: Arthritis and allied conditions, ed. 9, Philadelphia, 1979, Lea and Febiger.

27. McCarthy, D.J.: Calcium pyrophosphate crystal deposition disease: Pseudogout, articular chondrocalcinosis. In McCarthy, D.C., editor: Arthritis

and allied conditions, ed. 9, Philadelphia, 1979, Lea and Febiger.

28. McCarthy, D.J., Kohn, N.N., and Faires, J.S.: The significance of calcium pyrophosphate crystals in the synovial fluid of arthritic patients: the "pseudogout syndrome," Ann. Intern. Med. **56**:711-737, 1962.

29. Moskowitz, R.W., Howell, D.S., Mankin, H., and Goldberg, V., editors: Textbook of osteoarthritis, Philadelphia, 1983, W.B. Saunders Co.

30. Pearson, C.M.: Polymyositis, Ann. Rev. Med. **17**:63-82, 1966.

31. Poss, R., Ewald, F.C., Thomas, W.H., and Sledge, C.B.: Complications of total hip replacement arthroplasty in patients with rheumatoid arthritis, J. Bone Joint Surg. **58A**:1180, 1976.

32. Robinson, H.S.: Functional and social deficits: consequences of time and disease, In Ehrlich, G.E., editor: Total management of the arthritic patient, Philadelphia, 1973, J.B. Lippincott Co.

33. Rodnan, G.P.: Progressive systemic sclerosis (scleroderma). In McCarthy, D.C., editor: Arthritis and allied conditions, ed. 9, Philadelphia, 1979, Lea and Febiger.

34. Rodnan, G.P., Schumacher, N.R., and Zvaifler, N.J., editors: Primer on the rheumatic diseases, ed. 8, Atlanta, 1983, Arthritis Foundation.

35. Schmid, F.R., editor: Infectious arthritis, Clin. Rheum. Dis. **4**:1-241, 1978.

36. Schwartz, M.D., Slavin, G., Ward, P., and Ansell, B.: Muscle biopsy in polymyositis and dermatomyositis: a clinicopathological study, Ann. Rheu. Dis. **39**:500-507, 1980.

37. Sokoloff, L.: Pathology and pathogenesis of osteoarthritis, In McCarthy, D.J., editor: Arthritis and allied conditions, ed. 9, Philadelphia, 1979, Lea and Febiger.

38. Thompson, M., Anderson, M., and Wood, P.H.N.: Locomotor disability: a study of need in an urban community, Br. J. Prevent. Social Med. **28**:70-71, 1974.

39. Wood, P.H.N.: The challenge of arthritis and rheumatism, London, 1977, British League against Rheumatism.

40. Wood, P.H.N.: Epidemiology of rheumatic disorders. In Scott, J.T., editor: Copeman's Textbook of the rheumatic diseases, ed. 5, New York, 1978, Churchill Livingstone.

41. Wood, P.H.N.: An evaluation of criteria for polymyalgia rheumatica, Ann. Rheum. Dis. **38**:434-439, 1979.

42. Wyngarden, J.B., and Kelley, W.N.: Gout and hyperuricemia, New York, 1976, Grune and Stratton, Inc.

43. Yu, T.F., and Berger, L.: Impaired renal function in gout, Am. J. Med. **72**:95-100, 1982.

chapter 6

CLINICAL NEUROLOGY IN THE GERIATRIC PATIENT

Peter Tsairis

Nervous system disorders are among the most common causes of disability in the elderly patient. As a person ages, certain neurologic diseases or certain sets of neurologic symptoms and signs—for example, a gait disorder, mental deterioration, dizziness, strokes, and peripheral nerve disorders—become more frequent. In many instances these patients have multiple problems; therefore the approach to neurologic evaluation of these patients must be quite different from that used with younger populations. In the elderly symptoms and signs frequently have multiple causes. Furthermore, psychosocial and environmental factors usually weigh more heavily on the older person. Neurologic diseases account for about 50% of the incapacitation seen in patients over the age of 65.[1]

The purpose of this chapter is to provide an insight into the neurologic assessment of these patients and to acquaint the orthopaedic physician with the most common neurologic disorders seen in this age-group.

NEUROLOGIC ASSESSMENT OF THE ELDERLY PATIENT

Like any other discipline of medicine or surgery, the evaluation of any adult, young or old, includes a careful history, examination, and a series of laboratory studies. In evaluating or assessing the neurologic status of the elderly, orthopaedic physicians must adopt diagnostic strategies appropriate to both the variations in individual performance and the numerous factors that may contribute to a deficit. Ideally, the orthopaedist should be able to distinguish between normal and abnormal neurologic function commensurate with the patient's age. The physician must also determine whether any neurologic symptoms or dysfunction is a result of aging of the nervous system, previous damage to the nervous system, or a specific disease state. It is important to develop techniques to differentiate normal from abnormal, especially in the preoperative evaluation of these patients. For example, if a patient has pain and gait dysfunction resulting from severe osteoarthritis of the hip, it would be pointless to correct the problem if there is clinical evidence of severe impairment of gait function because of nervous system disease, which in effect would not allow the patient to become mobile even after such a surgical procedure. It is also extremely important to identify other features of the patient's condition that contribute to his her disability. For example, there is no point in correcting a deformity that limits function if a patient has a movement disorder or other problems with coordination, severely impairing function of the involved limb.

Normal versus abnormal function

Simply stated, normal function is regarded as the mean performance on a given test plus or minus two standard deviations for the given age of an individual. This concept of normalcy has many problems. Compared with young adults, the older person has a less homogeneous pattern of performance. Certain neurologic findings commonly seen in the older person (for example, mild gait ataxia, limb tremors, diminished or absent ankle jerk reflexes, or even an extensor plantar response) may be normal variants resulting from attrition of neural elements in the nervous system with aging. In another sense, normal function may designate those elderly patients who are functioning independently and are free of any known diseases. In general the concept of normalcy is difficult to fully define in an older person, and therefore through training and experience the physician must recognize basically two problems: first, that in some older patients normal involution of the nervous system masquerades as a disease state and second, that other patients may conceal their neurologic disease in the guise of the normal aging process of the nervous system. These distinctions are of extreme importance in the neurologic assessment of the elderly patient.

Neurologic history

Neurologists spend a considerable amount of time in recording each neurologic complaint and obtaining the standard history related to the primary illness. On the other hand, orthopaedists have much less time to spend on the neurologic history. Nevertheless, they should establish if there is any history of neurologic injury such as:

Stroke

Head trauma

Encephalitis

REVIEW OF NEUROLOGIC SYSTEMS

- *Head and mental function*
  Psychologic disorders, memory change
  Dizziness/vertigo
  Headaches
  Blackout spells
  Amnesia episodes
- *Cranial nerves*
  Disorders of special senses: anosmia, amaurosis, diplopia, hearing loss, tinnitus
  Facial weakness/numbness
  Bulbar dysfunction: dysphagia, dysarthria, dysphonia
  Neck weakness
- *Gait function*
  Balance problems
  Weakness/stiffness of arm or leg
  Clumsiness of arm or leg
- *Motor system*
  Adventitial movements of limbs: tremor, involuntary spasms, fasciculations
  Focal limb weakness, wasting
- *Sensory system*
  Numbness, tingling, coldness of limbs
  Radicular pain symptoms
- *Autonomic system*
  Sweating abnormalities
  Sphincter dysfunction
  Sexual dysfunction
  Gastrointestinal dysfunction

Tumors

Confusional states related to previous surgical procedures

Seizures

Peripheral nerve disorders

Myopathy

Dementia

An attempt should be made to review the neurologic system with specific inquiries concerning mentation and functions of the head, cranial nerves and neuromuscular and peripheral sensory systems (boxed material). In obtaining the neurologic history of these patients, the orthopaedist may be confronted with a number of special problems that make it difficult to distinguish between real disease and involutional changes caused by aging of the nervous system. For example, the patient may have a memory loss that makes it difficult to obtain an accurate history. The individual may be unaware of this intellectual deficit or may deny it. The history therefore can be obtained only from the patient's family. Those patients who admit to memory loss or intellectual impairment are often depressed and less likely to be significantly demented. It must be remembered that any impairment of memory is most frequently recognized by either the patient or family members as the initial deficit in most forms of dementia. If it can be determined that dementia does exist, then additional questions must be asked to try to get to the underlying basis of the problem. In addition, many of these elderly patients have some impairment of special senses that may have a significant effect on the patient's capacity to absorb new information. It is not uncommon for a deaf patient to be regarded as demented and a visually impaired elderly patient considered to have a balance disorder.

Neurologic examination

The neurologic examination of the elderly patient is no different from that of any other patient. However, in assessing these patients the standards of performance need to be adjusted in accordance with the patient's age, with particular attention to certain areas. The areas that should be of spe-

cial interest to the orthopaedist are memory function; assessment of vision and hearing; gait analysis; peripheral neuromuscular function, including testing of muscle strength; evaluation of reflexes and sensory function, particularly vibratory sensation; presence of cervical or cranial bruits; and last, and analysis of the patient's sleep patterns.

Assessment of cognitive function

Assessment of cognition is time-consuming. Many elderly patients may complain of impairment of memory, and this complaint may actually include other disorders of cognitive function as well. The elderly patient may be depressed, have diminished energy, or show decreased initiative, all of which may affect assessment of cognitive function and lead to suspicion of a cognitive disorder (pseudodementia).[18] In a situation where the physician is unsure of a cognitive disorder, documentation of the problem may be obtained by a battery of psychometric tests as objective measures. A standard battery of these tests that has proved to be of value in assessing cognitive functions was developed by Reitan at the Mayo Clinic.[28]

Most would agree that the incidence of dementia increases with advancing age. It is estimated that mild dementia occurs in the elderly population in a range from 2.6% to 15%.[14] In the over-80 age-group, the risk of moderate or severe dementia is between 15% and 20%.[5]

Evaluation of special senses

It is well documented that visual and hearing abnormalities occur with advancing age. Pupillary responses may be diminished or absent, ocular motility may be slowed, and upward gaze impaired. Similarly, high-frequency hearing loss may increase in the elderly population, usually beginning after age 50. There may also be diminution of taste and smell sense, but this is less well documented. Impairment of other cranial nerve functions are not common in the normal aging process and, if seen, may be indicative of specific disease states. Sometimes it may be difficult to distinguish between dysarthria secondary to neural dysfunction from that resulting from dental pathology.

Gait analysis

As with impairment of mental functions, disorders of balance and stability are among the common complaints of the elderly. For the orthopaedist this is not a rare problem although it is sometimes difficult to assess. One must keep in mind the role of mechanical changes because of arthritic joints and other musculoskeletal dysfunction, which contribute in a significant way to the restricted motility of these patients. The elderly patient with a hesitant, broad-based, small-stepped gait should alert the physician to the possibility of Parkinson's disease. These patients may also have a stooped posture and diminished arm swing. These changes are believed to result from central, probably extrapyramidal, deterioration. Another central nervous system disorder cauing gait dysfunction occurs with frontal lobe deterioration. These patients may have difficulty getting started and complain of their feet "sticking to the ground." They may display axial or limb rigidity or mild paratonic rigidity (active resistance to passive stretch), usually in association with other evidence of frontal lobe release signs (active snout or suck reflex, accentuated grasp reflex). Disorders of peripheral neuromuscular dysfunction may also cause gait disturbance. Patients with weakness in the proximal or distal muscles of their legs will display weakness in getting out of chairs or climbing stairs and may at times fall with prolonged ambulation. The neurologic examination may be normal or abnormal in the form of absent reflexes or diminished distal sensory function. Some of these patients may complain of aching discomfort in their legs, which is nonspecific and diffuse, and have what is characteristically termed pseudoclaudication of neurogenic origin. Lumbar spinal stenosis resulting from degenerative osteoarthritis of the spine may account for this problem (see Chapter 11).

Elderly patients with the problem of falling abruptly are often referred to a neurologist for evaluation. The nervous system dysfunction may be only one cause of the problem. In my experience most falls in the elderly population result from a combination of factors, including dysfunction of the vestibular system, cardiovascular disease (postural hypotension because of autonomic dysfunction or cardiac arrythmias), cerebral vascular insufficiency, specifically of the vertebrobasilar system, and drug-related incidents. It is therefore important to remember that arthritic and lumbar spine disorders may not be the only factor in the genesis of falling episodes in the elderly population.

Reflexes in the elderly

Diminution or absence of the ankle jerks may occur in 10% of the patients over the age of 60.[12] These reflex changes may occur in the absence of any typical peripheral neuropathy or sometimes may be a subclinical finding in indolent diabetes or nutritional neuropathy. The plantar reflexes may be mute or extensor in about 5% of the population group, and superficial abdominal reflexes are often absent.[12] These findings are normal variants; however, if they occur in association with other signs of nervous system dysfunction, then a careful neurologic examination is warranted.

Sensory functions

The most common abnormality of sensation in the group above the age of 60 is diminution of vibratory sensation, particularly in the lower extremities. Hobson and Pemberton report that about a tenth of individuals at age 60 and a third to a half beyond the age 75 have abnormalities in vibration or increases in the thresholds for touch and pin prick.[12] These increases may result from changes in skin and connective tissue. Cortical perception—namely, stereognosis, graphesthesia, and double simultaneous stimulation—ordinarily remains intact in the elderly group.

Vascular abnormalities

In a patient who has falling episodes, it is critical to examine the cervical and cranial vessels by auscultation. If bruits are detected, then this would imply significant stenosis of extracranial circulation to the cerebrum, a possible etiology for these falling episodes.

COMMON NEUROLOGIC DISORDERS OF THE ELDERLY PATIENT
Dementia

In the total evaluation of the elderly patient, physicians often spend little time in assessing cognitive function. Much has been written about the cognitive changes occurring with normal aging of the brain. These alterations in function are incompletely understood, as are the forms of cognitive function secondary to toxic, metabolic, or psychiatric disturbances. It is sometimes difficult, even for the neurologist, to determine where normal neuronal attrition ends and Alzheimer's disease begins.

The cognitive profiles of common dementing illnesses are only now beginning to be carefully elucidated. Neuropsychologic testing consists of assessing five basic areas of mental function:

Language
Memory
Attention
Visual-spatial ability
Conceptualization

This assessment can be used to help differentiate the effects of normal aging, delirium, depression, and dementing illnesses and to develop appropriate treatment measures. Numerous standardized tests have been developed for examining each of these areas in relative isolation from one another. These tests are useful because they assess cognitive functions individually and can be used to develop the profile of spared and impaired functions. In a clinical situation this is most useful not only for assisting with diagnosis of an individual patient suspected dementia but also for providing guidance regarding management of the patient. For the orthopaedist preoperative assessment of cognitive function in elderly patients is essential. It is not uncommon to see an elderly patient show signs and symptoms of a dementing illness following a surgical procedure, and knowledge of preoperative cognitive function may prevent unnecessary postoperative diagnostic studies.

Major types of dementia. Findings in several studies[11,23] suggest that among patients referred for evaluation of possible dementia, over one half will show signs of a cortical degenerative process or Alzheimer's disease (boxed material). Dementia resulting from depression, the toxic effects of alcohol, and microvascular infarcts are the next three most common diagnoses. Normal pressure hydrocephalus is the most common potentially reversible neurologic disorder causing dementia. Dementia secondary to drug effects, nutritional disorders, metabolic disease, and other systemic diseases is less common; it is frequently detected by the internist and treated without further referral. About 25% of patients have a potentially treatable disorder, particularly those dementias caused by depression, hypothyroidism, or normal pressure

---

CAUSES OF DEMENTIA	
Common causes:	*Less common causes:*
Alzheimer's or Pick's disease	Drug toxicity
Multiinfarctions	Nutritional disorders
Normal pressure hydrocephalus (NPH)	Hypothyroidism
Depression	Remote effect of cancer
Parkinson's disease	
Alcoholism	

hydrocephalus. It is important to remember that treatable cases of dementia definitely exist in sufficient number to warrant a close evaluation of all patients with progressive deterioration in intellectual function. For a more comprehensive view of the major types of dementia, the reader is referred to Alexander and Geschwind's chapter on dementia in the elderly.[2]

Acute confusional states (delirium)

Acute confusional states or delirium is a transient organic brain syndrome of acute onset and is characterized by cognitive impairment, disturbances of attention, abnormal psychomotor behavior, and disturbance of the sleepwaking cycle. These patients may have a fluctuating course from moment to moment or day to day, and usually the syndrome is of brief duration lasting less than 2 weeks. Metabolic alterations such as hyponatremia, uremia, or hepatic disturbances are well-known systemic conditions that may produce acute confusional states and are frequently correctable. Other elderly patients may become disoriented and confused at night because of unfamiliar surroundings in a hospital ("sundowning") or following a surgical procedure for reasons that are not entirely clear. The toxic effect of anesthesia on a brain already compromised by a dementing illness may be quite profound and disable the patient for several weeks. It is also not uncommon for elderly patients with mild dementia to develop an acute worsening during a febrile episode or acute delirium following a myocardial infarction.

Delirium following metrizamide myelography is not usual, especially in the elderly person. The most frequently reported signs and symptoms are agitation, fluctuating levels of awareness, impaired memory, disorientation, and occasional hallucinations and paranoid delusions.[29] Other less common but serious adverse effects reported with this water-soluble dye are seizures, transient aphasia, and mild clonus. All of these side effects have been observed more commonly after cervical and thoracic myelography than after lumbar myelography. Typically, these sequelae appear with-

in the first 24 hours after the procedure and persist as long as 4 to 5 days after onset. Phenothiazines, tricyclic antidepressants, central nervous system stimulants and monoamine inhibitors (which all lower seizure threshold) should be avoided in all patients receiving metrizamide. In my experience elderly patients are frequently dehydrated when they come into the hospital and should be adequately hydrated for at least 12 hours before metrizamide myelography. There is some evidence that adequate hydration for at least 12 hours before and after metrizamide myelography may prevent these side effects.

It is important to remember the relationship of the alteration of mental status to the underlying metabolic derangement. For example, when the underlying condition of metabolic alteration is corrected, the patient'a mental status should return to normal, or another cause must be investigated. The usual duration of an acute confusional state averages 1 to 2 weeks, but on occasions it may last as long as a month. In a few cases the delirium state may be followed by dementia that may or may not be reversible.

An acute confusional state in an elderly patient usually signals the onset of an exacerbation of an underlying physical illness which in itself may be life threatening or terminal; therefore the prognosis of delirium is guarded. In a strict sense delirium is a transient disorder of mental function and alertness, and its outcome should be full resolution with return to the premorbid psychologic state. In some cases, however, the delirium may lead to a comatose state or death or result in permanent organic brain damage. The following is a list of the most common and important etiologic factors associated with delirium in the elderly (for a more comprehensive analysis see the article by Lipowski[21]):

Alcohol and drug withdrawal

Metabolic/endocrine disorders (hyponatremia and acid-base imbalance; organ failure, hypoglycemia, thyroid dysfunction, vitamin B deficiency)

Drug toxicity (narcotics, anticholinergics, cimetidine)

Cardiac disease (congestive heart failure, arrhythmias)

Systemic infections (septicemia, meningoencephalitis, pulmonary and urinary tract infections)

Cerebrovascular disorders (infarction, hemorrhage, vasculitis)

Trauma (hip fractures, fat emboli, head injury, surgery)

Cancer (remote effect or metastases, especially carcinoma of lung)

Metrizamide myelography

Disorders of locomotion

A wide variety of disorders of locomotion can occur in the elderly patient. Some are relatively stereotyped and characteristic, although nonspecific to the aging process per se (the so-called "senile gait").

Other abnormalities of gait function in late life are associated with specific neurologic diseases: Parkinson's disease, multiinfarct dementia, agitated depression with or without associated drug effect, degenerative cortical diseases (Alzheimer's type of senile dementia, Steele-Richardson-Olszewski syndrome), and a treatable condition discussed earlier, normal pressure hydrocephalus.

A gait disorder may be one of the earliest findings in normal pressure hydrocephalus and frequently precedes the mental changes. These patients complain of a slight insecurity of balance and need assistance in the form of a crutch or the arm of a companion for gait stability. Characteristically, they complain of stiffness in their legs, and on observation their steps are slightly shortened and the base widened, similar at times to the type of gait seen in Parkinson's disease. There is usually no tremor, rigidity, or slowness of coordinated movements, however. These patients are unable to walk a straight line tandemly, raising the possibility of some form of midline cerebellar ataxic syndrome, but again there is no intention tremor, heel to shin ataxia, or irregular slowing of alternating movements characteristically seen in cerebellar diseases. Occasionally, these patients have drop attacks during which they remain full conscious but may be unable to arise for several minutes unless assisted. Fig. 6-1 shows a CT scan of the head in an

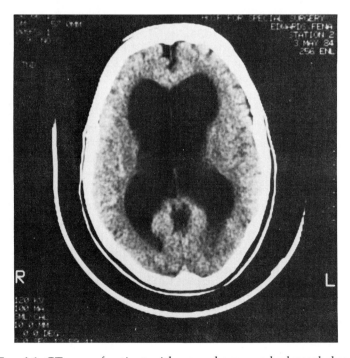

FIG. 6-1. CT scan of patient with normal pressure hydrocephalus.

elderly female patient who consulted an orthopaedist for gait dysfunction and painful hips. This patient had nocturnal urinary incontinence and only mild abnormalities of memory and other cognitive functions, all of which may be present in this syndrome. Gait ataxia was the most disabling part of her illness. This patient was referred to a neurosurgeon and had an excellent result following a ventriculoatrial shunt with almost complete resolution of her gait symptoms and incontinence within 10 days. The anatomic basis of the gait disorder of normal pressure hydrocephalus has not been established; some believe that is mainly a disorder of frontal lobe connections with basal ganglia.

The typical gait of Parkinson' disease was described earlier. These patients develop a stiff gait with short steps, sometimes referred to as a shuffling gait, and have associated slowing of normal body movements with little if any arm swing. In the severely demented patient who is receiving neuroleptic drugs for depression and agitation, a similar type of gait may be seen. Some of these patients have Parkinson's disease and have become demented or depressed as a result of their disease. Usually the parkinsonian patient will develop the locomotion disorder earlier, that is, before the onset of signs of dementia or depression. It must be remembered also that many of the phenothiazines and other neuroleptic drugs can induce symptoms of Parkinson's syndrome.

Gait dysfunction is an early change in the Steele-Richardson-Olszewski syndrome and a late change in the Alzheimer's type of senile dementia. With the first syndrome the gait becomes similar to that of Parkinson's disease, but these patients may experience sudden falling, and they state that they have a feeling of toppling forward. These individuals frequently suffer from fractures as a result of crashing to the floor suddenly. Characteristically, they show abnormalities of vertical gaze and dystonia of the axial and sometimes limb musculature. In the Alzheimer's type of senile dementia, memory failure and cognitive functions are impaired early, before any gait disturbance. In advanced cases locomotion deteriorates to the point where patients, unable to walk or curl up in bed, become virtually paraplegic.

Those patients with multiinfarct diseases of the central nervous system have a variety of gait disturbances, depending on which part of the nervous system is most severely effected. They may have hemiparetic and quadraparetic signs or cerebellar deficits with associated memory loss and language dysfunction, which may be related or unrelated to vascular disease.

Movement disorders

Elderly patients display a variety of syndromes that involve abnormalities in the control of movement and the production of abnormal involuntary movements. Some of the movement disorders were discussed in the previous section. They may be of diverse etiologies and commonly occur in association with isolated central nervous system degenerative processes or with metabolic disorders associated with systemic illness. Cerebral vascular diseases, brain tumors, and infections of the nervous system may also produce a focal or diffuse movement disorder.

The most common form of movement disorder in the elderly is a tremor. Tremors can be classified as those that occur at rest (resting tremors), those that occur with maintenance of a specific posture (postural or essential tremors), and those that occur at the end of a purposeful motor act (intention tremors). A resting tremor most commonly occurs in Parkinson's disease. In most patients the tremor is less prominent during action than rest, and it disappears during sleep. The rate of tremor averages about 3 to 5 oscillations per second. The postural tremor refers to those abnormal movements that are most prominent in limbs maintaining a static posture against gravity. These types of tremors are most frequently seen in the complex of benign essential or familial tremors and are considered benign disorders of the central nervous system. Essential tremors usually involve distal parts of the upper extremities and are relatively rhythmic with a much more rapid oscillation frequency than parkinsonian tremors, usually between 5 and 12 oscillations per second. These essential tremors can start at any age, but they occur most frequently in patients over the age of 60. There may or may not be an associated family history of the disorder. The tremor may be aggravated by emotional stress and fatigue and relieved by alcohol ingestion. Postural tremors may also be seen in patients treated with tricyclic antidepressants—amitriptyline (Elavil) and doxepin (Sinequan)—or lithium therapy for depression and in patients undergoing alcohol withdrawal. Occasionally, a postural tremor may be earliest manifestation of thyrotoxicosis.

The intention tremor is a rhythmic involuntary movement of the fingers superimposed on a purposeful action, and it may be seen at its maximal at the termination of the movement. For example, a patient who is asked to touch the examiner's finger with an index finger will be unable to maintain a stable end-point posture. This type of tremor is often seen in patients with cerebellar diseases or multiple sclerosis. Occasionally, patients with Parkinson's disease may display both resting and intention tremors, especially during emotional stress.

Other types of abnormal movements that occur in the elderly are chorea, athetosis, dystonia, myoclonus, and hemiballismus. All of these abnormal movements may be caused by a variety of disorders affecting multiple levels of the neuraxis. For a more comprehensive analysis of the types of neurologic syndromes causing these movement disorders, see the chapter on movement disorders in the elderly by Klawans and Tanner.[19]

Brain tumors

Brain tumors of the elderly are not substantially different from those occurring in earlier adult life. Low-grade astrocytomas become increasingly infrequent with advancing years. Metastatic brain tumors, malignant and low-grade astrocytomas, pi-tuitary adenomas, and meningiomas are the most common intracranial tumors occurring in this age-group. The development of CT scanning has revolutionized the diagnosis of intracranial tumors. This technique has been especially helpful in evaluating all elderly patients with neurologic disease because of the considerable morbidity associated with more invasive procedures such as cerebral angiography and pneumoencephalography. Once the diagnosis of a brain tumor is made in an elderly patient, the treatment is dictated by the histologic type of the tumor, the general health of the patient, and the inherent toxicity of the specific treatment modalities. For example, an elderly patient in poor health because of coronary artery disease, who is discovered to have a small meningioma in the motor strip producing focal motor seizures, might best be treated conservatively with anticonvulsants rather than with surgery. All brain tumors in the elderly produce neurologic dysfunction by a variety of mechanisms. Neurologic deficit may occur as a result of tumor destruction of the brain, massive edema with or without associated hermination of cerebral contents, seizure activity, hydrocephalus from obstruction of the spinal fluid pathway, or deficit occurring as a result of hemorrhage of vascular compression of major vessels. The symptoms and signs associated with these changes may occur acutely or insidiously. In general, brain tumors may produce headache, changes in mental status, nausea and vomiting, focal or lateralizing motor and sensory signs, speech difficulties, gait ataxia, and seizures. On examination there may or may not be papilledema. Fig. 6-2 is a CT scan of an elderly male who awoke in the recovery room with a right hemiparesis after total left hip replacement. He had no antecedent history of any neurologic dysfunction that would lead to suspicion of an intracranial problem. Clinically, he was thought to have an intraoperative stroke, but the CT scan dictated otherwise. As shown in Fig. 6-2, he turned out to have a meningioma, which was completely removed, and the neurologic deficit fully re-

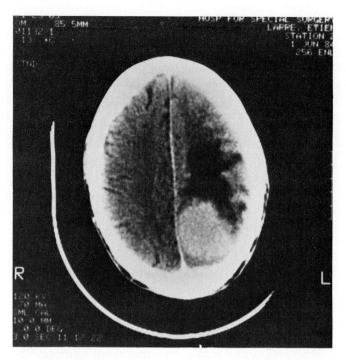

FIG. 6-2. CT scan of patient with meningioma.

solved. This case points out that some brain tumors like meningiomas may remain silent for many years until the patient is stressed by surgery or other medical illnesses.

Cerebrovascular diseases

Cerebrovascular diseases are one of the most common causes of disability and stroke in the elderly population. In various studies that have been reported in the literature, there is a direct relationship between the incidence of stroke and aging. This increasing incidence with age is applied to all forms of stroke and occurs in both sexes and all racial groups. Cerebral infarction is the most common stroke in the elderly group. Thrombosis or infarction of undetermined cause is the predominant factor in stroke genesis in those over 60 years of age. Embolism, and subarachnoid and intracerebral hemorrhages occur more frequently in younger people (under 50 years). Lacunar infarcts, which represent about 10% of all cerebrovascular accidents and are the least common variety of infarctions in all ages, seem to be more common in the older age population. This type of infarct develop primarily in hypertensive patients where there is a strong association with diabetes mellitus.[25] Although embolism accounts for at least a quarter of all strokes in the adult population, there seems to be no increased frequency of embolism in the older age-group when compared with individuals younger than 40 years old. Intracerebral hemorrhage occurs in all age-groups and usually in association with hypertensive cardiovascular disease. These hemorrhages occur predominantly in the deep portions of the cerebral hemispheres around the basal ganglia and also, less frequently, in the subcortical white matter and cerebellum. On the other hand, subarachnoid hemorrhage is a more common cause of stroke in the younger population and is usually a result of a rupture of a congenital berry aneurysm.

Transient ischemic attacks. Most transient ischemic attacks occur as a result of cerebral atherothrombosis or emboli from either extracranial or intracranial atherostenosis. Obviously, the clinical presentation of transient ischemic attack varies according to the vessel involved. These attacks are brief and usually reversible and may produce focal or nonspecific neurologic dysfunction. Patients with acute visual dysfunction or those who have developed sensory motor dysfunction, either in the arm or leg or both, with or without language impairment, usually have disease in the carotid system. Those with symptoms of dizziness, vertigo, hearing dysfunction, dysarthria, with or without associated contralateral sensory motor dysfunction in the limbs, usually have vertebrobasilar insufficiency. Headache and/or vomiting may or may not be an associated feature during ischemic attacks. Transient monocular blindness or so-called amaurosis fugax occurs as a sudden, unilateral, painless, and total or partial loss of vision that may last anywhere up to 15 minutes. Patients typically describe a "window shade" that descends or ascends until it obscures part of or the entire visual field.[26] In the transient ischemic attacks affecting the cerebral hemispheres there may be a combined sensory or motor deficit on one side. If the usually dominant left hemisphere is affected, there may be an associated aphasic deficit. Most transient ischemic attacks in the elderly occur in the distribution of the middle cerebral artery, which for the most part supplies circulation to the motor cortex controlling the face and arm. Ischemia in the anterior cerebral artery circulation, which is more rare, primarily affects motor and sensory function in the leg. Patients with these symptom complexes may have a loud bruit in the neck that may decrease in intensity with Valsalva's maneuver. This important point is useful in differentiation between a carotid bruit and a bruit originating in the external carotid artery circulation that does not change with this maneuver.

Carotid ultrasonography and/or digital intravenous angiography are useful diagnostic techniques in evaluating patients with carotid and/or vertebrobasilar atheromatous disease. Both these tests are noninvasive screening techniques use in evaluating these types of circulatory disorders. The computerized tomogram of the head or CT scan is more useful in assessing cerebral circulation from the standpoint of defining a small lacunar infarct or hemorrhage occurring as a result of a transient ischemic attack. All of these techniques are necessary in the evaluation of these patients before initiating any form of anticoagulation therapy.

Cerebral infarction. Elderly patients prone to cerebral infarction are those who have chronic hypertension, diabetes mellitus, or valvular disease of the heart. Clinical syndromes that occur as a result of occlusion of the internal carotid artery reflect an infarction from either failure of blood flow distally or embolization of the vessel. Embolization is probably more common and accounts for the majority of strokes resulting from atheromatous disease in the internal carotid artery circulation.[27] Emboli of cardiac origin usually result in identical clinical syndromes. Preoperative evaluation of the cardiac and circulatory systems of the elderly patient should be a mandatory part of orthopaedic evaluation. There is a higher incidence of stroke potential in any elderly patient with the aforementioned risk factors.

Lacunar infarction. The diagnosis of lacunar infarction is usually made on clinical grounds and varies according to the involved perforating artery. One of the most common causes of the lacunar syndrome is the occlusion of the lenticulostriate artery, which supplies the basal ganglia and the posterior limb of the internal capsule. This type of infarct leads to a pure motor hemiparesis involving the arm, leg, and face (and sometimes the trunk) and is accompanied by mild dysarthria without sensory deficit. There may be an associated visual field deficit, and if the infarct is severe in the dominant hemisphere, the patient may have an aphasia. Other syndromes in the territory of this vessel include the dysarthria–clumsy hand syndrome in which there is severe dysarthria and facial palsy with weakness of the tongue associated with clumsiness and mild weakness of the hand.[10] Pseudobulbar syndromes (inappropriate crying or laughing) associated with a gait disturbance in the elderly may occur as a result of a lacunar stroke involving the internal capsule. Pure sensory strokes caused by occlusion of perforating branches originating from the posterior cerebral artery, as well as focal weakness and ataxic syndromes resulting from occlusion of perforating pontine branches from the basilar artery, are other lacunar syndromes less commonly seen in the elderly. The CT scan may provide a positive diagnosis of lacunar infarction, especially if the CT scan is performed within a week to 10 days after onset of the syndrome.

Intracerebral hemorrhage. Arterial hypertension is the leading risk factor in the genesis of intracerebral hemorrhages. These type of hemorrhages characteristically occur during physical activity and, rarely, during sleep. A minor trauma in the elderly, especially patients taking anticoagulants, may be a factor in this type of stroke. In most cases the deficit is maximal at onset. It may be quite severe, causing coma or death within 24 hours. In these cases patients may have a very large hematoma with ventricular extension of the hemorrhage. In nearly 50% of cases the primary symptoms may be headache with or without vomiting. Seizures are uncommon manifestations of an intracerebral hemorrhage.

Peripheral neuromuscular disorders

With aging, neuromuscular performance deteriorates much like other organ systems. Some people age faster than others, depending on their level of activity. Aging of the neuromuscular apparatus results in slower movements and muscle contractions, loss of muscle bulk, and a decrease in strength. Several factors undoubtedly play a role in these changes, but there is evidence that the motor unit itself (lower motor neuron and all the muscle fibers that it innervates) undergoes a significant change. The physician diagnosing a patient with suspected peripheral neuromuscular dysfunction must seriously consider the normal aging process of the motor unit. Diseases affecting one or several parts of the motor unit are generally referred to as motor unit disorders or neuromuscular diseases. Specifically, these diseases are categorized as neuronal or anterior horn cell disorders, peripheral neuropathies, neuromuscular junction diseases, and myopathies. Weakness, atrophy, changes in stretch reflexes, and sensory dysfunction are major findings common to all of these disorders. The following outline, which precedes a full discussion of each disorder presents the most common type of neuromuscular diseases seen in the elderly population:

1. Neuronal diseases (motor neuron diseases, neuropathies, anterior horn cell diseases)
   a. Amyotrophic lateral sclerosis (ALS)
   b. Spinal muscular atrophies (neuronal type of peroneal muscular atrophy)
2. Peripheral neuropathies (polyneuropathy: sensory, motor, or mixed type)
   a. Diabetic polyneuropathy
   b. Uremic polyneuropathy
   c. Polyneuropathy of cancer
   d. Polyneuropathy associated with connective tissue diseases
   e. Polyneuropathy associated with plasma cell dyscrasias (multiple myeloma, dysproteinemias, paraproteinemias)
   f. Drug-induced and toxic neuropathies
   g. Nonhereditary amyloid polyneuropathy
   h. Ischemic polyneuropathy
   i. Mononeuropathies (diabetes, herpes zoster, trigeminal neuralgia, entrapment/compression neuropathies)
3. Neuromuscular junction disorders
   a. Myasthenia gravis
   b. Myasthenic syndrome, sometimes associated with bronchogenic carcinoma
4. Myopathic diseases
   a. Inflammatory myopathies (polymyositis-dermatomyositis syndromes, myositis associated with connective tissue diseases, infectious myositis)
   b. Endocrine myopathies (thyroid dysfunction and steroid toxicity)
   c. Drug-induced and toxic myopathies
   d. Genetic dystrophies (limb-girdle, oculopharyngeal, and distal type of dystrophy)

e. Miscellaneous disorders (ocular neuromuscular disease and ophthalmoplegia plus syndromes)

Neuronal or motor neuron diseases. Motor neuron diseases are progressive disorders of unknown etiology in which there is increasing weakness and wasting of muscles without sensory disturbances. The weakness and wasting may begin in one extremity, for example, manifested primarily as a painless foot-drop, or the disease may begin with distal asymmetric weakness and wasting associated with fasciculations and muscle cramps. In many cases the disease may remain in the lower motor neuron distribution and progress slowly over time with minimal to moderate disability. In some cases, when there is involvement of the cortical spinal tracts, the condition is termed amyotrophic lateral sclerosis (ALS). This subtype of motor neuron disease carries a poor prognosis. These patients have a much more malignant course and may die within a 2-year period from onset of symptoms. When there is involvement of the cortical spinal tracts above the medulla, these patients develop a speech disorder termed pseudobulbar palsy, or progressive bulbar palsy. These diseases are most common after age 50 and should be suspected in any elderly patient who complains of focal weakness or speech dysfunction. No method of treatment has been found to alter the course or progression of any of these diseases; therefore, only symptomatic measures are appropriate. These patients develop situational depressions that may be treated with one of the tricyclic antidepressants, which have anticholinergic properties that, at the same time, reduce excessive salivation sometimes seen with the bulbar forms of the disease. Orthopaedic aids may be helpful in controlling foot-drop. If there is difficulty in holding up the head, a wheelchair with head support may be necessary. The patient may survive for long periods with virtually no movement in the limbs and can be assisted with artificial respiration while in a wheelchair. The person who has difficulty swallowing may require a cricopharyngotomy or feeding gastrostomy.

Peripheral neuropathies. Morphologic and physiologic age-linked alterations in the peripheral nervous system have been extensively documented. For example, loss of vibration sense distally and depressed or absent ankle jerks are *not* uncommon in the aged. These findings alone are normal variants. Physiologically, it has been documented that there is a general decline in nerve conduction velocities as a person ages, presumably because of dropout of the faster conducting nerve fibers in the peripheral nerve. Brown[4] found an age-related fall in a number of motor units in the-nar muscles, which accelerates at midlife. Some of these elderly patients with clinically normal strength had only 50% of the number of motor units present during their younger years.

Peripheral nerves can be affected by a wide variety of inflammatory, metabolic, nutritional deficiency or toxic disorders, and trauma. Accurate diagnosis is important if specific therapy is to be applied. In a substantial proportion of elderly patients with peripheral neuropathy, cause cannot be determined, and therefore treatment is based on appropriate symptomatic measures. Clues to the diagnosis of peripheral neuropathies often lie in readily forgotten events occurring weeks or months before the onset of symptoms. In elderly people, inquiries should be made about recent viral or bacterial illnesses, use of new medications, excessive use of alcohol, systemic symptoms that might suggest occult malignancy, potentially toxic exposure to environmental pollution, pesticides or heavy metals, and the occurrence of similar symptoms in other family members. The symptoms of polyneuropathy in the elderly patient are manifestations of either altered sensory, motor, reflex, or autonomic functions, which may be symmetric or asymmetric, or various combinations of these functions. These manifestations usually appear in distal parts of limbs. Common symptoms that alert the physician to a possible peripheral nerve disorder are sensations of paresthesia or numbness, burning, coldness and crawling sensations, or exquisite sensitivity of the skin to touch.

Deep aching, cramping, or lancinating pains may occur, particularly at night and in an irregular pattern. The patients who have a feeling of walking on cotton or feel unsteady on their feet usually have an abnormality of deep sensation. Some patients may show pseudoathetotic movements of outstretched hands, which results from a loss of proprioception. Patients who are vulnerable to recurrent painless trauma with trophic ulcer formation should be alerted to the possibility that they have lost pain sense in their feet. Some patients may have clawed toe deformities, which are secondary to weakness and wasting of the intrinsic muscles of the feet.

In general, hyperpathic sensations represent an extreme example of a positive symptom. Negative symptoms of peripheral neuropathy result from the loss of sensation, with feelings of numbness and loss of proprioception leading to imbalance and difficulty walking (sensory ataxia).

Diabetic polyneuropathy. A distal, symmetric, predominantly sensory polyneuropathy is the most common variety of diabetic neuropathy seen in the elderly. Other less common varieties include proximal mononeuropathies, isolated cranial nerve palsies, and a symmetric autonomic neuropathy. The presence of any one of these neuropathic symptoms should raise the possibility of underlying diabetes. Two or more forms of these types of neuropathies may be encountered in the same diabetic patient. Sometimes the neuropathy is precipitated by the stress of an acute vascular event, for example, myocardial or cerebral infarction, surgery or sepsis. Most cases of diabetic neuropathy appear or worsen when the chemical disorder of the diabetic syndrome is poorly controlled. In other patients the neuropathy may be the first symptom of diabetes. In some the neuropathy may progress in spite of careful control of the blood sugar.

In some instances the pain of diabetic neuropathy may be quite severe, incapacitating, and misrepresented as a form of radiculopathy. For example, in patients with proximal mononeuropathies involving the femoral nerve, there may be a significant amount of pain. This lesion is a common sign of diabetic amyotrophy, which is believed to result from a more diffuse lesion in the lumbosacral plexus. These patients characteristically complain of constant pain that is worse at night and somewhat relieved by walking—symptoms not typical of a compressive radiculopathy. The syndrome of diabetic neuropathic cachexia is an extreme form of painful diabetic polyneuropathy.[9] This syndrome is most common in elderly men who have a mild distal sensory polyneuropathy and who experience acute pain in their limbs, anorexia, depression, profound weight loss, and insomnia. The results of routine malignancy tests prove negative. The syndrome may resolve completely in about a year, except for the underlying distal sensory neuropathy.

In the predominantly sensory polyneuropathies, meticulous care must be taken of the feet, which may easily be injured by minor trauma. These patients may have severe burning dysesthesia that is most prominent at night. The skin in their feet may ultimately break down to produce trophic ulcers, which are settings for serious necrotizing bacterial infections and osteomyelitis. Patients with long-standing diabetes and neuropathy may have an insidious painless destruction of metatarsophalangeal joints or other joints around the ankle. This may lead to striking deformities of the foot, the well-known Charcot's joint.

With diabetes, peripheral nerves may be vulnerable to entrapment or compression. The three most common compressive neuropathies seen in diabetic persons are the carpal tunnel syndrome, cubital tunnel syndrome resulting from entrapment of the ulnar nerve at the elbow, and compression of the peroneal nerve at the head of the fibula. Sensory dysfunction and pain may be the predominant symptoms in the diabetic patient with carpal tunnel syndrome. In some cases local decompression may be advisable to attempt correction of the sensory disturbances. Decompression of the ulnar nerve in the cubital tunnel or peroneal nerve at the fibula head are not commonly performed on diabetic patients.

Scrupulous control of chemical disturbances is considered particularly important whenever a diabetic neuropathy is first recognized. Some patients improve when they are treated with insulin and the blood sugars maintained within the physiologic range. With others, strict control has little effect on the polyneuropathy, especially if it has been of long duration.

The treatment of pain with diabetes is a difficult problem. Phenytoin (Dilantin) carbamazepine (Tegretol), or tricyclic antidepressants such as amitriptyline (Elavil) are sometimes effective in relieving pain or dysesthesia.

Uremic polyneuropathy. Chronic renal failure in the elderly population is not uncommon. These patients may develop a predominatly symmetric sensory polyneuropathy in the lower extremities. They may also experience distressing discomfort in the legs while lying in bed awaiting hemodialysis. Moving the legs or walking seems to relieve the discomfort, much like the patients with diabetic neuropathy (restless leg syndrome). Some uremic patients progress to severe sensory loss and paralysis of distal muscles.

The neuropathy may or may not improve with treatment of the renal disease. Maintenance hemodialysis may halt the neuropathy and improve sensation and/or strength, although this may take several months. The severe, established polyneuropathies generally respond poorly to dialysis. It is reported that the most effective treatment for uremic polyneuropathy is renal transplantation. Bolton et al.,[3] report dramatic improvement often beginning within weeks after renal transplantation.

Polyneuropathy of cancer. Among the many neurologic nonmetastatic manifestations that may be associated with carcinoma in the elderly, a relatively common disorder is a sensory motor polyneuropathy. The neuropathy may precede other evidence of carcinoma by several months or even years. Although carcinoma of the lung is the most common associated tumor, other organ system tumors are also involved. A motor neuropathy indistinguishable from motor neuron disease has been associated with bronchial carcinoma.[24] This neuropathy was reported to improve following resection of the tumor. In some instances the neuropathy improved in association with corticosteroid administration.[6]

A purely sensory neuropathy that can be very painful and is associated with a striking loss of cutaneous and deep sensations (ganglioneuritis) has also been reported in association with various types of cancer. These patients may have gait ataxia, dysesthesia and pseudoathetoid movements of the upper extremities that reflect a severe loss of proprioception. Small cell carcinoma of the lung is the primary tumor found in these patients. The neuropathy is progressive, despite treatment of the cancer. Recently, several elderly patients have been reported with this type of sensory neuropathy where no cancer was detected after an average follow-up of 7 years.[15]

Polyneuropathy associated with connective tissue diseases. Elderly patients with rheumatoid arthritis, mixed connective tissue diseases (features of systemic lupus erythematosis, scleroderma, and polymyositis), and various types of vasculitis (including polyarteritis nodosa and Sjögren's syndrome) are prone to various types of sensory-motor polyneuropathy, or entrapment neuropathies. Peripheral neuropathy has also been described in patients with cryoglobulinemia, whether in association with these disorders or in the essential mixed type of cryoglobulinemia of unknown cause. In systemic lupus erythematosus and polyarteritis nodosa, patients may develop either a mononeuritis multiplex or diffuse sensory motor neuropathy. In rheumatoid arthritis entrapment neuropathies occur commonly. Some rheumatoid patients have a distal sensory polyneuropathy, affecting the lower extremities, or they develop a mononeuritis multiplex, presumably a result of associated vasculitis.

Polyneuropathy associated with plasma cell dyscrasias (paraproteinemias and dysproteinemias). Chronic sensory motor polyneuropathies that are distal and relatively symmetric occur in typical multiple myeloma, predominately in middle-aged and elderly men. The neuropathy is usually progressive and may advance to almost complete quadriplegia, but occasional remissions have been reported. Bone pain and radicular pain from root compression are also characteristic of this type of neuropathy. Autonomic dysfunction is usually absent.

Waldenström's macroglobulinemia is a disorder mainly affecting the elderly. It is characterized by fatigue, weakness, anemia, bleeding, visual disturbances, lymphadenopathy and hepatosplenomegaly. In most cases the neuropathy develops after the systemic manifestations.

Another polyneuropathy that may be quite severe in the elderly group is that seen in association with osteosclerotic multiple myeloma (single or multiple). There is extensive multisystem involvement, including skin changes, finger clubbing, edema, diabetes mellitus, thyroid dysfunction, and hepatosplenomegaly.[13]

The neuropathies associated with paraproteinemias (benign monoclonal gammopathies) are present without any other evidence of malignant blood cell dyscrasias. The incidence of these gammopathies increases with age and is found in approximately 20% of people over 90 years of age.[20] IgG and IgA paraproteinemias have been reported in 10% of patients with peripheral neuropathy of unknown cause.[17]

The polyneuropathies associated with nonhereditary amyloidosis and cryoglobulinemias in the elderly are rare. For a further description and analysis of these types of neuropathies, the reader is referred to Kelley et al.[16] and Logothetis et al.[22]

Drug-induced and toxic neuropathies. Many medications are capable of causing neuropathy. It is not the purpose here to review all the medications known to produce diseases of the peripheral nervous system but to emphasize a few that are of special concern because of their relatively frequent use (boxed material).

Ischemic polyneuropathy. Polyneuropathy resulting from small and large vessel disease has been reported, but its clinical boundaries have not been clearly defined. Elderly patients with intermittent claudication may experience burning sensations in the toes or feet, which is worse at night, and on examination their pulses may be diminished or absent and skin may be dry and shiny. There is usually no motor dysfunction, and the sensory complaints are commonly limited to the legs.[7] Other patients may develop deep sensory loss in the feet, and occasionally there may be an isolated mononeuropathy in the distribution of the peroneal nerve. Many of the patients may come to ileofemoral bypass surgery with minimal if any resolution of their distal symptoms.

Common mononeuropathies in the elderly. Herpes zoster infection or shingles is a painful neuropathy in the acute stages. The pain may precede the vesicular skin eruptions in the dermatomal distribution

---

DRUG-INDUCED AND TOXIC NEUROPATHIES

Drug-induced:
  Gold therapy
  Isoniazid
  Hydralazine ? (caused by pyridoxine deficiency)
  Indomethacin
  Chloroquine
  Vincristine
  Phenytoin (Dilantin) (possible)
  Cimetidine (rare)
  Nitrofurantoin

Toxic conditions:
  Alcohol
  Pyridoxine deficiency
  Vitamin B_{12} deficiency

of the affected root or roots. These patients may have paroxysms of stabbing pain superimposed on a continuous burning sensation. Cutaneous sensibility is excessive to light touch and pin sensation, and patients will complain that they are not able to tolerate the friction of bed sheets or clothing. About 10% to 15% of patients develop a persistent dysesthetic condition known as postherpetic neuralgia. The frequency of this neuralgia increases with advancing age and is not uncommon following ophthalmic or thoracic zoster. Steroid therapy in the acute phases of the disease has reduced the incidence of postherpetic neuralgia. Other drugs such as amantadine (Symmetrel), carbamazepine (Tegretol), and levodopa have been used to treat this condition with variable degrees of effectiveness. The combination of a tricyclic antidepressant and phenothiazine has been effective in severe cases.

Trigeminal neuralgia is not an uncommon mononeuropathy afflicting the elderly population. Patients complain of paroxysms of lightninglike pain in the lips, cheek, or gums, usually on one side of the face. Slight stimulation of these areas may precipitate a paroxysm of pain (trigger zones). There are usually no other signs of neurologic dysfunction in this type of neuralgia.

The response to carbamazepine is dramatic and can be long-lasting. Some elderly patients cannot tolerate the drug or become refractory to the drug within 1 to 2 years of therapy; therefore, other treatment measures need to be tested. Surgical treatment on the fifth nerve may be required if carbamazepine therapy fails. Percutaneous radio frequency stimulation of the gasserian ganglion has been effective in over 80% of the refractory cases.[30]

Neuromuscular junction disorders

Myasthenia gravis. The fundamental defect in myasthenia gravis lies in the immune system, the defect in neuromuscular transmission is caused by antibodies to the acetycholine receptor at the postsynaptic membrane. Although myasthenia gravis may occur at any age, it is most common in young females and older males. The cus-

tomary symptom in the older person is ptosis, with or without diplopia. The symptoms wax and wane and may be worse at the end of a day. Sometimes the affected person may complain of easy fatigability, but there may not be any obvious muscle weakness in the limbs unless the examiner stresses the muscle with repetitive exercise. The course of the disease is difficult to predict; some cases progress steadily, others spontaneously remit or remain static. In general, the prognosis of the disease is confined to the extraocular muscles. The older patient with ocular myasthenia may respond poorly to anticholinesterase drugs, which are the mainstay in the treatment of the disease. Corticosteroids are indicated in affected patients who cannot be managed adequately with anticholinesterase medication.

The majority of cases are associated with thymic pathology. Thymic tumors are found in about 10% to 20% of the cases, and these patients have a less favorable outlook. Thymic pathology is not as commonly seen in the affected older patient.

Myasthenic syndrome, Lambert-Eaton syndrome.[8] This is an extremely rare disease, which is sometimes associated with bronchogenic carcinoma. The syndrome may antedate by several years the appearance of the cancer. Affected patients complain of painless proximal weakness, most commonly in the lower extremities, with easy fatigability. There is sparing of ocular muscles. In contrast to the patient with myasthenia gravis, there is on examination diminished or absent tendon reflexes, with symptoms and signs consistent with autonomic dysfunction. The response to anticholinesterases is minimal at best. The diagnosis is made by electrophysiologic studies, using techniques of repetitive peripheral nerve stimulation. The defect in this disease lies in the release of acetylcholine from the nerve endings, that is, abnormalities consistent with a prejunctional block similar to the defect that would arise from too much circulating magnesium or exposure to botulinum toxin.

Myopathic diseases. The most common disorders of voluntary muscles seen in the elderly are polymyositis, dermatomyositis syndromes, muscle weakness associated with endocrine or metabolic disorders, myopathies induced by drugs or toxins, and nonmyasthenic ocular neuromuscular disease or ophthalmoplegia plus. Occasionally, an elderly patient may develop a symptom of limb girdle muscle weakness on a genetic basis (limb girdle dystrophy) or a distal pattern of muscle weakness with myotonia (abnormal muscle relaxation), which is typical of myotonic dystrophy.

Inflammatory diseases (polymyositis-dermatomyositis syndromes). These acquired inflammatory diseases of muscle affect proximal muscles in a symmetric distribution, whereas the genetic dystrophies usually present as an asymmetric weakness of proximal muscles. In severe cases there may be dysphagia and facial weakness. In patients with dermatomyositis there may be an associated occult malignancy. There are also a number of reports of virus particles in specimens of muscle from patients with polymyositis, suggesting the possibility that this disease may result from hypersensitivity to a viral agent.

The natural history of these diseases is quite variable. In some the disease runs a self-limiting course with spontaneous recovery; in others it runs a relatively chronic progressive course, despite treatment with steroids or immunosuppressive agents, and results in mild to moderate degrees of disability. In those with associated malignancy, it may run a progressive course with involvement of respiratory and bulbar muscles and lead to a fatal outcome.

Most patients respond to corticosteroid therapy in moderate doses for a limited period of time. I cannot emphasize enough the possible hazards of overtreatment with steroids. Some patients may develop a steroid myopathy that supercedes the original myositis. Ideally, steroid therapy is given on an alternate-day basis to minimize side effects. Some patients respond poorly to steroids. In these situations the treatment may be supplemented by immunosuppressive drugs such as azathioprine or methotrexate.

Endocrine myopathies. Since corticosteroids are widely used in medical practice, the physician should be alerted to the fact that they may give rise to a syndrome of proximal muscular weakness (steroid myopathy). This myopathy is particularly likely to develop with fluorinated steroids such as triamcinolone. Affected patients will develop symmetric, proximal weakness and wasting in the pelvic girdle and on biopsy will show a selective atrophy of type II muscle fibers. The weakness will resolve as steroid therapy is withdrawn.

Occasionally, the elderly patient with occult thyrotoxicosis will develop a proximal myopathy, with or without wasting of the shoulder girdle musculature. This condition is generally reversed with adequate treatment of the thyroid dysfunction.

A painful proximal myopathy may also occur in association with hyperparathyroidism or in association with osteomalacia. The muscles from these patients would also show a nonspecific atrophy of type II fibers. If osteomalacia improves with administration of vitamin D and hyperparathyroidism, the myopathy may resolve with removal of the parathyroid adenoma.

Adult-onset limb-girdle dystrophy. Occasionally, an elderly patient will have a syndrome of limb-girdle muscular weakness and wasting that is slowly progressive and asymmetric in distribution. This type of myopathy may occur sporadically or appear as one of the genetic types of dystrophies that may have a variable expression in the same generation. A muscle biopsy is essential in making the correct diagnosis. Although most patients become extremely disabled and resort to wheelchairs for mobility, the disease does not shorten their life span.

References

1. Akhtar, A.J., et al.: Disability and dependence in the elderly at home, Age Ageing 2:102-110, 1973.
2. Alexander, M.P., and Geschwind, N.: Dementia in the elderly. In Albert, M.L., editor: Clinical neurology of aging, Oxford, England, 1984, Oxford University Press, Chapter 14.
3. Bolton, C.F., et al.: Electrophysiologic changes in uremic neuropathy after successful renal transplantation, Neurology 26:152-156, 1976.
4. Brown, W.F.: Method for estimating the number of motor units in thenar muscles and the changes in motor unit counts with aging, J Neurol. Neurosurg. Psychiatry 35:845-852, 1972.
5. Campbell, A., et al.: Dementia in old age and the need for services, Age Ageing 12:11-16, 1983.
6. Croft, P.B., et al.: Peripheral neuropathy of the sensory motor type associated with malignant disease, Brain 90:31-66, 1967.
7. Eames, R.A., and Lange, L.S.: Clinical and pathological study of ischemic neuropathy, J Neuro. Neurosurg. Psychiatry 30:215-218, 1967.
8. Eaton, L.M., and Lambert, E.H.: Electromyography and electrical stimulation of nerves in diseases of motor unit: observations on myasthenic syndrome associated with malignant tumors, JAMA 163:1117-1124, 1956.
9. Ellenberg, M.: Diabetic neuropathic cachexia, Diabetes 23:418-423, 1974.
10. Fischer, C.M.: A lacunar stroke: the dysarthria clumsy hand syndrome, Neurology 17:614-617, 1967.
11. Freemon, F.R.: Evaluation of patients with progressive intellectual deterioration, Arch Neurol. 33:658-659, 1976.
12. Hobson, W., and Pemberton, J.: The health of the elderly at home, London, 1955, Butterworth & Co. pp. 68-80.
13. Iwashita, H., et al.: Polyneuropathy, skin hyperpigmentation, edema, hypertrichosis in localized osteosclerotic myeloma, Neurology 27:675-681, 1977.
14. Jarvik, L.: Diagnosis of dementia in the elderly: a 1980 perspective. In Eisdorfel, Co., editor: Annual review of gerontology and geriatrics vol. I, New York, 1980, Springer Publishing Co.
15. Kaufman, M.D., et al.: Progressive sensory neuropathy in patients without carcinoma: a disorder with distinctive clinical and electrophysiological findings, Ann. Neurol. 9:237-292, 1981.
16. Kelley, J.J., et al.: The natural history of peripheral neuropathy and primary systemic amyloidosis, Ann. Neurol. 19:389-397, 1968.
17. Kelley, J.J., et al.: The prevalence of monoclonal gammopathy in peripheral neuropathy, Neurology 31:1480-1483, 1981.
18. Kiloh, L.G.: Pseudodementia, Acta Psychiatr. Scand. 37:336-351, 1961.
19. Klawans, H.L., and Tanner, C.M.: Movement disorders in the elderly. In Albert, M.L., editor: Clinical neurology of aging, Oxford, England, 1984, Oxford University Press, Chapter 21.
20. Kohn, J.: Benign paraproteinemias, J. Clin. Pathol. 8(suppl. 6):77-82, 1976.
21. Lipowski, Z.J.: Delirium updated, Compr. Psychiatry 21:190-196, 1980.
22. Logothetis, J., et al.: Cryoglobulinemic neuropathy: incidence and clinical characteristics, Arch. Neurol. 19:389-97, Oct. 1968.
23. Marsden, C.D., and Harrison, M.J.G.: Outcome of investigation of patients with presenile dementia, Br. Med. J. 2:249-252, 1972.
24. Mitchell, D.M., and Olczak, S.A.: Remission of a syndrome indistinguishable from motor neuron disease after resection of bronchial carcinoma, Br. Med. J. 2:176-177, 1979.
25. Mohr, J.P.: Lacunes, Stroke 13:3-11, 1982.
26. Pessin, M.S., et al.: Clinical and angiographic features of carotid transient ischemic attacks, N. Engl. J. Med. 296:358-362, 1977.
27. Pessin, M.S., et al.: Mechanisms of acute carotid stroke, Ann. Neurol. 6:245-252, 1979.
28. Reitan, R.M.: Changes with aging and cerebral damage, Mayo Clin. Proc. 42:653-673, 1967.
29. Schmidt, R.C.: Mental disorders after myelography with metrizamide and other water soluble contrast media, J. Neuroradiol. 19:153-157, 1980.
30. Sweet, W.H.: Treatment of facial pain by percutaneous differential thermal trigeminal rhizotomy, Prog. Neurol. Surg. 7:153-179, 1976.

part II
Musculoskeletal Dysfunction and Treatment

chapter 7

INTRODUCTION TO SURGERY IN THE GERIATRIC PATIENT

Thomas P. Sculco

Orthopaedic or any surgical intervention in the geriatric patient requires careful preoperative planning and consideration of possible medical, nursing, psychologic, and long-term planning problems. With the advent of comprehensive perioperative monitoring in these patients and new anesthetic techniques, surgical procedures that had previously been deemed too dangerous are now performed on a regular basis. The orthopaedic surgeon is well acquainted with the elderly patient who falls, incurring a fracture to the hip, and in whom, because of the nature of the injury and the morbidity from prolonged bed rest, surgery is urgent. These patients require not only expeditious and expert surgery but also thorough monitoring and attention to their needs as rehabilitation progresses, both in the hospital and after their return to the home or convalescent facility.

In addition to emergency surgery, major elective procedures that previously were not recommended in the geriatric patient are now undertaken, with a resultant improvement in the quality of life of these patients. This is particularly true in the field of orthopaedic surgery, in which the era of joint replacement arthroplasty has provided countless years of improved function to the geriatric patient. Furthermore, patients with disabling neurogenic claudication secondary to spinal stenosis have been helped significantly by spinal de-

compressions considered far too life-threatening only 10 years ago. Additional procedures on the failing musculoskeletal system performed on an elective basis continue to provide improved independence and function to these elderly patients.

In the previous chapters of this text the main emphasis was on an overall view of geriatric patients who are to undergo orthopaedic surgery, be it elective or emergency. The orthopaedic surgeon must be aware of the major impact a particular operative intervention will have on the life of an elderly patient. The surgeon should be familiar with the pathophysiology of the aging skeleton, with the medical and anesthetic considerations, and, as importantly, with the psychologic effects of the invasive procedure on patients. The treating surgeon should be cognizant of the fear in the geriatric patient that the condition currently affecting his locomotion or function might become a permanent detriment to his independence.

All physicians who treat geriatric patients with musculoskeletal dysfunctions must develop their treatment plans in a comprehensive and yet individualized way. The physician must consider the diversity of forces acting on these patients, all of which play a role in their response to the proposed therapeutic regimen. These factors include such obvious considerations, in addition to the current disorder, as the patient's general medical health and functional ability. As important for successful recovery of the patient is the patient's ability to cooperate with the complicated physical therapy program that might be required. This is particularly true after rotator cuff repair or total knee arthroplasty. The final result will be greatly compromised and the patient and physician will be disappointed if rehabilitative guidelines cannot be followed. In the case of lower extremity reconstructive surgery the physician must consider the neighboring joints and their ability to allow ambulatory capacity after reconstructive joint surgery. In addition, the functional status of the patient's upper extremities must be considered if assistive ambulatory aids are to be necessary for walking after surgery.

In the geriatric patient undergoing orthopaedic surgery a thorough medical history is requisite. Too often the operating surgeon defers this to a medical colleague. However, it should be emphasized that major system dysfunction must be apparent and understood by the surgeon. As a rule, in the geriatric patient a medical consultation should be obtained routinely before surgery. Communication should be frequent between surgeon and internist to avoid confusing the patient as to what his therapeutic plan entails and what medications he is taking and why. The surgeon should be aware of alterations in medical management and be able to assess their impact on a particular perioperative plan of care. The surgeon must also be willing to work closely with the internist in correcting medical abnormalities that may require postponement of surgery or interfere with the recovery of the surgical patient.

A complete list of all medications being taken by the patient should be obtained and understood by the orthopaedic surgeon. Allergic reactions to particular medications must be known by the surgeon. Geriatric patients not uncommonly manifest idiosyncratic reactions to various medications, particularly analgesics and sedatives, and this should be known by the operating surgeon. Should the patient demonstrate an untoward reaction to a particular medica-

tion, careful documentation of this must be noted so that a subsequent similar reaction to the drug does not occur.

In the medical history obtained by the orthopaedic surgeon special attention should be given to previous operative procedures and problems related to these. Excessive hemorrhage during an operative procedure or prolonged urinary retention or ileus after prior operative procedures can alert the surgeon to the need for alterations in intraoperative or postoperative planning. The patient's response to anesthesia is of particular importance and the anesthesiologist should be encouraged to use regional anesthesia whenever possible in these patients. As a rule, unless procedures are quite lengthy, local anesthesia is well tolerated by geriatric patients and its use is strongly encouraged.

If there had been a question concerning anesthesia in the past, a preoperative anesthesia consultation should also be obtained. As a rule, regional anesthesia is strongly recommended in the geriatric patient for all orthopaedic procedures. Studies have demonstrated reduced blood loss and fewer medical complications with regional anesthesia, particularly after joint replacement surgery.[1] The patient may be sedated mildly if necessary and quickly aroused after surgery, making pulmonary clearance and mental orientation rapid.

The surgeon in planning the patient's postoperative care should consider a variety of factors. Generally no surgical procedure that will require prolonged immobilization in bed should be undertaken in these patients. The complications of extended bed rest in the geriatric patient are well known and have been described previously. It is advisable to have the physical therapist meet the geriatric patient before surgery both to encourage pulmonary therapy as well as to lessen the patient's anxiety about postoperative therapy. If the patient is to be considered for an extended care facility or for home nursing or physical therapy services, the social worker should be encouraged to see the patient preoperatively. Too often the surgeon waits until the time of discharge to alert the social worker that a complicated extended care facility will be necessary or that home care services are to be provided.

The geriatric patient provides a special challenge to the orthopaedic surgeon and requires a careful commitment to preoperative planning so that the hospital course and postoperative period are without complication. Relief from pain and improved function are the end results of well-conceived surgical endeavors in these patients. On the other hand, a major complication in the geriatric patient is catastrophic to both his recovery and any potential benefit from the surgical intervention.

In the latter sections of this text specific areas of musculoskeletal dysfunction will be addressed. The organization will be primarily on an anatomic basis, but special emphasis will be given to other topics that are of major concern to those who treat geriatric patients and that affect many areas of the skeleton. In each chapter the author will attempt to provide an overview of the effects of aging on the particular area of concern and discuss the more common afflictions and their nonsurgical and surgical treatment. In most instances the discussion of the surgical treatment will be particularly detailed in order to describe the author's preferred method of surgical treatment for given problems.

Reference

1. Sculco, T.P., and Ranawat, C.: The use of spinal anesthesia for total hip replacement, J. Bone Joint Surg. **57A:**173-177, 1975.

chapter 8
THE CERVICAL SPINE

J. William Fielding

The cervical spine, like the lumbar spine, is a common area of pathologic involvement in the geriatric patient. Pain from degenerative disease is generally localized to the neck area but may produce radicular symptoms and dysfunction. These patients may note interference with activities of daily living when the neck is painful and routine functions such as driving an automobile, reading, gardening, and overhead reaching are compromised.

Although degenerative disc disease is a frequent cause of pain in the elderly, infection, neoplasms, and rheumatoid disease can also affect this area. The radicular component of pain in the shoulder and arm may also be secondary to localized shoulder and upper extremity pathology and should be considered by the examiner.

This chapter will deal with a review of the anatomic characteristics of the aging cervical spine and features of the history and physical examination.

HISTORY

The geriatric patient will frequently seek a physician for relief of neck pain and stiffness with or without a radicular component. If the pain is radicular, associated neurologic manifestations of paresthesias, numbness, or weakness may be noted. The duration and intensity of pain assist in differentiating the chronic pain of a spondylosis from the often more acute pain associated with nerve root compromise, neoplastic involvement, and other causes. The medication necessary to relieve pain and the activity limitation produced by the pain also provide useful information about its severity.

The treating physician should ask if there is associated upper extremity dysfunction. A degenerative rotator cuff may produce referred pain into the cervical area. A carpal tunnel syndrome may refer pain and paresthesias into the forearm. A metastatic lesion in the shoulder girdle may produce pain in the trapezius, cervical spine, and upper extremities, suggesting a radicular problem. Similarly, a tumor at the apex of the lung can result in primary neck and radicular symptoms.

Possible trauma to the neck (e.g., from an auto accident or fall) should be considered in the geriatric patient. What may have seemed a trivial incident could have produced significant damage to the cervical area. Cerebral vascular disease may explain syncopal episodes, headache, and dizziness. Additionally, compromise of the vertebral artery may develop secondary to cervical spondylosis with similar symptoms.

The patient should be further questioned on changes in gait, weakness, or "electrical jolts" into the extremities. Such symptoms may be the earliest signs of cervical myelopathy.

RHEUMATOID ARTHRITIS OF THE CERVICAL SPINE*

The neck, and particularly the atlantoaxial joint, is a common target for rheu-

---

*This section is slightly modified from the American Academy of Orthopaedic Surgeons: Instructional course lectures, vol. 32, St. Louis, 1983, The C.V. Mosby Co.

matoid arthritis and is the most frequent area of spinal involvement. Berens[4] credits Walton for first describing cervical vertebral subluxations in the United States in 1889.

Various studies attest to the frequency of this condition. It was mentioned as early as 1890 by Garrod who reported neck involvement in 178 of 500 cases.[46] His observations as well as those of Walton are thought provoking since they were made well before the introduction of radiology by Roentgen in 1896. Conlon, Isdale, and Rose[10] in a retrospective study of 845 patients with rheumatoid arthritis found 60% had neck involvement varying from mild to severe. Bland et al.[6] in 1963 noted that 86% of 100 patients with definite or classic rheumatoid arthritis had radiologic signs of cervical spine involvement.

The most common cause of atlantoaxial subluxation is rheumatoid arthritis; it is perhaps the most easily identifiable radiologic sign of this disease in the neck. Mathews,[32] as well as Meikle and Wilkinson,[35] have noted it early in the disease process (Fig. 8-1).

Even though Bell[3] in 1830 first described C1-2 displacement, it was probably not until 1951 that Davis and Markley[13] first reported that rheumatoid arthritis could produce atlantoaxial subluxation and death from medullary compression. Various observers have attempted to elucidate its frequency in rheumatoid arthritis, most using 3 mm as the upper limit or normal.

Isdale and Conlon[26] reported that in a prospective study of 333 consecutive hospital admissions 25% of patients showed atlantoaxial subluxation. In one-fourth of these it was greater than 5 mm. Six years later 171 of the 333 patients were available for further study and these showed a marked increase in the rheumatoid features; surprisingly, there was no instance of serious neurologic complication. Fifty-nine of the original 333 died, 17 of whom had atlantoaxial subluxation, but in no case was death caused by this anomaly. The authors concluded that in the absence of neurologic vascular complications surgery seemed unnecessary.[26]

Mathews[32] in 1969, using the criterion of 3 mm or more as abnormal found atlantoaxial subluxation in 25% of 76 consecutive outpatients. Martel[29] in 1961, using lateral tomograms of necks in flexion, found this condition in 24 of 34 patients with neck discomfort or severe progressive disease. The same author examined 100 un-

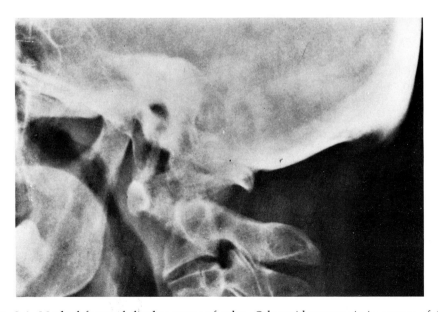

FIG. 8-1. Marked forward displacement of atlas. Odontoid process is in center of C1 ring.

selected clinic cases and found 34 incidences of atlantoaxial subluxation.

Sharp and Purser[45] in 1961 noted that atlantoaxial subluxation varied with the severity of the disease; it was approximately 1 in 30 in those with minimal evidence of rheumatoid arthritis, 1 in 15 of those with clinical evidence, and 1 in 5 of those with disease sufficiently severe to require hospitalization.[45]

Conlon et al.[10] in 1966 reported a correlation between vertebral luxations and widespread peripheral destructive lesions but indicated no correlation with the use of oral corticosteroids or disease duration. Mathews[32] in 1969 and Meikle and Wilkinson,[35] however, found that subluxation was related to disease duration and corticosteroid therapy.

Pathology

Unlike osteoarthritis, rheumatoid arthritis of the neck is a demineralizing destructive process. Osteopenia results in decreased bony density, which can often make radiologic assessment difficult.

Unlike degenerative spondylosis, rheumatoid arthritis of the neck affects mainly the upper cervical segments, and in the typical case little osteophyte formation and sclerosis at the vertebral end plates are found. In degenerative spondylosis the cervical spine becomes stiffer, whereas in rheumatoid arthritis it subluxes at several levels and may become unstable.

No bony interlocking occurs at occiput C1 and C2; joint strength depends on ligaments. These articulations are surrounded by synovial joints rendering them particularly prone to the synovial rheumatoid process.

The synovial joints between the transverse ligament and odontoid posteriorly and the anterior arch of C1 anteriorly are close to the synovial joints between the lateral masses of the occiput and C1 and between C1 and C2. Therefore, the upper cervical spine, and in particular the C1-2 articulation, is very vulnerable.

The cervicomedullary portion of the spinal cord lies at the C1-2 level where the potential for displacement is greatest. The vertebral arteries course through the foramen transversarium of C1 and C2 and can be compromised by abnormal atlantoaxial displacement. About 50% of cervical rotation takes place at C1-2, the canal of C1 rotating on the eccentric odontoid causing physiologic narrowing. To allow for this, the canal of the axis is large, approximately 3 cm in diameter, occupied equally by cord, odontoid, and free space—1 cm each.[16,51] Hence, some pathologic forward displacement of C1 is possible without cord compromise as the cord moves into the free space.

In the subaxial area some bony interlocking occurs at the facet joints, reducing the degree of displacement. Since the occiput-C1-2 complex is a series of synovial joints, destruction of the occipital condyles, lateral masses of C1, and the upper facets of C2 can cause the skull to settle downward with resultant upward translocation of the dens. This was described by Davis and Markley[13] in 1951 in a patient who died from medullary compression. Others have also recorded it as a cause of death[30,52,56] (Figs. 8-2 and 8-3).

In 1973, Rana et al.[39] presented eight cases of upward translocation of the dens without platybasia. Normally, the tip of the odontoid process should be no more than 4.5 mm above McGregor's line (a line from the upper surface of the posterior edge of the hard palate to the most caudal point of the occipital curve)[33] (Fig. 8-4). All of Rana's eight cases had the tip of the odontoid process 10 mm or more above this line. Two of the eight required surgery for acute neurologic problems that can occur from the frequent forward C1 shift in association with the upper displacement of the odontoid, which competes with the cord for space in the foramen magnum adding to cord and brain stem compromise.

Involvement of the odontoid process may lead to bony erosion and notching of the posterior aspect of the odontoid at the area of contact with the transverse ligament. The odontoid may be reduced to a narrow peg with little or no strength to an-

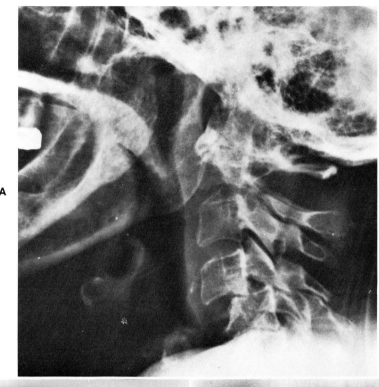

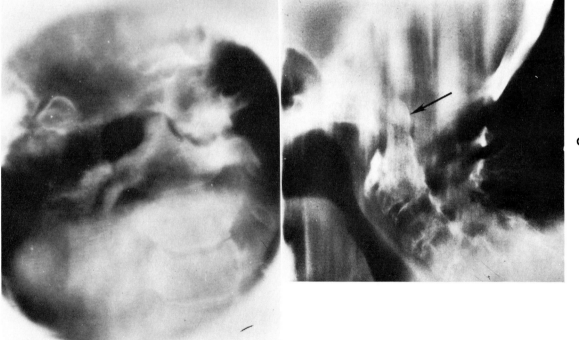

FIG. 8-2. A, Atlas "settled" on axis. Anterior arch of C1 is opposite upper portion of body of C2 and odontoid process is abnormally high, occupying space in foramen magnum. Posterior arch of C1 is markedly thin, and there is over 50% anterior displacement of C4 on C5. **B,** Advanced destruction of atlantoaxial articulation and odontoid process with lateral displacement of atlas on axis. **C,** Advanced destruction of atlantoaxial articulation with upward displacement of odontoid. (Courtesy Harvey L. Barish, M.D.)

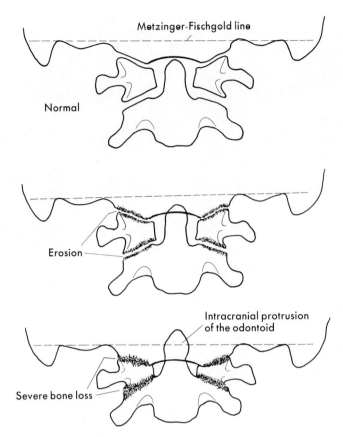

FIG. 8-3. Stages in destruction of atlantoaxial articulation with resultant settling of skull and upward displacement of odontoid process into foramen magnum. Fischgold and Metzger's line (a line drawn between the two digastric grooves on the anteroposterior laminogram of the skull) will pass well above odontoid tip (10.7 mm). It can be used to determine the degree of upper displacement of odontoid process. (From Fischgold, H., and Metzger, J.: Etude radiotomographique de l'impression basilaire, Rev. Rhum. Mal. Osteoartic. **19:**261-264, 1952.)

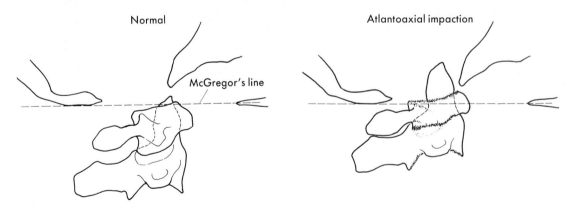

FIG. 8-4. Schematic representation of normal relationship of odontoid to base of skull and upward displacement of odontoid incident to destruction of atlantoaxial articulation. McGregor's line can be used for routine screening. Normally, tip of odontoid process should be no more than 4.5 mm above McGregor's line, which is drawn from upper surface of posterior edge of hard palate to most caudal portion of occipital curve of skull. (From McGregor, M.: The significance of certain measurements of the skull in the diagnosis of basilar impression, Br. J. Radiol. **23:**171-181, 1948.)

chor ligaments and protect the atlantoaxial joint (Figs. 8-5 and 8-6). This is compounded by the pathologic laxity of the transverse, alar, and capsular ligaments, with decalcification and weakening at the fibroosseous junction.

The disease process is compounded by osteopenia, which may be further aggravated by inactivity and the use of steroids often leaving the vertebra the same density as the soft tissues, which increases the problems of roentgenographic diagnosis. The posterior arch of C1 may be sclerotic or markedly thinned and unable to support an atlantoaxial fusion (see Fig. 8-2).

In the subaxial area the apophyseal joints are narrowed and eroded. The spinous processes tend to become sharp rather than "square-ended." The synovial process may involve the joints of Luschka. The intervertebral disc is involved by the same synovial process and the disc space narrowed without associated vertebral end plate sclerosis. One vertebra tends to "jigsaw" into its neighbor (Fig. 8-7). Later, multiple luxations at one, two, or more levels sometimes in stepladder fashion result from bony destruction and loss of ligament stability. Characteristically, these are rarely more than 3.5 mm and are more frequent in the upper regions of the spine (Fig. 8-8).

Meikle and Wilkinson,[35] in a study of 118 rheumatoid patients, found subaxial dislocation of greater than 1 mm in 26.3% of patients, end plate erosions in 15.3%, and narrowed discs in 72.9%.[35]

Park notes that 50% of loss of total height of the cervical spine is possible in patients with advanced rheumatoid arthritis.[38]

Neurologic complications

Compromise of the medullary cord by bony pressure from atlantoaxial subluxation may be compounded by pressure from the "wad" of inflammatory tissue in the synovial joint between the transverse ligament and the odontoid projecting backward against the cord.[12,15,21,34,40]

Involvement of the vertebral arteries may also cause neurologic signs. Crellin et al.[12] reported two such cases. In one pa-

tient the right vertebral artery was smaller than the left and was kinked at the level of the foramen transversarium of C4 and the axis.

An inflammatory arachnoiditis has been described in rheumatoid arthritis.[21] Dural fibrosis compressing the cord has been noted as well as vertebral artery thrombosis at the atlantoaxial level, which compromised the cervicomedullary blood supply.

The spinal cord tolerates gradual pressure better than acute compression. A narrowed cord may continue to function and the patient may be unaware of neurologic symptoms because of their gradual onset. Such a cord may be even more susceptible to trauma and may cease to function after a trivial injury (Fig. 8-9). Surprisingly, it is not always possible to correlate the degree of C1 displacement with either the presence or severity of neurologic findings, and this suggests that factors other than the subluxation may cause neurologic difficulties and the onset of these problems may be difficult to predict.[32,40]

Weissman et al. studied 194 patients with rheumatoid arthritis and atlantoaxial subluxation and settling of the skull and C1 on to C2. They noted that 24% of patients with 9 mm or more atlantoaxial subluxation developed spinal cord compression compared to only 2% with lesser degrees. Those patients with additional settling of the skull and C1 on C2 had an approximately 20% chance of developing cord compression compared with 7.3% of patients without this condition. Neurologic sequelae were more prevalent in men (24%) than in women (7.5%).[57]

Neurologic involvement in patients with rheumatoid arthritis usually occurs gradually but it may begin with alarming suddenness as with abrupt C1-2 displacement from minor trauma to an already weakened atlantoaxial complex (see Fig. 8-9).

Atlantoaxial displacement may vary from extreme mobility to relative fixation. In the latter instance, the gradual glacier-like slip of the atlas on the axis may be overlooked, leading to the erroneous conclusion that the displacement is "fixed" whereas it actually increases year by year.

Text continued on p. 92.

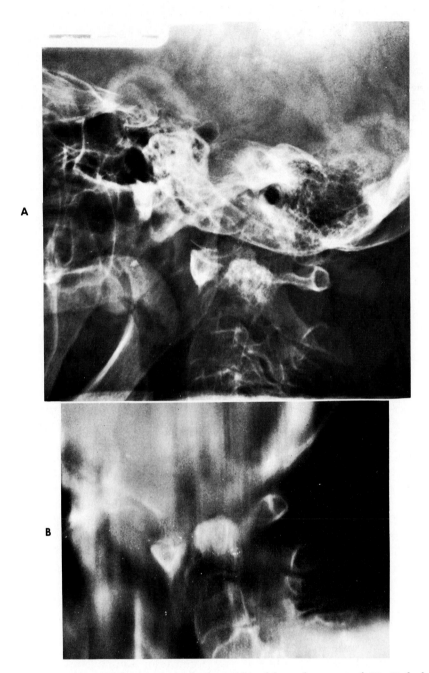

FIG. 8-5. A, Advanced destruction of odontoid and lateral masses of C1. Only base of odontoid is visible. Anterior arch of C1 is opposite body of C2 and there is destruction of posterior arch of C1. There is no visible bony continuity between base of skull and first and second cervical vertebrae. B, Advanced destruction of odontoid and lateral C1 masses of anterior arch of C1 opposite body of C2.

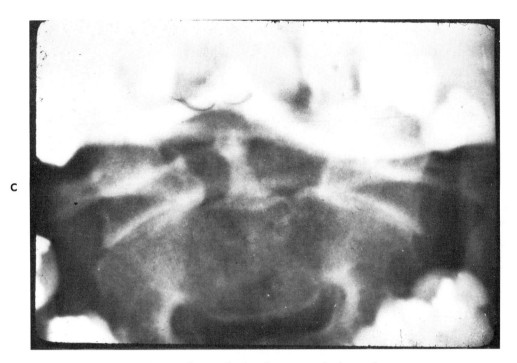

Fig. 8-5, cont'd. C, Advanced erosion of odontoid process.

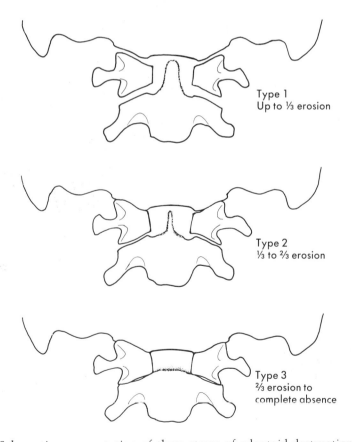

Type 1
Up to ⅓ erosion

Type 2
⅓ to ⅔ erosion

Type 3
⅔ erosion to
complete absence

Fig. 8-6. Schematic representation of three stages of odontoid destruction: Type 1—destruction of one third or less; type 2—destruction of one third to two thirds; type 3—destruction of more than two thirds.

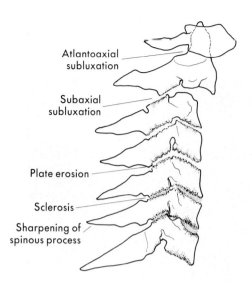

Atlantoaxial
subluxation

Subaxial
subluxation

Plate erosion

Sclerosis

Sharpening of
spinous process

Fig. 8-7. Schematic representation of effects of rheumatoid process on cervical spine. (Courtesy William Park.)

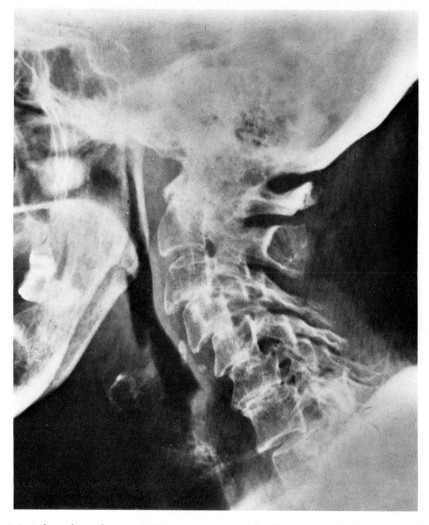

Fig. 8-8. Subaxial involvement. Disc spaces are markedly narrowed without significant sclerosis. End plates tend to "jigsaw" into one another, and vertebral spines are thinned and "sharpened." Subluxation from C3 to C6 has occurred in stepladder fashion.

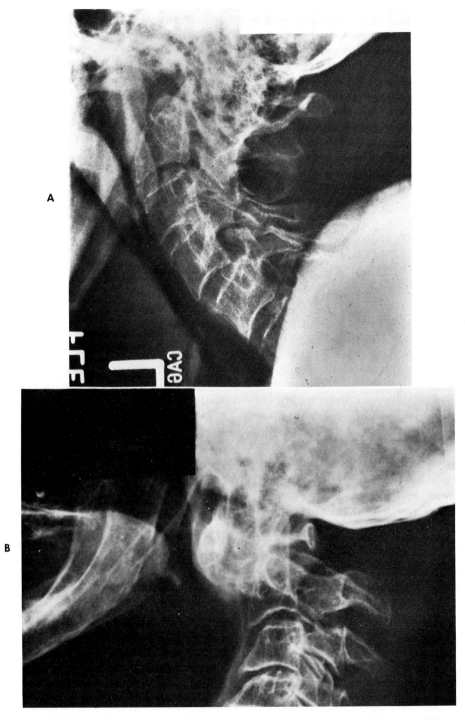

FIG. 8-9. A, Posterior displacement of C1 and C2 resulting from destruction of atlantoaxial joint and odontoid. B, Marked anterior displacement of C1 and C2 with quadraparesis and marked narrowing of space available for cord (distance between posterior aspect of odontoid and anterior aspect of posterior ring of C1).

Cord compromise may lead to weakness that may be mistakenly attributed to the crippling arthritic process in the peripheral areas. The disease produces weakness and painful deformed and contracted joints, making range of motion and strength evaluation difficult. Weakness may be a function of pain rather than neurologic damage. A dislocated and contracted great toe may not respond to the plantar reflex. Reflexes may be difficult to evaluate or even impossible to obtain, especially with joint stiffness. Other conditions found in the rheumatoid patient, such as a carpal tunnel syndrome, may mislead the examiner into believing that the patient has a cervical nerve root involvement when the fingers are numb.

Rana et al.[39] in 1973 stated that the neurologic picture confronting the clinician may be complex since progressive loss of reflexes suggests peripheral neuropathy; loss of consciousness on neck movement implies vertebral artery insufficiency; palatal weakness, deafness, tinnitus, vertigo, and facial paresthesias indicate intrinsic pontine vascular disease; and urinary urgency suggests parapyramidal tract involvement.

Neurologic problems can be produced by compression of the spinal cord, brain stem, or vertebral arteries, by vertebral displacement, or by inflammatory masses. The neurologic picture varies with the site and extent of compression. The following neurologic signs may be present:

1. Signs of spinothalamic tract involvement (decreased pain sensation)
2. Signs of the first two divisions of trigeminal nerve involvement (facial numbness, depressed or absent corneal reflex) because the spinal nucleus of this nerve is at the level of C2
3. Signs of pyramidal tract involvement (hyperactive reflexes, spasticity, and weakness)
4. Pontine signs such as palatal weakness
5. Fasciculation caused by involvement of the anterior horn cells
6. Signs of brain stem ischemia from vertebral artery occlusion or stenosis
7. Signs of urinary tract difficulty resulting from parapyramidal tract involvement

There are few reports of impaired position sense, indicating that the cord and brain stem damage is anterior and does not involve the posterior columns.

In addition to the neurologic problems, patients with rheumatoid arthritis usually complain of varying degrees of neck pain, limited motion, and crepitation.

If the atlantoaxial joint is involved or displaced, the patient may complain of neck pain radiating to the occiput. When the neck is flexed the patient may feel that his head is "slipping off" as C1 shifts forward on C2. This causes prominence of the spine of C2 in the posterior neck and difficulty looking upward with associated flattening of the occipitocervical curve.

Treatment

Surgery is rarely necessary for atlantoaxial or subaxial subluxation in the patient with rheumatoid arthritis[26] (Fig. 8-10). It is generally difficult to draw firm conclusions from the infrequent reports of surgical management. It is the consensus that nonoperative treatment is preferred. Smith et al.[49] gave strong support to this concept, and Isdale and Conlon[26] stated that in the absence of neurologic or vascular complications operative intervention was unwarranted. Ranawat et al.[41] noted that fusion was infrequently needed and performed in only 0.7% of a clinic population of nearly 2897. Ferlic et al.[15] reported only 12 cervical fusion operations in 1975. Others, however, have advocated surgery.[41] Between those two extremes lie the majority of patients where judgment plays the major role.

Conservative management generally consists of analgesics and soft or hard collars that may restrict motion, depending on their degree of rigidity. Collars do not prevent nor correct progressive subluxation or neurologic problems and may be poorly tolerated by some patients irrespective of their neck pain.[49] The same can be said of halter traction.

If the patient's condition will permit, surgery may be indicated in the following instances:

1. Intractable pain associated with vertebral luxation unrelieved by conservative treatment
2. Significant vertebral artery compromise
3. Significant spinal cord or brain stem compression especially if progressive
4. Progressive instability associated with pain or neurologic involvement

Surgical procedures generally take two forms, fusion or decompression of neural or vascular structures. If decompression produces instability, it may be combined with fusion. Anterior fusion may be associated with graft collapse in the soft osteoporotic bone and generally is reserved for postlaminectomy instability where posterior arthrodesis cannot be carried out. Posterior arthrodesis is preferable and may be done in the occiput to C1-2 area, the subaxial region, or both.

Excessive rates of complication and pseudarthrosis result from the generalized rheumatoid process, bony demineralization, and destruction of bony structure in the area to be fused. These patients poorly tolerate postoperative fixation devices, and the rate of fusion is low compared with that of other patients. Only six of Ferlic's 12 patients had solid union.[15] The fatality rate after surgery is high. Ranawat[41] reported 27%, Cregan[11] 33%, Crellin et al.[12] 27%, and Meijers et al.[34] 42%.

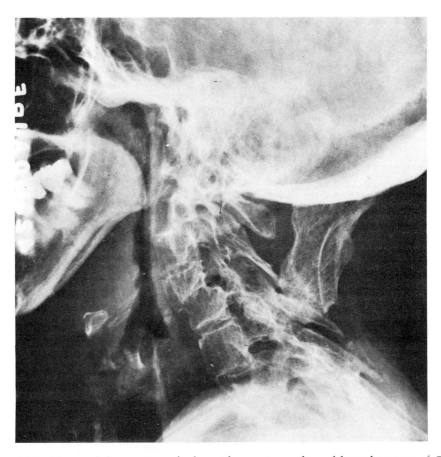

FIG. 8-10. Advanced destruction of odontoid, anterior arch, and lateral masses of C1. There is no connection between posterior C1 arch and lateral masses of C1. Posterior fusion had to be carried out from skull to lower cervical vertebra since it was impossible to obtain bony fusion posterior cervical arch of C1.

Before surgery, attempts to reduce displacement and maintain reduction include skull tong traction, halo devices, or both. Atlantoaxial fusion is generally carried out utilizing bone graft and wire fixation, as described by Gallie. Indications to include the occiput are absence or deficiency of the posterior C1 arch or atlantoaxial impaction. In the subaxial area, fusion is performed by the standard midline technique with or without wire fixation. Internal stabilization has been enhanced by the use of wires or wire mesh incorporated in methylmethacrylate to avoid or minimize the hazards of external fixation. In a series of 11 patients where this technique was used, the pseudarthrosis rate was 18% and complications included wound dehiscence and late instability below the fusion mass.[9]

ANKYLOSING SPONDYLITIS

Unlike rheumatoid arthritis, which results in joint destruction, ankylosing spondylitis results in joint fusion. In the cervical region this often produces ankylosis from occiput downward (Fig. 8-11).

Pathology

Postmortem studies have suggested an initial inflammation, followed by ossification of joint capsule and articular cartilage resulting in ankylosis. In the spine the vertebral bodies tend to become "square"; os-

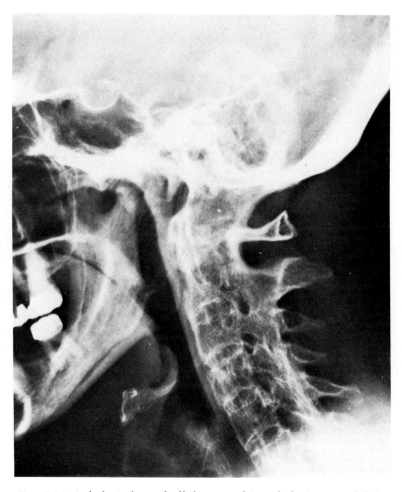

FIG. 8-11. Ankylosis from skull downward in ankylosing spondylitis.

sification of ligaments and disc tissue follows.

Clinical features

The onset is insidious, usually associated with unremitting low back pain and morning stiffness decreasing during the day and recurring in the evening. The sacroiliac joints are usually involved early in the disease, a finding that explains the initial area of symptoms.

In the cervical region, the pain, stiffness, and limitation of motion associated with a flexion deformity usually cause patients to seek medical advice. Patients may compensate for these symptoms by simultaneously flexing hips and knees to obtain a horizontal line of vision.

O'Driscoll et al. report that lateral flexion is the most common movement restricted; further restriction is proportional to the degree of ankylosis.[36]

Surgical management

If the patient's position is satisfactory, and the cervical spine completely fused, there is little that surgery can offer.

Surgical intervention may by necessary in unacceptable cervical flexion deformities, fractures, and atlantoaxial displacements.

Fixed flexion deformity. Probably the commonest complication of this disease is unacceptable fixed cervical flexion.

Cervical osteotomy, as described by Mason et al.,[31] Urist,[55] and Simmons,[48] has been found to provide satisfactory correction. Simmons recommends that the procedure be performed under local anesthesia, with the patient in the sitting position, with the halo ring and halo jacket applied. A laminectomy is performed at the C7 level extending upward into C6, and downward into D1 with local appropriate resection of the C7-D1 facets. The spine is then manually fractured at the C7-D1 level with the patient under temporary general anesthesia and the proper correction obtained. The halo ring is then fastened to the body jacket. Osteotomy of the C7-D1 level is recommended because the vertebral canal is wid-

er in this region and also because the vertebral arteries enter the foramen transversarium at C6, above osteotomy site. The neurologic and other hazards of this operation should be known to the patient before surgery to aid in the surgical decision.

Fractures. The rigidity of the spondylitic cervical spine unprotected by ribs or abnormal musculature renders it particularly vulnerable to trauma. The force of a blow cannot be absorbed by mobile cervical segments and the ankylosed spine may behave in a manner similar to a long bone. The fractures are usually transverse, occur at the level of a disc space, and are generally at the midportion of the neck. Woodruff and Dewing[60] in 1963 reported 20 cases, five were above C5, and 15 below. Since a degree of osteoporosis is present, the spine may fracture easily with minimal pain and the patient may not recall the injury.

Simmons has noted the significance of such injuries in patients with severe flexion deformities. In 40 patients presenting for cervical osteotomy with unacceptable flexion deformity, 36% had evidence of previous fractures and in 31% the fracture contributed significantly to the deformity.[47] Such fractures may go unnoticed for a variety of reasons. First, the fracture may spontaneously reduce without displacement; second, the patient may not recall the incident, and also fracture may be difficult to detect, particularly in the lower portions of the cervical spine in an individual where x-ray positioning is difficult. Hudson[23] reported correcting a flexion deformity at the site of a fresh fracture dislocation between C5 and 6, in a patient without significant neurologic or vascular injury.

Not all fractures of the ankylosed cervical spine are benign: some have a very poor prognosis. The normal flexibility of the neck is eliminated by the ankylosing process. Therefore, all motion takes place at the fracture site. This is in close proximity to the vulnerable vertebral arteries and spinal cord as described by Taylor and Blackwood[53] (Fig. 8-12).

Bohlman[7] in 1979 described eight fractures in patients with ankylosing spondylitis. Three were above C5, and five were at C5 or below. All had cord lesions and five died. Others have noted problems with these injuries.[5,20,22]

Woodruff and Dewing[60] presented 20 cases of ankylosing spondylitis with fracture. They made four observations:

1. Fractures may be caused by relatively slight trauma since the fused rigid spine affected by osteoporosis cannot give with stress. In none of their cases was the blow considered severe and in one the weight of the head alone was thought sufficient to cause fracture.

2. The ankylosed spine breaks like a solid long bone and the vertebral body compression is not a feature since the line runs transversely. Hence every fracture is complete, which increases the chance of dislocation and spinal cord injury.

3. Mortality is high; of their 20 patients

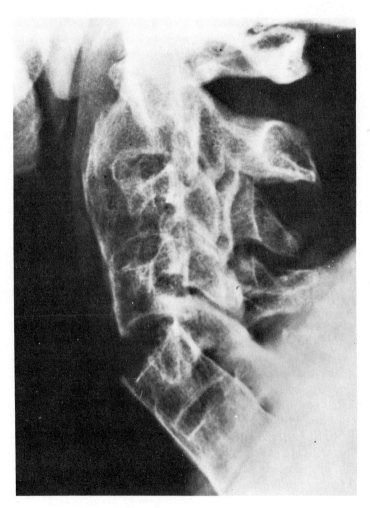

FIG. 8-12. Cervical spine fracture in ankylosing spondylitis.

9 died within a short time. Generally, the degree of displacement correlated with the severity of the spinal cord injury. They also noted that gross malalignment can be found with minimal or no cord impairment.

4. Treatment will vary with the clinical situation. They recommended "neutral traction."

Atlantoaxial displacement. Jefferey[27] reports that the incidence of this complication in the literature is as high as 90%, cau-

tioning that this high percentage may reflect the severity of the disease in patients referred to the hospital. He indicates that in his own experience atlantoaxial subluxation in ankylosing spondylitis is uncommon, an opinion I share. This complication would suggest that this joint is unfused, particularly prone to trauma, or both.

Surgical arthrodesis is probably the safest method of management though it will sacrifice rotary motion at the atlantoaxial joint (Fig. 8-13).

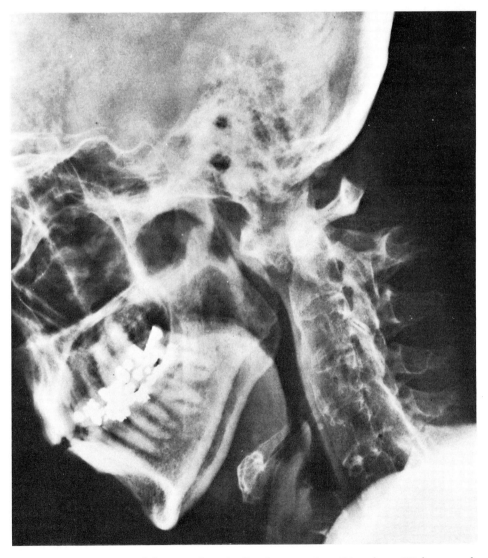

FIG. 8-13. Cervical spondylosis or chronic disc degeneration. Discs from C3 downward are markedly narrowed with sclerosis and spurring of adjacent surfaces of vertebral bodies and narrowing and sclerosis of articular facets.

Cervical Spondylosis*

In this condition the cervical disc pro gressively degenerates, hence the synonym "chronic cervical disc degeneration." Among its many other appelations are cervical osteoarthritis, spondylitis, chondroma, and chronic herniated disc.[44]

Key in 1831 and Gowers in 1892 clearly described bars and ridges arising from the intervertebral area projecting backward, narrowing the spinal canal as a potential cause of spinal cord compression[19,28] (Fig. 8-14).

Wilkinson reports that Pallis, Jones, and Spillane in 1954 stressed that cervical spon-

*This section is reproduced from Creuss, R., and Rennie, W.: Adult orthopaedics, New York, 1984, Churchill-Livingstone.

dylosis was common in elderly people.[8,58] They found 50% of people over 50 years and 75% over 65 years had typical radiologic changes of cervical spondylosis. Forty percent of people over 50 had some limitation of neck movement and some had neurologic abnormality; neurologic signs often preceded symptoms.[37]

Pathology

The degeneration starts in the intervertebral disc and subsequently affects the adjacent osseous structures.[14,58]

Wilkinson in 1960 studied the cervical spines of 17 patients at autopsy and reported that the primary lesion was a degeneration of intervertebral disc and that the bony lesions were secondary to this[58]

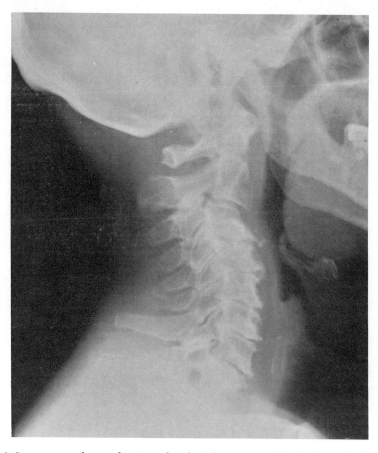

FIG. 8-14. Large osteophytes that interfered with passage of food through pharynx and esophagus. Patient's complaint was difficulty swallowing.

The discs that constitute about 20% of the length of the cervical vertebral column[59] gradually narrow and the length of the neck decreases (Fig. 8-14). Secondary proliferative changes occur in the adjacent surfaces of the vertebral body, joints of Luschka, and facet joints, the latter simultaneously losing their articular cartilage. Since the cervical discs are generally wider anteriorly than posteriorly, they contribute to the normal cervical lordosis, which tends to be reduced when disc degeneration is present.

DePalma and Rothman[14] in 1970 reported their detailed study of 70 autopsied cervical spines from persons whose age ranged from 38 to 95 years. They noted that degeneration affected the entire cervical spine and was generally age related. Seventy-two percent of individuals of the specimens over 70 years had severe abnormalities and the C5-6 level was the most frequently involved, followed by C6-7, with the C2-3 level least involved. The marked narrowing of the disc was associated with fissures extending into and becoming continuous with fissures and joints of Luschka. Nuclear material extruded under the longitudinal ligament into the joints of Luschka and even into the adjacent vertebral bodies. The joints of Luschka were markedly altered in the lower three levels, most frequently at the C5-6 region.

The intervertebral foramen is bounded posteriorly by the articular facets, and anterior and medially by the intervertebral disc, joints of Luschka, and adjacent vertebral bodies. Involvement of any or all of these structures will compromise the intervertebral foramina. DePalma and Rothman's studies found that when the intervertebral foramina were compromised, the joints of Luschka, the discs, and the apophyseal joints were each involved in 75% of the cases.[14] They also reported that spontaneous bony ankylosis was invariably associated with resorption of the osteophytes surrounding the foramina.[14] This observation has also been made by Robinson and Smith[43] following anterior cervical interbody fusion.

Symptoms

Friedenberg and Miller[17] in 1963 correlated x-ray changes with symptoms in two groups of patients, one symptomatic and the other asymptomatic.

In the asymptomatic group 25% of patients in the fifth decade and 75% in the seventh decade showed degenerative changes. The narrowing between C5-6 and C6-7 was higher in the symptomatic group but there was no difference between the two groups in the changes elsewhere in the spine (joints of Luschka, posterior articular processes, etc.). One must exercise caution, therefore, in attributing cervical symptoms to degenerative disc change.

It is reasonable to assume that symptoms and cervical spondylosis are mechanical in origin: neck pain and headache from altered biomechanics and neural and vascular complaints from mechanical compression.

Brain and Wilkinson[8] divided symptoms of cervical spondylosis into five groups which may occur singly or in any combination. The following list shows the order of their frequency.

1. Neck pain
2. Headache
3. Radicular symptoms
4. Spinal cord symptoms
5. Symptoms of vertebral vascular ischemia

Two more are added:

6. Visceral pressure symptoms
7. Symptoms from involvement of the sympathetic system

Acute symptoms are not characteristic of this condition. Generally, the symptoms in cervical spondylosis are as insidious in their appearance as the pathologic changes are in their development. The radiculopathy is chronic, and the myelopathy and symptoms of headache and neck pain develop gradually. Acute symptoms may occur in previously asymptomatic cervical spondylosis or may aggravate the characteristically chronic preexisting symptoms. These acute problems generally arise as a result of acute disc protrusion from sudden trauma or inflammatory process.

Neck pain and headache

It is well known that there is often a discrepancy between findings and complaints; severe changes are sometimes unassociated with significant symptoms.[17]

In chronic cervical degenerative disc disease, pain is usually comparatively mild, occasionally severe, generally aggravated by activity, worse in the morning, and associated with stiffness with varying degrees of restriction of cervical motion. Severe roentgenographic changes are not always associated with a concomitantly severe limitation of motion. Fifty percent of cervical rotation occurs at the atlantoaxial articulation which is rarely involved by the spondylitic process.[14,16] Considerable flexion and extension take place between the occiput and C1, C2 and C3, and C3 and C4, which are also infrequently involved.[14,16]

Headache is generally in the occipital region, and like neck pain is worse on awakening but decreases during the remainder of the day.

Radicular symptoms

The emerging nerve roots are compressed in the bony foramina by a combination of factors. Hypertrophic changes from the adjacent surfaces of the vertebral bodies, joints of Luschka, and articular facets. This may be compounded by extrusion of some intervertebral disc material, and the settling of one vertebra on the other with imbrication of the articular facets. Since the nerve root occupies 20% to 25% of the foraminal space, considerable narrowing must occur before radicular symptoms develop.[18]

The main symptom found is pain al-

TABLE 8-1
Summary of radicular symptoms

Nerve root	Disc level	Symptoms	Weakness: reflex change
C3	C2-3	Pain and numbness in back of neck, particularly around mastoid process and pinna of ear	No readily detectable weakness or reflex change except by EMG
C4	C3-4	Pain and numbness in back of neck, radiating along levator scapula muscle and occasionally down anterior chest	No readily detectable weakness or reflex change except by EMG
C5	C4-5	Pain radiating from side of neck to shoulder top; numbness over middle of body of deltoid muscle (axillary nerve distribution)	Weakness of extension of arm and shoulder, particularly above 90 degrees; atrophy of deltoid muscle; no reflex change
C6	C5-6	Pain radiating down lateral side of arm and forearm, often into thumb and index fingers; numbness of tip of thumb or on dorsum of hand over first dorsal interosseous muscle	Weakness of biceps muscle; depression of biceps reflex
C7	C6-7	Pain radiating down middle of forearm, usually to middle finger, though index and ring finger may be involved	Weakness of triceps muscle; depression of triceps reflex
C8	C7-T1	Pain down medial aspect of forearm to ring and small finger; numbness can involve small finger and medial portion of ring finger; numbness rarely extends above wrist	Weakness of triceps and small muscles of the hand; no reflex change

Adapted from Rothman, R.H., and Simeone, F.A.: The spine, Philadelphia, 1975, W.B. Saunders.

though occasionally weakness and sensory disturbances in the area supplied by the involved nerve are reported. Radicular symptoms are summarized in Table 8-1.

Myelopathy

It has been well established that cervical spondylosis results in narrowing of the cervical vertebral canal. Cervical myelopathy is considered by Brain and Wilkinson[8] to be one of the commonest disorders of the spinal cord during and after middle life. This is caused mainly by posterior vertebral body spondylitic protrusions gradually indenting the anterior aspect of the spinal cord. Hughes[24] has pointed out that such indentation may not be associated with clinical or microscopic evidence of myelopathy.

Myelopathy, characterized by demyelination of the lateral columns, degeneration of the dorsal columns, nerve cell damage in the grey matter, and marked cavitation was noted in some of Wilkinson's 17 cases of cervical spondylosis studied at autopsy.[8,58,59]

It would seem reasonable that clinical findings of myelopathy would be justified by degeneration of the long tracts and destruction of the anterior horn cells at the area of indentation. Hughes' observation of occasional indentation of the cord without clinical or pathologic evidence of myelopathy would indicate that in some instances the cervical spinal cord is relatively resistant to gradual pressure and may continue to function.[24] In such cases, however, minor trauma to the already compromised cord may precipitate the onset of symptoms. Hyperextension injuries have been described as causing cord damage as a result of pinching of the cord between a bulging disc and spondylotic bar anteriorly and infolding of ligamentum flava posteriorly.[50] Recurrent trauma has also been indicted in the production of myelopathy, with percentages varying from 47 to 16.[42,59]

Characteristically, the symptoms are insidious with disability occurring over months or even years with dysesthesia, weakness, and difficulty with the hands. The patient may complain of difficulty buttoning clothing, while in the lower extremity complaints of weakness and difficulty walking are often the presenting symptom. Involvement of the corticospinal tract will result in hyperactive deep tendon reflexes, a positive plantar response, weakness, loss of coordination, clonus, and depressed or absent abdominal and cremasteric reflexes. Involvement of the anterior horn cells at the level of the involvement will result in weakness in the upper extremities at this level. Sphincter control is rarely absent.

In summary, the onset of myelopathy is insidious and may be present for months or years before a diagnosis is made. The symptoms and findings in the lower extremities are the result of an upper motor neuron lesion from involvement of the corticospinal tract, with varying degrees of involvement of the afferent pathways. In the upper extremities, in addition to cord signs, a lower motor neuron lesion may be present from direct compression of the anterior horn cells from the spondylitic bar.

Symptoms of vascular ischemia

The vertebral arteries, "trapped" in the foramin transversarium from C6 to C1 can be affected by intervertebral motion and can be narrowed by osteophytes arising from the facet or neurocentral joints. Brain and Wilkinson[8] in 1967 reported angiographic evidence of temporary impairment of blood flow by simple head rotation, and Hutchinson and Yates[25] demonstrated distortion and narrowing of the vertebral arteries by osteophytes.

It is reasonable to deduce that individuals in this age group may well have atheromatous changes in the vertebral arteries. Thus head movement may restrict circulation to an extent that syncope, loss of consciousness, "drop attacks," and strokes may occur.

Visceral symptoms

On rare occasions large osteophytes projecting anteriorly from cervical vertebral bodies may directly compress the esophagus or trachea with resultant difficulties in swallowing solid food comfortably. In these instances, anterior resection should be considered.

Symptoms from involvement of the sympathetic nervous system

Some patients with cervical spondylosis may have a constellation of vague and indefinite symptoms. The validity of these complaints is suggested by the frequent repetition of similar symptoms from patient to patient. Among them are migratory headaches, dizziness, visual blurring, change in voice characteristics, and a sensation of separation from the environment. Barré[2] reported these symptoms in 1926.

In the years since these were first described, few articles have confirmed Barré's original description, which may indicate that the cause of such symptoms remains vague.

PHYSICAL EXAMINATION

The examination of a geriatric patient with suspected problems in the cervical spine must encompass not only the neck but also the upper and lower extremities. The gait pattern should be observed. Spasticity or imbalance can indicate disorders in the central nervous system including cervical myelopathy from spondylosis. The posturing of the neck should be noted for head position and spinal alignment. Atrophy of the upper back, shoulder girdle musculature, and upper extremity should be noted as well as muscle spasm. Active range of cervical motion is followed by passive motion. The physician should record ranges in flexion-extension, lateral bending, and rotation. Upper extremity range of motion should also be tested.

Areas of tenderness may be localized to the occiput, neck, trapezius, shoulder as well as the elbow, wrist, and hand. These "trigger points" can at times manifest the radicular component of the patient's pain.

The neurologic examination of the cervical spine and upper extremity should include strength, sensory, and reflex testing, as well as vibratory and two point discrimination. Hyperreflexia suggests the presence of myelopathy and should be evaluated in upper and lower extremities.

RADIOGRAPHIC EVALUATION

Plain radiographs of the cervical spine generally provide adequate information to confirm the diagnosis made from history and physical examination. Anteroposterior, lateral, right and left oblique, and open mouth radiographs are suggested. Flexion-extension cervical spine films may be added if instability is suspected.

The anteroposterior film demonstrates the uncovertebral joints and degenerative changes that can be seen early, before development of osteophytic spurs. As the spondylitic condition progresses, obliteration of this joint takes place and on the oblique views of the cervical spine encroachment of the intervertebral foramen can become quite marked.

The lateral radiograph is useful for identifying specific changes in the disc and areas of instability. The most common site of disc degeneration is in the lower cervical spine. As disc degeneration progresses osteophyte formation occurs anteriorly and beaking is noted from the adjacent anterior margins of the vertebral body in the area of the anterior longitudinal ligament. Although on occasion bony ankylosis may occur spontaneously across a disc space, it is quite rare.

Computed tomography adds a further dimension in demonstrating the extent of lateral recess and central stenosis. Myelography is generally reserved as a prelude to surgery in those patients who have been unresponsive to attempts at conservative treatment.

DIFFERENTIAL DIAGNOSIS

The geriatric patient's dysfunction may be caused by a variety of problems. The most common is degenerative disc disease with concomitant cervical spondylosis. Although unusual because of the degeneration of the intervertebral disc, frank herniation can occur.

In addition, tumors may arise in the cervical spine or be metastatic to this area. In the geriatric patient whose host resistance may be poor and whose nutritional state has been compromised, infection in the disc space, though rare, should be considered.

Shoulder inflammatory problems can produce retrograde pain to the neck. Occasionally carpal tunnel syndrome or de Quervain's tenosynovitis can refer pain to the wrist, forearm, and elbow area.

Vascular compromise as a source of radicular pain as found in the thoracic outlet compression syndromes is rare in the geriatric patient. Compromise of the vertebral artery system, however, can be the source of headache, dizziness, and syncope in the older age group.

Purely radicular symptoms may occur in the anterior chest area. If the pain is left-sided and aggravated by activity, it can appear quite similar to the angina caused by arteriosclerotic cardiovascular disease.

TREATMENT

The vast majority of geriatric patients with degenerative disease affecting the cervical spine will recover with conservative treatment. This generally consists of medication, heat, a collar, and reduction of activity. Since the condition is chronic, recovery may be slow and incomplete. Thus a discussion with the patient is recommended concerning the cause and prognosis of the illness and the rationale for the treatment.

Most patients are treated on an ambulatory basis with some type of immobilization. The idea is to rest the involved tissues. The weight of the head is supported by these inflamed structures. Rest in bed, eliminating axial loading of the cervical area, is recommended in the early stages if symptoms demand.

Various cervical collars have been developed to "support" the neck and reduce motions. The soft foam cervical collar is the best tolerated but does little to immobilize the cervical spine or to support the head. It does, however, provide some "protective feedback" to the central nervous system and this may be its main advantage. A plastic cervical collar with protective foam and chest and chin supports is more rigid and may better serve to reduce symptoms. If pain and spasm are severe, the patient should be encouraged to wear the plastic collar full time, using the soft collar at night. As symptoms improve, a gradual weaning from the collar should take place. Paracervical muscle weakness, already present in most of these patients with chronic neck symptoms, may be aggravated by the protective collar and, therefore, it should be removed as early as possible.

At night, a contoured "cervical pillow" can also be used to prevent excessive neck flexion and rotation.

Medications

The pain in patients with cervical spondylosis is generally based on muscle instability, spasm, and inflammation within the facet and uncovertebral joints. Secondary nerve root irritation and inflammation may develop. Medications should be given to deal with the components of the painful cycle. Analgesics, such as codeine, may be needed to control the pain when it is severe. In milder degrees of pain, milder analgesics are helpful. The constipating and gastrointestinal side effects of codeine can be a severe problem to the geriatric patient and a stool softener with a mild laxative may be necessary.

Antiinflammatory medication is used to reduce the active inflammatory component of the pain. Indomethacin, phenylbutazone, and others are generally effective, but gastrointestinal dysfunction may occur. Better tolerated nonsteroidal antiinflammatory medications such as ibuprofen or naprosyn, may be administered and may be better tolerated if taken with food or an antacid.

Muscle relaxants tend to reduce the pain and paracervical spasm. However, this category of medication works by depressing the central nervous system and untoward reactions including drowsiness, confusion, and lethargy can occur. Cyclobenzaprine, one of the medications in this group, has proven effective; additionally, methocarbamol can be used. Most patients will sleep better if these medications are taken late in the evening.

Local injection of Depo-Medrol in areas of trigger points may be used if indicated. On occasion, injection of these somatic areas provides prolonged relief.

Exercises

During the acute phase of cervical spondylosis, range of motion exercises can be performed within the range of comfort. As the pain and spasm subside, more active exercises can be carried out. Most patients will be more comfortable putting the neck through a range of motion in a warm shower or during the application of heat.

Further exercises should be begun as neck pain and mobility improve. A series of flexion-extension and rotary isometric exercises can be performed by using the heel of the hand against the forehead or occiput area.

If a collar has been necessary on a full-time basis for an extended period, exercises should begin slowly and the patient progressively "weaned" from the collar.

Local treatment

Moist heat, liniments, and gentle massage can reduce the spasm in the paraspinal soft tissues with reduction in pain and improved range of motion. This will be transient, however, and these local treatments should be continued if they reduce and improve patient function. To apply heat a towel immersed in warm water and squeezed dry can be applied around the neck.

Physical therapy

A physical therapist can instruct the patient in basic care of the neck, as well as exercise programs, cervical traction, and counseling. Activities, such as driving, working for long periods at a desk, painting ceilings and walls, are to be avoided. Also, lifting or overhead reach is to be avoided.

Intermittent cervical traction can be used generally with the neck in slight flexion. The traction force should be limited to 12 to 15 pounds and should be discontinued if it causes pain. If the patient finds significant improvement of the radicular symptoms, a home traction unit can be used on a daily basis.

Hospital care

In patients who do not respond to conservative measures as ambulatory patients, admission to the hospital can be considered to ensure rest. Neurologic consultation, electrodiagnostic and myelographic studies can be performed if symptoms demand. More frequent cervical traction can also be implemented with increasing duration. Hydrotherapy is also helpful as well as ultrasound and diathermy.

Surgical treatment

Surgical consideration, while rarely necessary, is generally reserved for patients with intractable pain, progressive neurologic deficit, cervical myelopathy, or radiculopathy. The choice of procedure and level of surgery are usually determined by clinical and radiographic findings, electromyogram, myelogram, and/or CT scan.

Myelopathy in cervical spondylosis is generally caused by posteriorly projecting osteophytes arising from the adjacent posterior borders of the vertebral bodies compressing the anterior cord. This may also be associated with posterior bulging of the degenerated disc, sometimes referred to as a "hard disc." Rarely does the chronically degenerated disc herniate. If the involvement is limited to one or two levels, anterior decompression may be carried out. Since considerable bone may have to be removed to gain access to the osteophyte, an anterior fusion might be necessary. Nerve root compression may occur in the foramina by osteophyte formation with or without associated disc pressure, and this condition is also usually managed by an anterior removal of the disc and osteophytes with or without fusion.

If the myelopathy results from involvement over two or more segments, decompressive laminectomy is advised with or without foraminotomy depending on the condition of the nerve roots and facets.

References

1. Ball, J.: Enthesopathy of rheumatoid and ankylosing spondylitis, Ann. Rheum. Dis. **30**:213-222, 1971.
2. Barré, J.A.: Le syndrome sympathique posterieur, Rev. Neurol. (Paris) **33**:248-249, 1926.
3. Bell, C.: The nervous system of the human body, London, 1830.
4. Berens, D.: Roentgen diagnosis of rheumatoid arthritis, Springfield, Ill., 1969, Charles C Thomas.
5. Bergmann, E.W.: Fractures of the ankylosed spine. J. Bone Joint Surg. **45B**:21-35, 1963.
6. Bland, J.H., et al.: Rheumatoid arthritis of the cervical spine, Arch. Intern. Med. **112**:892, 130-136, 1963.
7. Bohlman, H.: Acute fractures and dislocations of the cervical spine, J. Bone Joint Surg. **61A**:1119-1142, 1979.
8. Brain, L. and Wilkinson, M.: Cervical spondylosis and other disorders of the cervical spine, Philadelphia, 1967, W.B. Saunders Co.
9. Bryan, W.J., et al.: Methyl-methacrylate stabilization for enhancement of posterior cervical arthrodesis in rheumatoid arthritis, J. Bone Joint Surg. **64A**:1045-1050, 1982.
10. Conlon, P.W., Isdale, I.C., and Rose, B.S.: Rheumatoid arthritis of the cervical spine; an analysis of 33 cases, Ann. Rheum. Dis. **25**:120, 1966.
11. Cregan, J.C.F.: Internal fixation of the unstable rheumatoid cervical spine, Ann. Rheum. Dis. **25**:242-252, 1966.
12. Crellin, R.Q., Maccabe, J.J., and Hamilton F.B.D.: Severe subluxation of the cervical spine in rheumatoid arthritis. J. Bone Joint Surg. **52B**:224-251, 1970.
13. Davis, F.W., Jr., and Markley, H.E.: Rheumatoid arthritis with death from medullary compression, Ann. Intern. Med. **35**:451, 1951.
14. DePalma, A., and Rothman, R.: The intervertebral disc, Philadelphia, 1970, W.B. Saunders Co.
15. Ferlic, D.C., et al.: Surgical treatment of the symptomatic unstable cervical spine in rheumatoid arthritis, J. Bone Joint Surg. **57A**:349, 1975.
16. Fielding, J.W.: Cineradiography of the normal cervical spine, J. Bone Joint Surg. **39A**:1280-1301, 1957.
17. Friedenberg, Z., and Miller, W.: Degenerative disc disease of the cervical spine, J. Bone Joint Surg. **45A**:1171-1178, 1963.
18. Frykholm, R.: Cervical nerve root compression resulting from disc degeneration and root sleeve fibrosis, Acta Chir. Scand. Suppl. **160**:1-149, 1951.
19. Gowers, W.R.: Diseases of the nervous system, vol. 1, London 1892, Churchill, p. 260.
19. Gowers, W.R.: Diseases of the nervous system, vol. 1, London 1892, Churchill, p. 260.
20. Harris, L.S., and Adelson, L.: "Spinal injury" and sudden infant death: a second look, Am. J. Clin. Pathol. **52**:289-295, 1969.
21. Hauge, T.: Chronic rheumatoid polyarthritis and spondyloarthritis associated with neurological symptoms and signs occasionally simulating an intraspinal expansive process, Acta Chir. Scand. **120**:395-401, 1961.
22. Hollin, S.A., Gross, S.W., and Levin, P.: Fracture of the cervical spine in patients with rheumatoid spondylitis, Am. Surg. **31**:532-536, 1965.
23. Hudson, C.P.: Cervical osteotomy for severe flexion, J. Bone Joint Surg. **54B**:202, 1972.
24. Hughes, J.T.: Pathology of the spinal cord, London, 1966, Lloyd-Luke.
25. Hutchinson, E.C. and Yates, P.O.: The cervical portion of the vertebral artery: a clinico-pathological study, Brain **79**:319-331, 1956.
26. Isdale, I.C., Conlon, P.W.: Atlanto-axial subluxation: a six-year follow-up report, Ann. Rheum. Dis. **30**:387-389, 1971.
27. Jefferys, E.: Disorders of the cervical spine, London, 1980, Butterworths.
28. Key, C.A.: On paraplegia depending on disease of the ligaments of the spine, Guy's Hosp. Rep. **3**:17-34, 1838.
29. Martel, W.: The occipito-axial joint in rheumatoid arthritis and ankylosing spondylitis, Am. J. Roentgenol. Radium Ther. Nuclear Med. **86**:223, 1961.
30. Martel, W., and Abell, M.R.: Fatal atlanto-axial luxation in rheumatoid arthritis, Arthritis Rheum. **6**:224, 1963.
31. Mason, C., Cozen, L., and Addelstein, L.: Surgical correction of flexion deformity of the cervical spine, Calif. Med. **79**:244, 193.
32. Mathews, J.A.: Atlanto-axial subluxation in rheumatoid arthritis, Ann. Rheum. Dis. **28**:260-265, 1969.
33. McGregor, M.: The significance of certain measurements of the skull in the diagnosis of basilar impression, Br. J. Radiol. **21**:171, 1948.
34. Meijers, K.A.E., et al.: Dislocation of the cervical spine with cord compression in rheumatoid arthritis, J. Bone Joint Surg. **56B**:668-680, 1974.
35. Meikle, J.A.K., and Wilkinson, M. Rheumatoid involvement of the cervical spine: radiological assessment. Ann. Rheum. Dis. **30**(2):154-161, 1971.
36. O'Driscoll, S.L., Jayson, M.I.V., and Badley, H.: Neck movements in ankylosing spondylitis, Ann. Rheu. Dis. **37**:64-66, 1978.
37. Pallis, C.A., Jones, A.M., and Spillane, J.D.: Cervical spondylosis: incidence and complications, Brain. **77**:274-289, 1954.
38. Park, W.M.: Personal communication.
39. Rana, N.H., Hancock, D.O., and Hill, A.G.S.: Upward translocation of the dens in rheumatoid arthritis, J. Bone Joint Surg. **55B**:471-477, 1973.
40. Rana, N.A., et al.: Atlanto-axial subluxation in rheumatoid arthritis, J. Bone Joint Surg. **55B**:458-470, 1973.
41. Ranawat, C.S. et al.: Cervical spine fusion in rheumatoid arthritis, J. Bone Joint Surg. **61A**:1003-1010, 1979.
42. Ricard, A., and Masson, R.: Complications médullaires des discopathies cervicales (a propos de 24 cas operés), Rev. Neurol. **85**:420, 1951.
43. Robinson, R.A., and Smith, G.W.: The treatment of certain cervical-spine disorders by anterior removal of the intervertebral disc and interbody fusion, J. Bone Joint Surg. **40A**:607, 1958.
44. Rothman, R.H., and Simeone, F.A.: The spine. Philadelphia, 1975, W.B. Saunders Co.
45. Sharp, J., and Purser, D.W.: Spontaneous atlanto-axial dislocation in ankylosing spondylitis and rheumatoid arthritis, Ann Rheuma. Dis. **20**:47-77, 1961.
46. Short. C.L.: The antiquity of rheumatoid arthritis, Arthritis Rheum. **17**:193-195, 1974.
47. Simmons, E.H. Personal communication.
48. Simmons, E.H.: The surgical correction of flexion deformity of the cervical spine in ankylosing spondylitis, Clin. Orthop. Rel. Res. **86**:132-142, 1972.

49. Smith, P.H., Benn, R.T., and Sharp, J.: Natural history of rheumatoid cervical luxations, Ann. Rheum. Dis. **31:**431-439, 1972.

50. Stauffer, E.S.: Fractures and dislocations of the spine, Part 1, The cervical spine fractures. In Rockwood, C.A. Jr. and Green, D.P., editors. Philadelphia, 1975, J.B. Lippincott Co.

51. Steele, H.H.: Anatomical and mechanical considerations of the atlanto-axial articulation. In Proceedings of the American Orthopaedic Association, J. Bone Joint Surg. **50A:**1481-1482, 1968.

52. Storey, G.: Changes in the cervical spine in rheumatoid arthritis with compression of the cord, Ann. Phys. Med. **4:**216, 1958.

53. Taylor, A.R., and Blackwood, W.: Paraplegia in hyperextension cervical injuries, J. Bone Joint Surg. **30B:**245-248, 1948.

54. Todd, T.W., and Pyle, S.I.: A quantitative study of the vertebral column by direct and roentgenoscopic methods, Am. J. Phys. Anthrop. **12:**321-338, 1928.

55. Urist, M.R.: Osteotomy of the cervical spine: report of case of ankylosing rheumatoid spondylitis. J. Bone Joint Surg. **40A:**833, 1958.

56. Webb, F.W.S., Hickman, J.A., and Brew, D.S.J.: Death from vertebral artery thrombosis in rheumatoid arthritis. Br. Med. J. **2:**537-538, 1968.

57. Weissman, B.N.W., et al.: Prognostic features of atlanto-axial subluxation in rheumatoid arthritis patients, Radiology **144:**745-751, 1982.

58. Wilkinson, M.: Brain. **83:**589, 1960.

59. Wilkinson, M.: Cervical spondylosis, Oxford University, DM Thesis, 1959.

60. Woodruff, F.V., and Dewing, S.B.: Fracture of the cervical spine in patients with ankylosing spondylitis, Radiology **80:**17-21, 1963.

chapter 9
THE SHOULDER

Russell F. Warren

Shoulder pain in older patients is a frequent problem that confronts the community orthopaedist. Unfortunately, residency training in this anatomic area is often deficient so that many patients are managed as if they simply have bursitis, with little attempt having been made to arrive at a specific diagnosis. The diagnosis of bursitis in the shoulder is often used as a nonspecific term much as internal derangement was used in the past as a diagnosis for knee problems. In this chapter I will discuss the more common diagnoses that are seen in the shoulder clinic at The Hospital for Special Surgery in terms of their recognition and management.

Shoulder pain may be a result of intrinsic or extrinsic causes. Probably in no area is there greater confusion created by referred patterns of pain. In considering the source of shoulder pain, we have found that there is a tendency for certain problems to be age related. The impingement syndrome is the commonest diagnosis made in our clinic, and it may be seen in its various stages in all age groups. The common diagnoses are as follows:

15 to 35 years
  Impingement syndrome stage I
  Subluxation
  Dislocation
  Acromioclavicular (AC) joint trauma
  Strains
35 to 55 years
  Impingement syndrome stage II
  Adhesive capsulitis
  Calcific tendonitis
Over 55 years
  Impingement syndrome stages II and
    III

AC joint arthritis
Sternoclavicular (SC) joint arthritis
Osteoarthritis, rheumatoid arthritis
Adhesive capsulitis

INCIDENCE OF SHOULDER PAIN

As mentioned previously, the impingement syndrome stage II, progressing on to full-thickness rotator cuff tear, is the most frequent problem seen in our clinic. While calcific tendonitis and adhesive capsulitis are occasionally seen in older patients, they are more common in the 45 to 55 age group. Arthritis of the AC joint frequently occurs in older patients, and it may be a distinct component of the impingement syndrome. SC joint arthritis may initially occur as a lesion in older patients with marked prominence of the medial clavicle secondary to subluxation of the SC joint. Osteoarthritis of the glenohumeral joint, while infrequent, may occur as a primary diagnosis or it may be secondary to shoulder instability. Rheumatoid arthritis and avascular necrosis may involve the shoulder joint and must be considered in the differential diagnosis. Instability is infrequent in older patients, but there is a small group of patients in whom recurrent dislocations are a problem.

IMPINGEMENT SYNDROME

The impingement syndrome is a term used by Dr. Charles Neer,[9] which basically includes diagnoses previously called bursitis or supraspinatus syndromes. In the young the impingement syndrome may be seen as the result of overuse or acutely fol-

107

lowing an injury. More commonly, it is seen in older patients in whom degeneration of the supraspinatus tendon and associated soft tissue swelling, bursa inflammation, and acromial thickening have developed over time.

Neer described the impingement syndrome as consisting of three basic stages. Stage I, consisting of inflammation and edema of the rotator cuff, occurs in patients in the second to fourth decades. It is generally reversible and is not visible on x-ray films. Stage II represents a progressive process in the tissues of the rotator cuff, and it frequently develops in the fifth to sixth decades. It is characterized by progressive cuff degeneration with fibrosis and partial tears. Often it is helped by conservative treatment, but surgery is resorted to frequently. Stage III of the impingement syndrome represents end-stage destruction of the soft tissues with rupture of the rotator cuff. In turn, this may progress on to a final stage IV, or cuff arthropathy, in which following cuff destruction degeneration of the glenohumeral joint ensues (Fig. 9-1).

Pathophysiology of the impingement syndrome

Anatomy. The tissue passing through the subacromial space has to function repeatedly within a confined space defined by bony structures, which limits the expansion of these soft tissues. This space is defined superiorly by the acromion and the AC joint, inferiorly by the humeral head and greater tuberosity, and medially by the coracoid. The coracoacromial ligament completes the arch running from the inferior surface of the acromium to the coracoid. (Fig. 9-2). It is constructed in a Y-shaped configuration (Fig. 9-3). Its function is unclear, but it appears to play a role in preventing superior migration of the humeral head if the rotator cuff is grossly deficient.

Within the subacromial space lies the bursa, which may be grossly thickened in patients with impingement or degeneration of the rotator cuff. The insertion site of the supraspinatus tendon on the greater tuberosity should be noted. Note that its path lies directly beneath the AC joint.

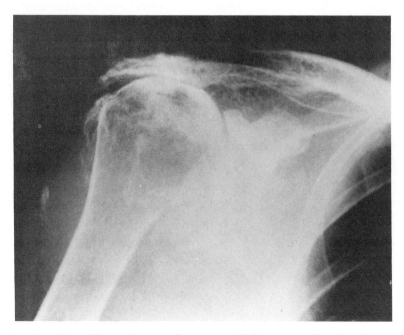

FIG. 9-1. X-ray film end stage of rotator cuff disease—cuff arthroplasty.

The impingement syndrome is characterized by progressive degeneration within the supraspinatus. This appears to be the result of several factors at work simultaneously: (1) The circulation to the rotator cuff is unidirectional with no flow traversing the tide mark on the insertion site of the supraspinatus. (2) The vessels within the supraspinatus are sensitive to postural changes of the arm. As McNab[10] has previously demonstrated, with the arm adducted to the side the vessels within the supra-

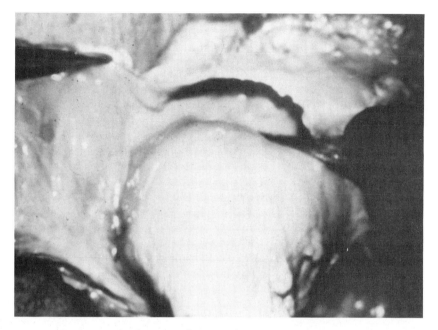

FIG. 9-2. Anatomy of subacromial space, demonstrating coracoacromial arch.

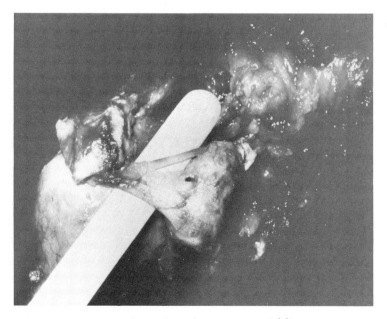

FIG. 9-3. Y configuration of coracoacromial ligament.

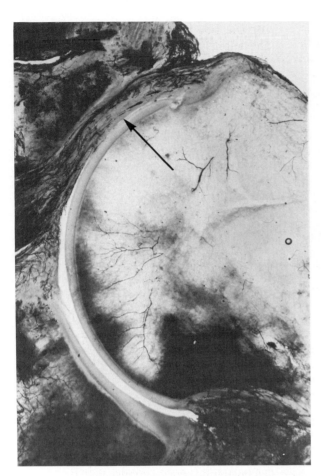

FIG. 9-4. Sagittal section of human shoulder illustrating vascular supply to rotator cuff (Spalteholz technique). Arrow indicates area of decreased vascular supply to rotator cuff. (Study by Steven Arnoczky and Russell F. Warren.)

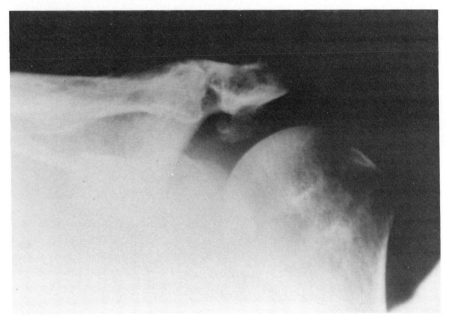

FIG. 9-5. X-ray film demonstrating spur formation from anterior aspect of acromiom.

spinatus are empty of dye, but with abduction the vessels fill (Fig. 9-4). However, it appears that with progressive abduction they are again compressed. (3) With normal arm elevation the pressure within the subacromial space will increase, possibly placing the circulation in jeopardy. (4) Any alterations in the bony architecture that narrow the subacromial space will affect the pressures within the soft tissues. Previously, Neer[9] had noted the development of an anteriorly directed osteophyte arising from the anterior third of the acromion. It is my impression that this osteophyte is generally a result of chronic traction or a sign of impingement rather than a cause of impingement per se (Fig. 9-5). It lies directly within the coracoacromial ligament, but at its origin it can result in thickening of the anterior portion of the acromion, further compromising the subacromial region. Obviously, any inferior spurring of the AC joint will have a similar effect.

Overall, it appears that with repeated use a process of inflammation and edema develops in the rotator cuff, which progresses to a point where the circulation to the cuff is altered. This results in a further decrease in the ability of the cuff tissue to handle the effects of repeated use. In time, the collagen fibers undergo degeneration that progresses to tearing of the rotator cuff. In fact, the onset of a tear is generally a slow, progressive process that goes on for some time before a sudden completion of the process. In many patients no specific event was ever associated with the development of a tear. In others, a sudden fall on an outstretched arm or, for example, in New York City a lurching subway while holding an overhead strap may complete the process. This is not to say that cuff tears may not occur acutely as in dislocations; however, the process is usually a progressive one.

With these alterations in the rotator cuff, the surrounding tissues, including bone, will gradually demonstrate their effects. The bursa becomes thickened with a markedly increased elastic component. With superior migration of the humeral head, the acromion reacts by losing its normal inferior convexity and becoming concave (Fig. 9-6). Pathologically, new bone formation is seen within the acromion (Fig. 9-7). The coracoacromial ligament becomes scarred, then sharing in the degenerative process.

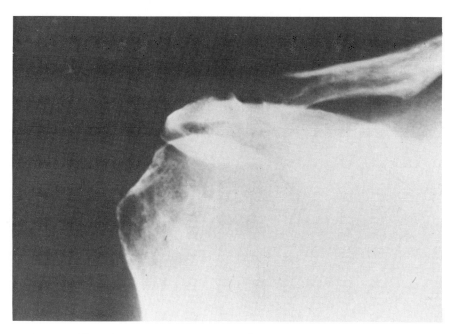

FIG. 9-6. X-ray film of acromion in patient with impingement process; acromion has become concave, as opposed to more normal convexity.

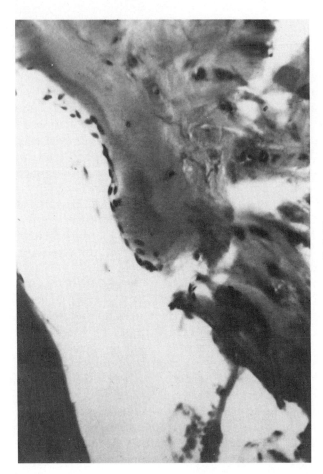

FIG. 9-7. Hematoxylin and eosin stain demonstrating new bone formation in acromion of patient with impingement syndrome.

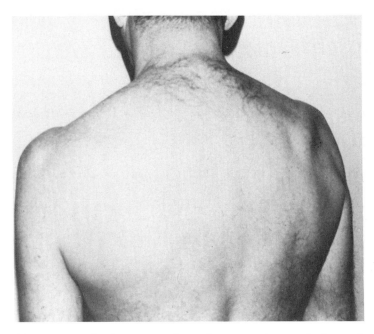

FIG. 9-8. Oblique view of infraspinatus fossa demonstrating marked atrophy of infraspinatus in patient with large rotator cuff tear.

The AC joint normally begins a degenerative process in the second decade, resulting in spurs at its inferior aspect. Thus, in treating the impingement syndrome, one should look at the condition as a continuum in which the patient may come to the physician at any given time with a variety of pathology present.

The success of treatment will depend on recognizing the level of disease present and tailoring the approach for the more advanced stages. Similarly, the patient has to share in developing this treatment approach since activities that he previously found were easy to engage in may have to be altered or carried out in moderation.

Recognition of impingement syndrome stages II and III

Patients are generally in the fifth to sixth decades, and come to the physician with pain and discomfort from overhead activities. Less commonly, an acute injury may have precipitated the problem. Patients will notice pain at night and will find that lying on the shoulder is painful. Generally, they will have pain directly at the humeral head or pain referred to the area of the deltoid tuberosity. Occasionally, referred patterns will be more distally positioned, although this seems to be more common in patients with complete cuff tears. Many patients will suggest that playing tennis or paddle ball started their problems, while others note that working overhead started their pain. Patients may also note clicking in the shoulder with elevation: In time weakness may become a significant complaint. In evaluating a patient one should ask questions that can be used to evaluate cervical or chest complaints since these can frequently complicate a diagnosis by causing pain that is referred to the C5-6 area. Conversely, shoulder problems rarely, if ever, cause chest pains; if pain is referred proximally from the shoulder, it is generally along the trapezius area and not to the spinous processes or interscapular area.

Clinical examination

In examining the shoulder region, one should first notice any atrophy of the shoulder muscles. Localized atrophy is more characteristic of cervical root dysfunction or of a full-thickness cuff tear than of impingement syndrome stage II (Fig. 9-8). A swelling over the humeral head may be noted in some patients with large cuff tears in which the bursa is filled with fluid directly from the glenohumeral joint.

Inspection should indicate the prominence of the AC or SC joint as possible sources of pain. Next, the patient should demonstrate his active motion while standing. Flexion is recorded as 0 to 180 degrees; abduction also is recorded from 0 to 180 degrees. Internal rotation at the side is measured to the highest spinous process that the thumb will reach, while external rotation is from 0 to 90 degrees. External rotation can be noted in the young at the 90 degree position as well, but often this cannot be evaluated in the elderly.

In evaluating active elevation if it is less than 180 degrees, one should determine if passive elevation is possible or if a contracture is present. As the arm is elevated, the shoulder is palpated for crepitation. As the elevated arm is lowered, any weakness or a drop as the shoulder passes through a painful arc region is noted. Generally this occurs at 80 to 100 degrees of abduction.

In addition, the examiner should note any weakness of shoulder elevation while viewing the patient from behind as he abducts the arm. Does he initially shrug the shoulder? This shrugging mechanism is typically seen in full-thickness cuff tears and is an attempt by the patient to position the glenoid under the humeral head to facilitate elevation of the arm. The movement can be subtle, but it is a sensitive indicator of rotator cuff dysfunction. The drop sign is frequently referred to as being present in cuff tears, but it may be absent even with large tears if they developed over a period of time. In noting the strength of the arm, one should particularly look for a weakness in external rotation, which is present in large cuff tears because the infraspinatus attachment site is torn off the tuberosity. A useful sign that Jobe[7] has observed is for the patient to hold the arm at 90 degrees of abduction in the plane of the

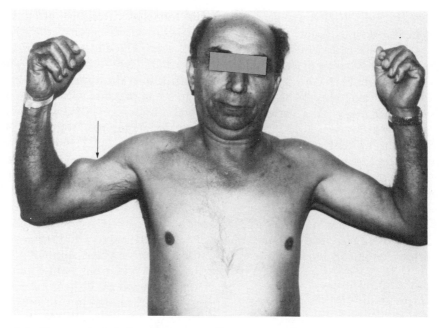

FIG. 9-9. Characteristic bulge of contracted biceps secondary to rupture of long head of biceps.

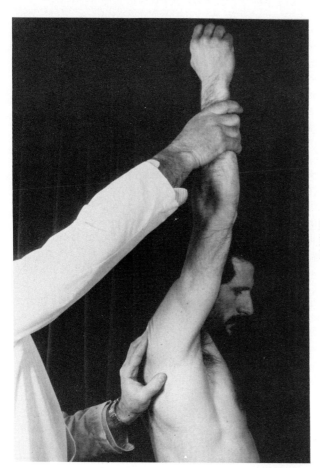

FIG. 9-10. Impingement sign performed by passive forward flexion of arm, producing pain as arm approaches full flexion.

scapula while the arm is internally rotated to check for resistance. Weakness of the supraspinatus, Jobe feels, is detected by this maneuver.[7] In palpating the shoulder region one should carefully note any tenderness at the AC joint, since this may be a component of the impingement process. Humeral head tenderness should be observed. Often tender areas on the cuff may be elicited by extending the arm to bring the supraspinatus out from under the acromion. Tenderness along the coracoid and biceps tendons occurs frequently. Similarly, one should note the biceps tendon while the biceps is contracted against resistance. A ruptured long head of the biceps is often associated with a full-thickness rotator cuff tear (Fig. 9-9).

The impingement sign, as described by Neer,[9] and the abduction test are helpful in making a diagnosis of the impingement syndrome. The impingement sign is elicited by passively elevating the arm in forward flexion to its maximum (Fig. 9-10). If the test is positive, pain is produced in the last 10 to 15 degrees of elevation. The abduction test is performed by elevating the arm to 90 degrees in the plane of the scapula

and internally rotating the arm so that the greater tuberosity passes under the coracoacromial arch; this again results in pain (Fig. 9-11). If shoulder motion is significantly restricted, these tests cannot be performed.

The impingement test basically consists of injecting the subacromial space with 10 ml of lidocaine (xylocaine) and repeating the impingement sign and abduction test to see if the pain is eliminated. This is a helpful test that should be positive with flexion at either 180 degrees or at 90 degrees of abduction if the diagnosis of impingement is to be made. The adduction test is useful for AC joint complaints. It involves forcing the arm across the chest, noting any pain at the AC joint (Fig. 9-12). At times, pain will preclude active or passive arm elevation, but following injection elevation can be performed, allowing one to rule out the diagnosis of frozen shoulder and to consider impingement as the etiology.

The impingement syndrome stage II may be associated with some mild losses of motion or occasionally by marked losses in which an adhesive capsulitis has developed. Conversely, full-thickness cuff tears

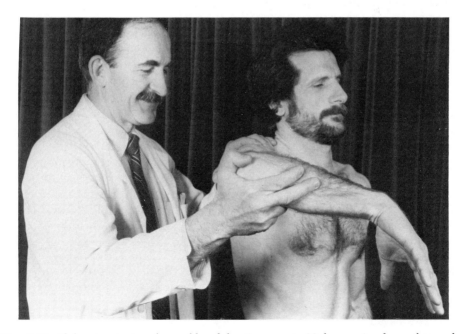

FIG. 9-11. Abduction test performed by abducting arm to 90 degrees in plane of scapula. Internal rotation will produce pain as tuberosity passes under coracoacromial arch.

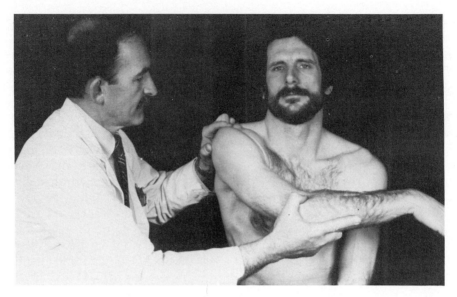

Fig. 9-12. Adduction test; positive result suggests disease involving the acromioclavicular joint.

will generally allow a full range of motion, but on occasion a patient will be seen who has a cuff tear along with a fixed limitation of motion.

When passively rotating the arm, one should palpate the subacromial space for crepitation since a thickened bursa is frequently present and this may result in crepitation. In addition, the edges of a torn cuff will thicken and produce a sudden jump in this region as the arm is rotated.

In completing the examination, the examiner should carefully assess the function of the cervical spine since pain from disc disease at the C5-6 level may mimic rotator cuff disease. In contrast, referred patterns of pain in cuff disease may mimic cervical disease by producing pain in the forearm and even in the hand, with vague parasthesias being noted. In the diagnostic workup lesions within the supraclavicular fossa or apex of the lung should be considered. As previously noted, chest lesions and occasionally diaphragmatic lesions may result in shoulder pain.

Radiology

In evaluating patients for the impingement syndrome, x-ray films will often show obvious signs of impingement. These gen-erally consist initially of sclerosis of the greater tuberosity and acromion followed by spurring of the anterior inferior surface of the acromion (Figs. 9-5 and 9-6). Often this is confused with calcific tendinitis unless the films are viewed closely under a hot light. In time, progressive changes develop as the rotator cuff fails and the humeral head migrates superiorly. McNab has noted that if the subacromial space is less than 1 cm wide, one should be suspicious of a rotator cuff tear; less than 5 mm is diagnostic. I would essentially agree with this, but one must be careful of the angle at which the x-ray film is taken. If it is not tangential to the acromion, the measurement is inaccurate. With increasing force on the acromion, the normally convex inferior acromial surface becomes increasingly sclerotic and in time concave (Fig. 9-6). The AC joint should be evaluated for inferior spurs and cystic changes of early degeneration.

Management of impingement syndrome stages II and III

In setting up a program of conservative treatment the physician has to direct therapy toward (1) decreasing the local inflammation, (2) relieving contractures, (3) increasing strength, (4) educating the patient about the problem and about altering the activities that may increase his complaints.

To diminish the inflammation acutely if the inflammation has been a short-term problem, I prefer to use oral anti-inflammatory agents such as indomethacin (Indocin), 25 mg four times a day for 2 weeks. During this time activities should be diminished. Patients are instructed to avoid sports during this period and to avoid overhead positions with the arm except during exercise periods. Icing down for 15 to 20 minutes after stretching or strengthening programs will help to decrease discomfort.

Stretching is started after a few days of anti-inflammatory medication. The goal here is to restore as comfortably as possible the shoulder motion because contractures will create abnormal force requirements in the rotator cuff and perpetuate inflammation. Stretching is performed three times a day for 15 minutes emphasizing full forward flexion, external rotation, and internal rotation. Stretching exercises are followed after 2 weeks by strengthening exercises. Basically these are aimed at improving the strength of the rotator cuff. Initially they are performed with a spring exerciser and the patient should work on rotation with the arms at the side. The deltoid muscle is worked in flexion, avoiding abduction because pain is more rapidly produced in that position. Flexion is initially limited to 90 degrees. The trapezius and rhomboid muscles are also strengthened. Over 4 weeks as improvement develops some activities may be resumed.

Patient education is important because patients may be performing activities that are specifically creating their problems. Thus in middle-aged tennis and paddle ball players an alteration of the serve may be required. By facing the service line and opening their stance, the patients will decrease some of the overhead motion. Their serves will be less powerful with more of an emphasis on spin and placement, but such changes often will allow the patients to resume participation in these sports.

The majority of patients can be managed with this approach. However, if there is no improvement or on occasion in severe acute situations, injections of lidocaine and anti-inflammatory agents into the subacromial space are required. Generally I will repeat this in older patients up to a maximum of three injections. Following injections patients' activities will be decreased for 3 to 4 weeks because the tendon is further weakened at this time. During this period the stretching and strengthening programs are gradually begun.

If the program fails to achieve success over a 6-month period, the patient may be a candidate for surgery. Surgery in this situation consists basically of an acromioplasty with excision of the coracoacromial ligament. AC joint resection is at times required.

Generally to be a candidate for surgery a patient should fulfill the following criteria: The patient should (1) have a condition that has been refractory to conservative treatment for 6 months; (2) have a positive impingement sign or abduction sign; (3) have mild limitations of motion; (4) have a positive impingement test with some improvement being noted following a subacromial injection.

In evaluating a patient at this stage the question of arthrography often arises. Frequently small and even large rotator cuff tears may be present and they may appear as an impingement syndrome stage II with little or no obvious weakness. Standard x-ray films may show superior migration of the humeral head or only sclerotic changes of the greater tuberosity and acromion. Arthrography is helpful in planning surgery and in discussing the postoperative program for the patient since it varies considerably if a large cuff tear is present and only mildly if a small tear is noted.

Surgery for impingement syndrome stage II

In performing surgery for this problem a variety of approaches have been recommended. The procedure that is critical to the success of surgery is a well-performed acromioplasty. Previously some authors had recommended that an acromionectomy be performed on these patients. While this may alleviate the patient's pain, in some cases it may lead to much larger problems for which there is little solution. If an acromionectomy is performed, the deltoid muscle may detach. In addition it may significantly weaken the deltoid by decreasing the moment arm for the deltoid. Therefore acromionectomies are to be avoided. In contrast, acromioplasty is directed toward the anterior third of the acromion where thickening and spurring are frequently seen. At the time of surgery, attention must be directed to all components of the subacromial space, and surgery should be performed for each pathologic site.

Incision. Generally I have utilized Neer's superior approach to the shoulder for treating impingement in either stage II or stage III full-thickness cuff tear) (Fig. 9-13, *A*). This approach allows excellent visualization with minimal damage to the deltoid.

In detaching the deltoid from the anterior acromion, the lateral acromion is left alone unless further dissection is necessary to repair the rotator cuff (Fig. 9-13, *B*). The deltoid is detached with a bovie, leaving a rim of soft tissue on the acromion. As the dissection is carried medially, one should beware of entering the AC joint unless a resection is planned. After release of the anterior deltoid, the deltoid fibers are split distally for approximately 1½ inches, since further dissection may damage the axillary nerve. Generally this is started at the AC joint and continues in the plane of the muscle fibers (Fig. 9-13, *B*). The bursa is then noted; it may be markedly thickened. Inferior traction on the arm will allow for visualization of the subacromial space. A periosteal elevator is used to dissect any soft tissue off the inferior acromial surface, the bursa is partially excised, and the cuff

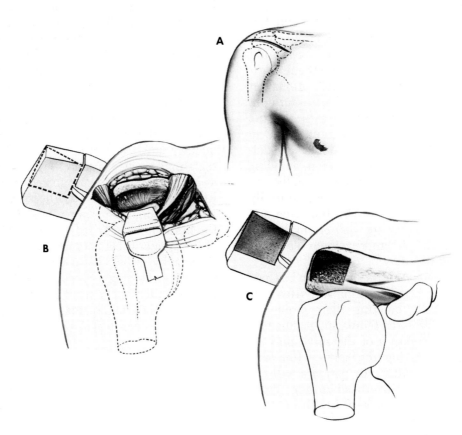

FIG. 9-13. Acromioplasty. **A,** Superior incision for acromioplasty or rotator cuff repair. **B,** Outline of bone to be removed from anterior half of acromion. **C,** In performing acromioplasty one attempts to avoid acromioclavicular joint. If there are spurs under the joint, these may be smoothed off with a burr.

is noted. An osteotome is used to perform the acromioplasty, inclining it at an oblique angle to miss the AC joint, unless the AC joint is to be excised and directed posteriorly in a slightly oblique manner to avoid injuring the AC joint (Fig. 9-13, *B* and *C*). The osteotome should initially be straight, then replaced by a curved one to enter the subacromial space at the midpoint of the acromion. The tendency is to take too little bone and to remove an inadequate portion of the acromion. It is important to remove enough laterally in patients where hypertrophic bone has developed along the lateral edge of the acromion. A curved rasp is used to smooth off the surface, or a power burr can be used to facilitate this aspect of the surgery. In performing an acromioplasty the surgeon has to be sure that the rotator cuff is not attached to the acromion as may be the case in large cuff tears. There is no exact measurement of how much bone to remove. Generally when surgery is completed one should be able to insert an index finger into the subacromial space easily when the arm is in an adducted position.

The inferior surface of the AC joint may be hypertrophic and thickened. If it is, then debridement of the inferior surface with a burr will smooth off this site. However, if the patient had preoperative pain at the AC joint, then excision of the outer 1.5 to 2 cm of the clavicle is indicated. In addition, if the acromioplasty has significantly violated the acromioclavicular joint, then resection may have to be performed.

Decompression of the AC joint is often critical for success but I do not think it should be performed routinely. Removing portions of the clavicle further weakens the attachment site of the deltoid; thus as little bone as possible should be excised. Generally I find that 2 cm is adequate although this will vary with the angle of the joint and the size of the calvicle.

AC joint resection is performed by dissecting anteriorly and posteriorly on the clavicle. An attempt is made to preserve the soft tissue attachment for deltoid reattachment. In removing the clavicle, care must be directed toward protecting the supraspinatus, which lies directly beneath the AC joint. After inserting retractors about the clavicle, a power saw is used to cut the clavicle so that it has a slight obliquity in the direction of the acromion. Generally, more bone is removed inferiorly and posteriorly from the clavicle. It is important to remove enough bone posteriorly because the edge of the acromion may come in contact with the clavicle here during adduction and elevation. To check for the adequacy of the resection, one inserts an index finger in the space created and abducts the arm to 90 degrees, then adducts the arm, making sure that there is no contact between the acromion and the clavicle.

When an acromioplasty has been performed, the rotator cuff will be well visualized. If an AC joint resection was added, visualization of the cuff will be even better. In fact, Bateman has suggested that this be used as a method of gaining exposure for large rotator cuff tears.

Next the position of the coracoid is evaluated. Rarely there are patients in whom the coracoid comes into intimate contact with the lesser tuberosity during internal rotation. If this is present, then removing the tip of the coracoid and reattaching the conjoined tendon is indicated.[12]

Once the rotator cuff and bursa have been exposed, further excision of the bursa is indicated if it is grossly thickened. It will repair over time. In evaluating the cuff, surgeons are frequently initially fooled by the thickened bursa, which can lie over a rotator cuff tear. Surgeons may assume that the tissue is tendinous and try to use it in a cuff repair. In impingement syndrome stage II the cuff is intact but often degenerating. If a cuff tear is suspected but none is noted, then injecting the joint with saline and looking for a leak will be helpful. Generally, in this situation I do not operate on the rotator cuff unless a full-thickness tear is seen. If an arthrogram has demonstrated a partial-thickness tear underneath the cuff, then incising the cuff at the suspected site may be beneficial followed by repair of the defect. Prominence of the greater tuberosity may be secondary to hypertrophy or an old fracture of the greater tuberosity. In this situation resecting a portion of the

tuberosity will further decompress the subacromial space.

The coracoacromial ligament frequently
becomes thickened and undergoes degeneration during this process. In patients in
whom an aromioplasty has been performed,
resecting more ligament is not required
since the acromial attachment has already
been removed.

Biceps pathology has frequently been reported as a common cause of shoulder complaints. It has been my experience that this
is rarely an isolated situation since it is generally a component of the impingement
syndrome.[4] As such, decompression of the
space is sufficient to decrease the pressure
and subsequent inflammation of both the
cuff and the biceps. If concern has been
raised regarding the biceps, then the biceps
is carefully exposed and if it is markedly
inflamed, it is then tenodesed in its groove.
This has infrequently been required.

Rotator Cuff Tears (Impingement Stage III)

Rotator cuff tears in older patients are a
common problem and is frequently poorly
managed. Conservative therapy will help
some patients, but age alone is certainly not
a contraindication to surgery. The patients'
complaints and findings will vary considerably, depending on the rate of progression
of the tear and the ability of the patient to
compensate for a torn cuff. In patients over
the age of 50, rotator cuff tears are generally
the end stage of an impingement syndrome
with resultant cuff degeneration. The tear
then generally occurs as a result of a sudden
overload on the tendon. Although dislocations are less common in patients over the
age of 50, when they do occur there is a
high incidence of cuff tear. Therefore, if a
patient's pain does not clear up quickly after reduction, an arthrogram should be performed during the second week after the
injury.

Often a patient will have a recent injury
of the shoulder superimposed on a history
of recurrent shoulder pain; the patient may
have had previous injections for "bursitis."
Generally these patients are in their late
fifties or sixties. If they are in good health
and physically active, I feel that early surgery should be considered as opposed to a
wait- and-see approach. This is particularly
true if they have had impingement-type
symptoms for some time. It appears that
rotator cuff surgery performed before 3
weeks after a tear has significantly better
results than surgery performed at later
dates.[2] It is true that some patients placed
on an extensive exercise program will significantly improve their condition in terms
of both strength and pain. Generally,
though, when examined these patients are
found to have distinct ranges that are weak
and they have some persistent although
mild complaints. The problem with waiting is that when the cuff tear extends further, repair becomes particularly difficult
and this accounts for many of the poorer
results from surgery. Tears that are operated on early allow easier tissue apposition
with more predictable results in terms of
pain and strength improvements. In addition, it appears that acromioplasty performed at the time of repair may aid in preventing further cuff degeneration.

In selecting patients for surgery, there is
one extreme where there has been a massive cuff tear with loss of tissue and the
humeral head rides superiorly and comes
into contact with the acromion. Examination will demonstrate marked weakness on
attempted elevation; in particular there is
loss of external rotation power. These patients' pain may improve following surgery
but functional improvements will be unpredictable. In evaluating a patient it is important to assess the function of the infraspinatus since marked weakness indicates
an extensive cuff tear with detachment of
the infraspinatus. If joint degeneration has
developed, then one is dealing with a cuff
arthropathy and a total shoulder replacement will have to be considered (Fig. 9-1).

In addition, patients need to be made
aware of the extensive rehabilitation program that is necessary after cuff surgery. If
they are unable to comply with this program, then cuff repair is probably not warranted. At times in elderly patients with
extensive tears and impingement pain, at-

tention can be directed to the impingement by using acromioplasty as the main component of surgery. These patients may experience significant pain relief although strength will not improve.

Arthrography

Patients in the fifth through seventh decades with persistent pain that is either undiagnosed or from suspected cuff tears should have an arthrogram to confirm the presence of a tear and to provide more information on the size of the tear. Double-contrast arthrography is the preferred method and this may be combined with tomography to further clarify the degree of soft-tissue destruction. In evaluating cuff tears rotation views plus axillary and postexercise films are important. In addition, it is often helpful to observe the dye injection under fluoroscopy to note small leaks. In making a diagnosis of cuff tears extravasation of dye from poor needle placement and dye within the biceps tendon sheath must be considered to avoid a false positive diagnosis.

Anteroposterior views will generally show dye penetration through the cuff into the bursa (Fig. 9-14). This bursa dye is best seen in the internal rotation view because the biceps tendon sheath moves medially, eliminating it as a source of confusion. Similarly an axillary view will demonstrate dye crossing the neck of the humerus, indicating dye in the subdeltoid bursa. Exercise will pump dye from the joint into the bursa and aid in making the diagnosis. It should be noted, though, that arthrography can miss tears of the cuff if the bursa is markedly thickened producing a flap over the defect. This has occurred in surprisingly large tears. Tomography, as noted by Matsen,[8] when combined with double-contrast arthrography often provides an excellent impression of the remaining rotator cuff. At times standard films will give similar pictures. By using these radiologic techniques the surgical approach and postoperative program can be planned more intelligently.

Partial tears of the cuff may be seen in which the dye extends into a defect from below. Generally these patients have come to the physician with impingement syndrome stage II.

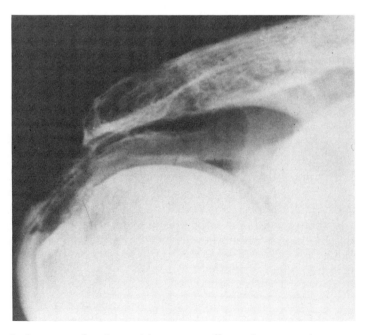

FIG. 9-14. Arthrogram of patient with rotator cuff tear demonstrating extravasation of dye into subdeltoid bursa. Rotator cuff is outlined by dye.

Rotator cuff surgery

Essentially rotator cuff surgery is approached similarly to surgery for impingement problems and cuff repair is simply a component of the surgery. Acromioplasty is routinely performed in the older population. AC joint resection is reserved for those with clinically symptomatic degeneration. If there is significant inferior spurring of the AC joint, then a high-powered burr can be used to smooth off the inferior surface. In addition, it should be realized that in large cuff tears resection of the AC joint will allow better visualization of the supraspinatus and facilitate repair.

Rotator cuff tears generally start at the supraspinatus and extend posteriorly to involve the infraspinatus. As the tear increases in size, the head migrates superiorly with increased stress on the infraspinatus. Rarely, the subscapularis will start to tear and detach from the lesser tuberosity. The biceps tendon will start to subluxate or dislocate medially as the subscapularis detaches. In repairing rotator cuff tears, it is impressive how often a tear that a resident will think is impossible to close initially will, with effort and patience, become one that can be closed. In general, tears that are less than 1 cm in length or width are repaired by simply advancing the edges to close the defect. Generally there is no tendon remaining on the greater tuberosity. Repair is best carried out by approximating the tendon to bone just lateral to the articular surface. In Fig. 9-15 sutures are placed and the cuff is pulled laterally. If any time has passed since the tear, the cuff may have retracted to some degree. Dissection in cuff tears is carried out medially along the subscapularis, posteriorly along the infraspinatus, and superiorly along the supraspinatus tendon. It is extremely important to dissect and free the rotator cuff from all adhesions superficially and within the joint. In small to moderate tears dissection outside the cuff is sufficient, but in large tears dissection along the glenoid rim may be required, including freeing the capsule from the labrum to gain length (Fig. 9-16). Having freed the cuff, its length is then noted, and the site for attachment is judged

with the arm at the side. It is important that the arm not be required to abduct to perform the repair or, as the arm is adducted to the side, even after healing there will be a significant potential for the cuff to avulse from the humeral head. Thus the arm is adducted and the site for cuff attachment is noted in both large and small tears. The surface of the humeral head is freshened with an osteotome to create a wide bleeding surface for the tendon to repair to rather than relying on the edge of the tendon to repair to the bone (Figs. 9-17 and 9-18).

The lateral cortex of the humeral head is preserved to prevent the sutures from pulling out of the bone (Fig. 9-17, C). In advancing the cuff to close the defect, a bulge may occur in the tendon as the circular defect is closed to form a straight surface; thus a Z-plasty may be required to close the defect (Fig. 9-15, C and D).

A common question is how much cuff should be excised to encourage healing of the defect. Generally the tendons at the site of the repair have poor circulation for a large distance so that only a trimming of the edges of the defect is performed.

Drill holes are placed in the humeral head, preserving a good island of cortical bone to prevent the sutures from pulling out (Fig. 9-17, C). Generally nonabsorbable sutures are used, but as longer lasting absorbable sutures become available these would appear to have some advantages.

In performing the tendon reattachment it is important to restore the proper length-tension relationship for the tendon to function well. In some cases this is obviously impossible and probably contributes to surgical failures because the tendons have been overstretched and thus will not function well or because conversely the tendon is understressed, resulting in a lax tendon.

Thus, in advancing the infraspinatus superiorly and laterally in a large tear the arm position is important since a reattachment with full internal rotation will result in little power of external rotation after a neutral position has been reached. Generally I will select a neutral position of rotation for reattachment of either the infraspinatus or sub-

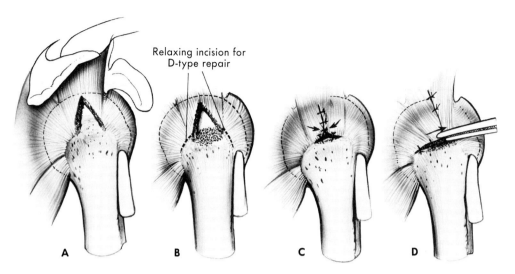

FIG. 9-15. A, Relatively small (less than 2 cm in long axis) tear, which often will form a V shape as the supraspinatus retracts. **B,** Preparation of bony bed to receive tendon. This area is roughened to bleeding bone and is made as broad as possible to promote tendon reattachment. **C,** V tear may be converted to partial Y and advanced laterally with or without relaxing incision. **D,** If V tear is long and difficult to close, one edge may be advanced to fill defect hinging on apex of tear. This will require a relaxing incision.

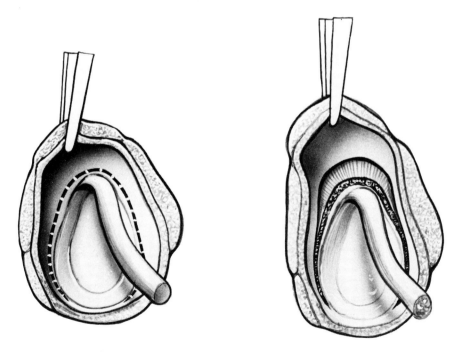

FIG. 9-16. Relaxing incision of capsular attachment to labrum may be necessary if rotator cuff tear has become fixed in a retracted position. Release combined with lysis of superficial adhesions will allow even longstanding tears to be advanced.

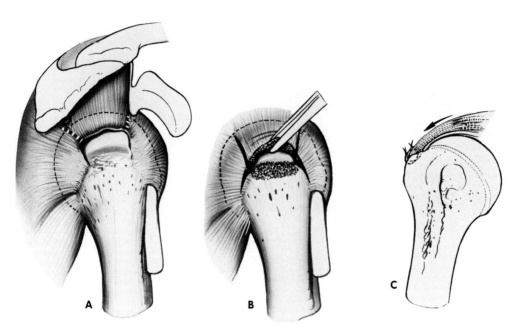

FIG. 9-17. **A,** Moderate-sized tear (2 to 5 cm in long axis). This tear may be difficult to close and require extensive dissection on both sides of rotator cuff. **B,** Relaxing incisions parallel to fibers of cuff to coracoid and spine of scapula may be required to advance retracted segment. This is combined with capsular release. **C,** Tendon is advanced to bone bed and attached with nonabsorbable sutures placed through cortex.

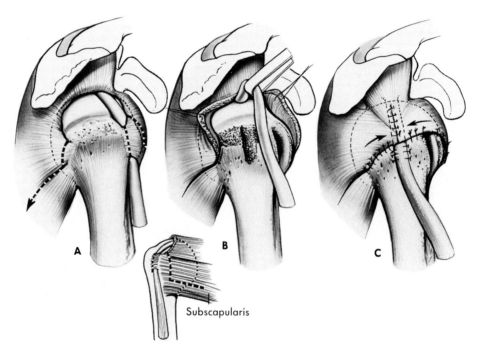

FIG. 9-18. **A,** Large (longer than 5cm in long axis) rotator cuff tear. To close this defect, cuff must be released posteriorly, freeing infraspinatus from teres minor. Anteriorly subscapularis is incised at junction of the lower third. **B,** Repositioning of biceps tendon into more posteriorly positioned groove to aid closure of defect. **C,** Superior advancement of infraspinatus and subscapularis to biceps tendon. This leaves a defect anteriorly and posteriorly.

scapularis. (After completion of the repair, the arm is placed through its range of motion to check the adequacy of the repair.) If the attachment is too tight, then a different attachment should be selected so that the tendon will not pull out with the arm adducted or rotated.

It should be noted that before repair in some patients with cuff tears, a degree of adhesive capsulitis may have developed. While it has been said that a frozen shoulder excludes the diagnosis of a cuff tear, this is not always true. In performing a repair in these patients the shoulder should be manipulated before the repair to restore motion. If this is not done, restoration of motion may be extremely difficult following surgery.

After completing the repair, the deltoid is reattached, with attention paid toward pulling the deltoid to the acromion edge and superior surface rather than under the acromion. A good firm reattachment is critical and sutures through bone are often required.

Postoperatively patients with smaller tears are managed with their arm in a sling, but if a moderate or large tear was noted with significant cuff retraction then a splint is used. The splint has several advantages in that it is generally preferable for tendon healing to take place in a relaxed position and, as McNab[10] has demonstrated, the circulation through the tendon is better with some abduction of the arm. Finally it is my impression that those patients able to tolerate a splint generally improve their motion more rapidly because passive motion may be initiated from the brace during the early phase of healing.

Large cuff tears

In dealing with rotator cuff tears certain patterns are observed but there is wide variation from patient to patient. Large tears, heralded by the "bald head sign" as the subacromial space is opened and measuring more than 5 cm in the long axis, are challenging to the surgeon. In approaching these tears an organized approach is necessary including (1) complete decompression of the subacromial space and, if nec-

essary, AC joint ressection; (2) release of all adhesions from the rotator cuff to the bursa, deltoid, coracoid, and acromion; (3) release of the attached capsule from the glenoid margin within the joint (Fig. 9-16); (4) insertion of traction sutures in the remaining cuff with dissection along the infraspinatus, supraspinatus, and subscapularis from within the joint avoiding the suprascapular nerve. Having freed the cuff an assessment of cuff deficiency is made. Several options then exist in closing the defect: (1) Leaving the defect open is advocated by Rockwood[11] in elderly debilitated patients, the concept being that the pain will diminish as a result of the acromioplasty but function will not change. This is an option to use at times in selected patients. (2) The biceps tendon can be used to fill the defect (Fig. 9-18, B). Often the biceps will thicken as the cuff tear increases in size. It appears that the biceps is active in stabilizing the humeral head by acting as a depressor. Therefore I try to avoid disturbing the biceps, but at times this tendon is useful for filling the defect, thus facilitating repair. This is accomplished by removing the biceps from the groove and placing it in a new groove at the center of the defect; it is then tenodesed in the new groove (Fig. 9-18, B). The remaining cuff can then be approximated to this tendon. In essence one is attempting to pull the cuff back up over the head to allow the cuff to exert its depressor actions. This technique works best in long, wide splits of the cuff in which marked retraction is preventing opposition. (3) Fascial grafting can be attempted using the fascia lata. This tissue has a tendency to stretch with time and is generally avoided, but Bateman has advocated its use as a suture to aid in filling the defect. (4) Freeze-dried allografts have been advocated by Neviaser with some success noted; however, I have had no experience with these. Some have advocated the use of bovine allografts to fill large defects, but the material presently available appears insufficient for filling the defect. (5) Advancement of the supraspinatus as advocated by Debeyre et al.[3] requires complete elevation of the muscle-tendon unit, but the advancement is limited by the neurovascular bundle; thus I will release the muscle to the superior edge of the glenoid but have not advocated a complete release for fear of compromising its functions. (6) In general, the preferred method is to transfer portions of the cuff to provide superior coverage. This may be accomplished posteriorly with the infraspinatus and anteriorly with the subscapularis. (Fig. 9-18).

If the subscapularis is advanced superiorly, its lower third is left attached (Fig. 9-18, B). Loss of this internal rotator is permissible since three rotators remain. The inferior aspect is left behind to prevent anterior inferior instability. It is migrated proximally and posteriorly. Posteriorly, the infraspinatus is dissected both inside and outside of the joint, detaching it from the teres minor and leaving the capsule in place if possible. It is then detached from the head and advanced superiorly to meet the edge of the supraspinatus and subscapularis (Fig. 9-18 C). This approach often is combined with biceps transfer and has been particularly successful at closing large defects. Often only a partial transfer might be sufficient, but even a completely bald head can generally be closed by this method.

Postoperative programs

In impingement syndrome stage I, if only the coracoacromial ligament was excised, then motion may be started promptly, especially when the muscle was left attached to the acromion. Generally this is the situation only in young patients in their second and third decades.

In patients over the age of 50 impingement is generally in stage II, and I have found that acromioplasty possibly combined with an AC joint resection is required. In these patients passive motion is started on the fourth day after surgery and progresses to active-assisted motion by day seven. The attachment site of the deltoid is the only tissue at risk and if it has been well attached motion is actively pursued. Generally at 8 weeks a strengthening program for the deltoid is instituted using flexion and initially avoiding abduction because that will generate higher pressures in

the subacromial space. In time, as full elevation is achieved, active abduction with weights is used but only to about 60 degrees of abduction.

Rotation exercises are started with a spring exerciser at 4 weeks since these tissues are not at risk. By 8 weeks, strengthening exercises in rotation are added at an elevated position.

Recovery following an acromioplasty with or without an AC resection is slow and will take a minimum of 4 to 6 months. Therefore, patients need to be well prepared preoperatively for the effort required on their part during the rehabilitation phase.

Following cuff repair the progression of therapy will vary with the anatomy of the tear, the quality of the tissues, and the success of the repair. Under anesthesia the arm should be placed through a range of motion to determine the stress on the repair. Thus, in a small tear a full arc of motion may be possible initially and the therapist can strive for this over the first 2 to 3 weeks. In others there may be confidence in the repair only for rotation to a 0-degree position and elevation to 90 degrees for the first 6 weeks. I feel it is important to start a passive exercise program with these patients as soon as possible after the initial swelling has started to decrease. Thus, for a patient with a large tear in which a brace has been utilized the arm will be passively moved three times a day in a previously determined plane of motion starting on the fourth or fifth day postoperatively. Generally the brace will be removed at 6 weeks and the arm will gradually be weaned from the sling. During the ensuing 6 weeks further motion is restored. It would not be until 3 to 4 months after surgery that strengthening programs would be started in those patients with these large global tears. Therapy in these individuals is continued for 6 to 9 months, with many patients requiring a year to optimize their result. In between these extremes are the tears of a moderate size of from 2 to 5 cm in which the tissues are available and approximated with some difficulty. There will still be variations, depending on the surgeon's confidence in the repair, as to the progression of the therapy.

BICEPS TENDINITIS, SUBLUXATION, AND RUPTURE

Lesions of the biceps have frequently been referred to as a source of shoulder pain. While on occasion it appears that a biceps problem is the main factor causing the pain, generally it is a component of the impingement syndrome. There are thus many patients in whom biceps tendinitis is simply an aspect of the impingement problem. Similarly, biceps rupture is commonly associated with rotator cuff tears, and if attention is solely directed toward managing the biceps rupture, the rotator cuff tear will be neglected and frequently it becomes the patient's main complaint.

In an attempt to evaluate the success of procedures for the biceps we have previously reviewed a small group of patients who underwent biceps tenodesis for tendinitis and subluxation. Overall the failure rate was approximately 35% with a high rate of failure being found in younger patients and in those in whom the coracoacromial ligament was not incised. Those who did well were older and had excision of the coracoacromial ligament, a procedure that partially treated a probable impingement problem. At review we found that the failures usually resulted from impingement problems, or in young patients they were the result of subluxations of the shoulder that had been misdiagnosed.[4]

Subluxation of the biceps tendon was a popular diagnosis during the 1960s and 1970s. Our review demonstrated that the diagnosis was often inaccurate preoperatively with no unusual movement being seen at surgery. However, biceps subluxation or dislocations can on occasion occur with a rotator cuff tear or rarely in a violent external rotation injury to the arm. More commonly, subluxation occurs in older patients who have a large tear that involves the subscapularis in addition to the supraspinatus, thus allowing the biceps tendon to slip medially. Biceps dislocation has also

occurred acutely, such as in a 30-year-old man who was involved in a wrestling match in which there was a violent external rotation of the arm. This resulted in a tearing of the attachment site of the subscapularis and medial migration of the biceps tendon, which then became fixed in a new groove. Arthrography using a bicipital groove view was helpful in demonstrating the displaced tendon. At the time of repair the biceps tendon was found to be fixed in a new position medial to the bicipital groove.

Ruptures of the long head of the biceps tendon occur frequently in patients in their sixties and seventies. In contrast to distal biceps lesions, such a rupture may occur slowly and progressively, with the patient not even being aware that it has occurred. Generally the patient will have first been diagnosed as having an impingement problem, and an incidental rupture of the long head with a prominent bulge of the biceps will be noted. Such a situation is treated as an impingement problem and the ruptured tendon generally is ignored (Fig. 9-9).

Ruptures of the long head of the biceps can be seen acutely, as noted previously, and they present a problem in management. Ruptures may be a result of pathology within the groove, such as an osteophyte or old tuberosity fracture, but more commonly they result from degeneration of the tendon; thus they are frequently associated with rotator cuff inflammation or rupture. If a heavy load is placed on the biceps, an acute rupture may occur. If such patients are in their sixties or seventies, then observation is generally the treatment of choice. Frequently a patient will have had shoulder complaints for some period before the rupture. The patient should be examined for a rotator cuff tear as well as for elbow function. I have found, as have other researchers, that the patient will gradually recover excellent elbow function but that shoulder complaints may develop or increase over time.[13] When elbow flexion was evaluated using a Cybex isokinetic device, minimal strength deficits were found in patients 1 to 2 years after rupture of the long head of the biceps. Patients should be told though that this rupture is part of a degenerative process involving the shoulder and that a cuff tear may be present or may develop over time.

In the occasional patient in his forties who is active in overhead sports and who has an acute biceps rupture, an arthrogram should be performed. If a cuff tear is present, then I feel that early reattachment of the long head tendon with acromioplasty and cuff repair should be performed rather than waiting for the patient to develop increasing complaints over time. If the surgeon waits, the cuff repair will be harder to perform and reattachment of the long head of the biceps at its proper length will no longer be possible. In addition, there are occasional patients who develop chronic pain in the biceps bulge that is refractory to any specific treatment presently available. Thus, while surgery may represent overtreatment in older patients, I feel that in those who are younger and who are using the arm vigorously for overhead activity that surgery is indicated.

There is a small group of patients who will have primarily biceps tendonitis, but as stated before an impingement syndrome is generally the underlying cause. These patients will have pain along the bicipital groove with local tenderness. Speed's test of resisted flexion of the arm may be positive, but Yergason's sign is often unreliable. The examination for impingement should be carefully performed.

If it is felt that the inflammation is primarily along the biceps, then oral anti-inflammatory agents or in some severe cases local injections of steroids will often provide dramatic relief. Generally I limit the patient to three such injections. Following the injection, the patient's activities should be curtailed for 3 to 4 weeks since otherwise rupture of the long head could occur.

In those patients whose conditions are refractory to treatment or who only gain temporary relief, tenodesis often combined with an acromioplasty or at least excision of the corocoacromial ligament may be helpful.

Surgery

Biceps tenodesis may be performed by simply roughening the bicipital groove and suturing the tendon in place. If the proximal tendon is free within the joint, then it is excised and the distal tendon is tenodesed in the groove. The easiest way to do this is to roll the tendon into a ball. Following this, a keyhole is created in the bicipital groove with a narrow slot distally (Fig. 9-19). After placing satisfactory tension on the tendon, the tendon is placed into the groove. The ball at the end of the tendon will stabilize it in the groove and allow early elbow motion.[5] Postoperatively the shoulder motion will be dependent on the rotator cuff and not on the biceps. A sling will support the elbow for 2 weeks but full elbow motion is allowed daily. Any weights in the hand should be avoided for 6 weeks.

Tenodesis to the coracoid has been suggested in the past but probably should be avoided since theoretically with muscle contraction it would force the humeral head proximally and increase impingement symptoms.

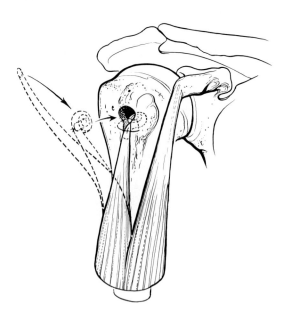

Fig. 9-19. Keyhole tenodesis of long head of biceps. Rolling detached biceps tendon into ball and inserting into distal aspect of keyhole will fix tendon in place, allowing early elbow motion. (From Froimson, A.I., and Oh, I.: Keyhole tenodesis of biceps origin at the shoulder, Clin. Orthop. **112:**245-249, 1974.)

TOTAL SHOULDER REPLACEMENT
Glenohumeral joint disease

Pathology of the glenohumeral joint advancing to a degree necessitating replacement is relatively uncommon compared to the knee and hip. Destruction following trauma is frequent but that is not within the scope of this chapter.

A variety of conditions may affect the glenohumeral joint including rheumatoid arthritis, osteoarthritis, and avascular necrosis. Rheumatoid arthritis will frequently involve the shoulders and progress to a severe destructive process including not only the glenohumeral joint but also the acromioclavicular joint and the rotator cuff. Often other joints are involved and the shoulders are left alone until little can be offered because of gross soft tissue destruction as well as marked bone loss at the glenoid. Overall it would appear better to be more aggressive in treating shoulder degeneration in rheumatoid arthritis once it has become significant rather than waiting for end-stage arthritis. In managing patients with rheumatoid arthritis of the shoulder, a patient's general status as well as the shoulder lesion are noted. Generally there is marked proliferation of the synovium followed by destruction of the articular cartilage, capsule, and rotator cuff as well as the AC joint. In the past synovectomy and subsequently synovectomy with hemiarthroplasty were attempted to improve the condition of these patients.

Previous reviews found these procedures to be only moderately successful.[9a] Over the past 10 years total shoulder replacement has evolved to a point where it is helpful in most of these patients with severe disease.

In selecting patients for total shoulder replacement, regardless of the etiology, one must assess certain aspects initially. Basically shoulder replacement is used in patients with severe pain secondary to rheumatoid arthritis, osteoarthritis, necrosis, or an old trauma.

Total shoulder replacement consists of three basic designs with increasing degrees of contraint: (1) nonconstrained—Neer, DANA, Bectal; (2) semiconstrained—Fenlin, Neer with superior coverage; (3) fully constrained—POST, Beuchel, Cristina. With increasing degrees of constraint the requirement for a functioning rotator cuff diminishes, but the chances of loosening and prosthesis failure increase. It appears that for the majority of patients a nonconstrained prosthesis, such as the Neer II, is sufficient (Fig. 9-20). In patients with a deficient cuff some degree of increasing constraint established by partially covering the humeral head may be helpful. Finally, in patients with a nonfunctional cuff but good bone stock, a fixed fulcrum device may be considered if the risks of loosening are understood.

A careful examination to establish rotator cuff function followed by arthrography when indicated will provide information regarding the quality and function of the cuff. Overall we have found a 25% in-

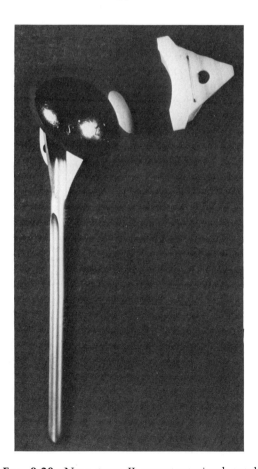

FIG. 9-20. Neer type II nonconstrained total shoulder replacement.

cidence of rotator cuff tears in our rheumatoid arthritis patients having a total shoulder replacement.[8a] In addition, a functioning deltoid is imperative regardless of the degree of constraint. In patients with cervical disease, particularly involving C5-6, this is an important consideration. Electromyograms will help differentiate these patients, particularly where there has been previous trauma.

Bone stock assessment is critical. Generally there is a sufficient humeral head but glenoid deficiency is common in rheumatoid arthritis patients. Protrusio of the glenoid is common and necessitated trimming of the glenoid stem in 20% of our initial rheumatoid arthritis patients. An x-ray evaluation is critical since views taken at 90 degrees to the scapula and axillary views are required to evaluate properly the depth of the glenoid. In measuring from the joint space to the base of the coracoid, a depth of 2 cm is normally present. If protrusio is present then trimming of the stem, a bone graft, or a custom glenoid may be required. In some patients it may be impossible to insert a glenoid and only a hemiarthroplasty is inserted.

In selecting rheumatoid arthritis patients for surgery, consideration of their weight-bearing status as well as elbow and shoulder function are important. There are patients with severely involved hips and knees who following total knee and hip replacement still need crutches. Total shoulder replacement with a Neer design has allowed crutch walking, but using a more constrained prosthesis would be hazardous at best. Patients with severely disabled elbows may benefit from total elbow replacement before the total shoulder replacement since a severely painful elbow will interfere with the exercise program following replacement of the shoulder more than the converse.

In osteoarthritis the bone stock is generally excellent as is the condition of the rotator cuff. In patients with cuff arthropathy (Fig. 9-1) in which there was initially a cuff tear that has become massive, with resulting migration of the humeral head to the acromion and subsequent destruction of the articular surface, there is massive loss of soft tissue as well as joint destruction.

Osteoarthritis may be secondary to old fractures and this is a particularly difficult group of patients to work with because the soft tissue that envelopes the humeral head has frequently been destroyed or is difficult to reestablish. However, in patients with degeneration secondary to shoulder instability the results of total shoulder replacement are uniformly excellent since the soft tissues are present and of good quality. Degenerative arthritis may be secondary to a previous infection and this should be considered in the differential diagnosis. Depending on the time since infection and the patient's present status, joint replacement may be considered but often fusion is a better choice.

Avascular necrosis has been seen in approximately 50 patients to date and it is generally secondary to the steroids used for a variety of diseases, most commonly lupus erythematosus as well as rheumatoid disease. The patient in approximately one third of the cases will progress to a severe destructive disease requiring joint replacement. Often this replacement can be of the hemiarthroplasty type unless there has been significant glenoid destruction.

Overall, total shoulder replacement has been found to be an increasingly effective procedure when carried out for the correct conditions and when accompanied by adequate soft tissue and bone stock. When there is a deficiency of the rotator cuff, the patients will generally notice significant pain reduction but only partial strength and motion gains. Pain relief after surgery has been significant in all diagnostic groups, with 90% of the patients having no pain at rest or minimal pain with activity.[1] Functional improvements have been significant resulting in improved hygiene and functions of daily activity in most patients. A few patients have even resumed heavy lifting and sports such as handball and tennis.

Total shoulder replacement technique

Total shoulder replacement is often a difficult procedure that demands considerable experience in rotator cuff surgery before one should attempt it in difficult rheumatoid and old trauma patients. Generally the surgery is performed with the patient elevated 30 degrees and with his arm free on a short armboard at the side.

A long deltopectoral incision facilitates exposure. This incision allows the elevation of a portion of the distal deltoid attachment and preserves the clavicular origin (Fig. 9-21, *A*). Previously superior and posterior approaches have been utilized, but these patients had poorer motion on follow-up examinations.

After exposing the subscapularis it is incised, leaving some soft tissue on the humeral head for reattachment (Fig. 9-21, *B*). The head is exposed and then using a power

saw it is excised at the edge of the articular surface (Fig. 9-21, *C* and *D*). If there has been bone loss, then this procedure is modified. It is important to restore the normal version of the humeral head. This is done by placing the elbow at 90 degrees with the arm at the side and then externally rotating it approximately 40 degrees, which is comparable to the angle that the head faces posteriorly (Fig. 9-21, *C* and *D*). This allows for a straight posteriorly directed cut that creates the proper angle. The shaft is then reamed distally and the trial prosthesis is inserted. The rotator cuff if torn may be repaired before the joint is incised if there are small tears or at the completion of the procedure if a large tear is present.

Next attention is directed toward the

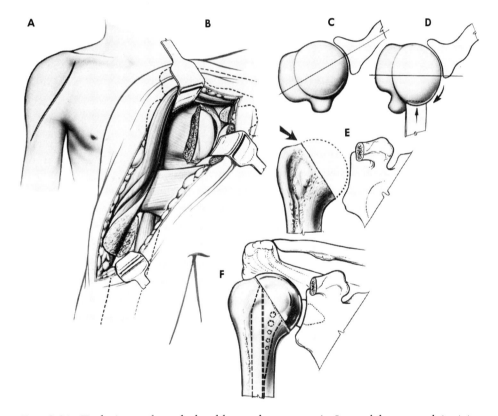

Fig. 9-21. Technique of total shoulder replacement. **A,** Long deltopectoral incision allows visualization without detaching deltoid origin. **B,** View obtained after subperiosteally dissecting off a portion of deltoid insertion on humerus. This will not preclude early motion program. **C,** Degree of retroversion of humeral head. **D,** With arm externally rotated same number of degrees, a straight posteriorly directed cut will provide proper angle of version for humeral component. **E,** In cutting humeral head there is a tendency to remove too much bone inferiorly at neck. **F,** Humeral prosthesis should be postioned such that its proximal border is just above greater tuberosity, and not inferior to it.

glenoid. The glenoid is approximately 20 by 40 mm and it allows little margin for error when inserting a prosthesis. Excellent exposure must be obtained. We use a set of retractors that facilitate this exposure. Both the anterior and posterior margins are defined so that the angle of glenoid version is noted. All soft tissue from the glenoid surface is removed. The bone of the coracoid is palpated and then a burr is utilized to create a centering slot for the stem of the glenoid (Fig. 9-22). This slot must be well centered and reach the superior aspect of the glenoid. It should not be too wide or it will allow toggling of the prosthesis. A power burr facilitates reaming, but a curved cuvette is often helpful and it is less likely to penetrate the cortex. If glenoid penetration occurs, a bone plug fashioned from the humeral head will help avoid poor cement pressurization.

In preparing the surface of the glenoid, it should be curetted to subchondral bone but this bone must be preserved or the glenoid will be weakened and its pullout strength diminished. If the bone stock of the glenoid is deficient, then a bone graft fashioned from the humeral head will aid in glenoid fixation (Fig. 9-22, *C*). The trial prosthesis is then inserted and the cuff is pulled to its attachment site. Motion is checked for capsular adhesions or contrac-tures, which should be released now if that was not completed initially.

The glenoid is inserted first followed by the humerus. Attention to detail at the time of glenoid preparation and insertion are critical if the 80% incidence of glenoid lucent lines found in our review is to be reduced. A water pic is helpful and an absolutely dry surface is imperative. The notch in the glenoid is extended into the bone of the coracoid to improve cement fixation. After the glenoid is inserted, a cement restrictor is placed in the humerus followed by the cementing of the humeral component. In inserting the humeral component, the superior aspect of the prosthesis must be at or slightly proximal to the greater tuberosity if impingement problems are to be avoided (Fig. 9-21, *E* and *F*). Following this the rotator cuff is reattached. One of the problems that has been encountered after surgery is the result of AC joint arthritis that was not treated at the time of the total shoulder replacement. Such arthritis has necessitated subsequent AC joint resection. Damage to the AC joint is particularly common in rheumatoid arthritis and it demands treatment either in the form of resection or removal of inferior osteophytes.

Impingement may result from an improper placement of the humeral compo-

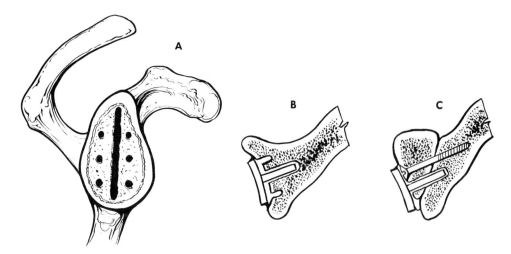

FIG. 9-22. A and **B,** Preparation of slot for glenoid. **C,** If bone is deficient, then graft is prepared from humeral head and attached before slot is made.

nent that leaves the greater tuberosity prominent. In addition, if there is a prominent acromial spur or a rotator cuff tear, then acromioplasty should be performed. Persistent stiffness following surgery is often a result of inadequate capsular release, particularly in the axillary recess, at the time of surgery. The capsule here is often contracted and thickened and if it is left untreated the patient cannot abduct the arm. Release of the capsule must be performed carefully to avoid the axillary nerve.

Loosening of the glenoid has been noted but this is generally a reflection of cement technique and bone stock. Lucent lines are present in approximately 80% of patients but they are generally nonprogressive. Glenoid loosening has been seen in two of our patients. Humeral lucent lines are less common (25%) than glenoid lines, but loosening can occur and has necessitated revision in one of our patients.

Postoperatively, patients are held in a sling and swathe for 3 to 4 days and then passive exercise is started within the limits determined at surgery. Generally flexion and external rotation are started initially and abduction is avoided. The sling is discarded by 7 days after surgery and active assisted exercise is added at 2 weeks progressing to full active exercises at 6 weeks. Stretching is a component of this program for 6 to 9 months with strength training starting at 6 weeks and progressing over the next 6 months. The rehabilitation is much more difficult than that following total knee or total hip replacement and the patient should be forewarned. But with good tissues and a cooperative patient good results can be anticipated. Pain relief is predictable in 90% of the patients but functional and motion improvements are de- termined by the quality of the soft tissues as well as the ability to restore the function of the rotator cuff. Thus a more limited goal in these patients is advisable.

References

1. Bade, H., Warren, R.F., Ranawat, C., and Inglis, A.E.: Long term results of Neer TSR, Paper presented to The American Academy of Orthopaedic Surgeons, annual meeting, 1983.
2. Cofield, R.: Rotator cuff tear: results of treatment, Paper presented to The American Academy of Orthopaedic Surgeons, annual meeting, 1983.
3. Debeyre, J., Patte, D., and Elmelik, E.: Repair of rupture of the rotator cuff of the shoulder with a note on advancement of the supraspinatus muscle, J. Bone Joint Surg. **46B**:436, 1949.
4. Dines, D., Warren, R.F., and Inglis, A.E.: Surgical treatment of lesions of the long head of the biceps, Clin. Orthop. **164**: 1982.
5. Froimson, A.I., and Oh, I.: Keyhole tenodesis of biceps origin at the shoulder, Clin. Orthop. **112**:245-249, 1974.
6. Hitchcock, H.M., and Bechtol, C.O.: Painful shoulders observations in the role of the tendon of the long head of the biceps brachii in its causation, J. Bone Joint Surg. **30A**:263, 1948.
7. Jobe, F.: Function of supraspinatus, Personal communication.
8. Matsen, F.: Arthrotomography to evaluate rotator cuff tears, Personal communication.
8a. McCoy, S., et al.: Total shoulder replacement in rheumatoid arthritis. Paper presented to The American Academy of Orthopaedic Surgeons, annual meeting, Atlanta, 1984.
9. Neer, C.: Anterior acromioplasty for chronic impingement syndrome in the shoulder, J. Bone Joint Surg. **54A**:41, 1972.
9a. Ranawat, C., and Inglis, A.E.: Hemiarthroplasty in patients with rheumatoid arthritis. (Unpublished.)
10. Rathbun, J.B., and MacNab, T.: The microvascular patterns of the rotator cuff, J. Bone Joint Surg. **52B**:540, 1976.
11. Rockwood, C. Acromioplasty without cuff repair in elderly patients. Presented to the Society for Shoulder and Elbow Surgeons, Rochester, Minn., 1983.
12. Warren, R.F., Dines, D., and Inglis, A.E.: Coracoid process as a cause of impingement. (In progress.)
13. Warren, R.F., and Otis, J.: Elbow strength after rupture of the long head of the biceps. Presented to the Hospital for Special Surgery alumni meeting, November 1978.

chapter 10
THE ELBOW, WRIST, AND HAND

SECTION I
Upper Extremity Fractures in the Elderly
William E. Burkhalter

WRIST FRACTURE

When one thinks of upper extremity fractures in the elderly, one immediately thinks of the fracture of the distal radius as described by Abraham Colles. This fracture, although extremely common, has been a source of frustration for all of us for a variety of reasons. Classifications of this fracture are all based on the presence or absence of displacement and the presence or absence of comminution with or without an interarticular extension. In addition, recently Frykman[4] has talked about the association of Colles' fractures with fractures of the distal ulna. In addition to fractures of the radius and ulna, the distal radioulnar joint may be subluxated or frankly dislocated either volarly or dorsally. According to Gartland and Werley,[5] there is a definite indication for reduction of this fracture. They believed that functional loss paralleled anatomic distortion.

We are all aware of the cosmetic changes associated with shortening of the radius with or without radial deviation of the distal fragment. The radially deviated hand is weakened functionally as far as power grip is concerned. In addition, radial shortening results in subluxation of the distal radioulnar joint with articulation of the distal ulna and the carpus. Limitation of the wrist motion in the flexion-extension plane plus loss of forearm rotation may result. In addition, ulnar deviation of the wrist is impossible.

Although a multitude of methods of reduction have been advocated, the technique of closed reduction with static Chinese finger trap traction plus countertraction is still the method most widely used. This allows restoration of radial length and eliminates radial angulation and dorsal angulation of the distal radial fragment. Thus the fracture is relatively easy to reduce, but it is difficult to maintain this reduction.

In an attempt to reduce the three main radial deformities associated with Colles' fracture, the hand is placed in flexion with ulnar deviation and forearm pronation following reduction of the fracture by longitudinal traction. This is a relatively poor position for hand and finger motion and therefore considerable hand stiffness may follow this method of treatment.

Sarmiento[11] has stated that the brachioradialis is the major deforming force in this fracture and he also found that supination reduces the tension of the brachioradialis muscle. In addition, according to Sarmiento,[12] supination places the hand in a much more functional position, so that patients are better able to use their hand, which helps to prevent stiffness during union of the fracture. These fractures, especially in elderly patients, may have considerable comminution (Fig. 10-1). How does one prevent radial shortening during union of the fracture? Sarmiento thinks that brachioradialis relaxation plus ulnar deviation of the wrist are important. All methods of reduction have attempted to maintain radial length by forced ulnar deviation of the wrist and hand. Unless the immobilization is effective and prolonged, maintenance of the length in the presence of comminution is difficult.

Because of this, continuous static traction with pins and plaster has been widely used.[7,13] Small Steinmann pins or heavy Kirschner wires are placed through the base of the second and third metacarpals and the proximal ulna or the middle third of the radial shaft. Once length has been regained by the Chinese finger trap traction, length may be maintained statically with proximal and distal pins incorporated into the plaster cast. This skeletal distraction reduction method, however, requires considerable attention to detail. The pins placed in the dorsum of the hand are especially prone to complications since the pins must be maintained for a considerable time, which is usually 6 to 8 weeks, in the presence of motion. Loosening and infection are the most frequent complications. In addition to these, insertional or surgical complications can occur during placement of the pins. It is important to avoid the extensor digitorum communis and its paratenon during insertion as well as the fleshy portion of the first dorsal interosseous muscle. If either of these is wound up in the threaded ends during placement, considerable hand stiffness can result. If the pins are drilled into a position while the hand and forearm are in the Chinese finger trap, then the palm of the hand will be positioned as a flat structure. There will be no normal transverse or longitudinal arch. This flat palm position of the hand is a poor one for hand function, and these patients are already prone to hand stiffness. In addition, impaling tendons is easy in this position, especially the first dorsal interosseous and index extensor tendons.

Ideally, pin placement should be performed with the two pins at 60 to 70 degrees to each other. The flare at the second metacarpal can be palpated quite easily with the hand closed passively into a tight fist. Obviously pins are placed before the reduction

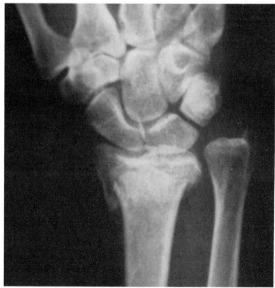

A

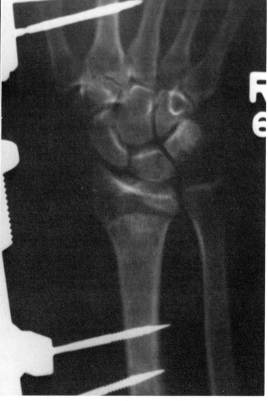

B

FIG. 10-1. **A** and **B,** Comminuted intra-articular fracture of distal radius in 70-year-old woman.

Continued.

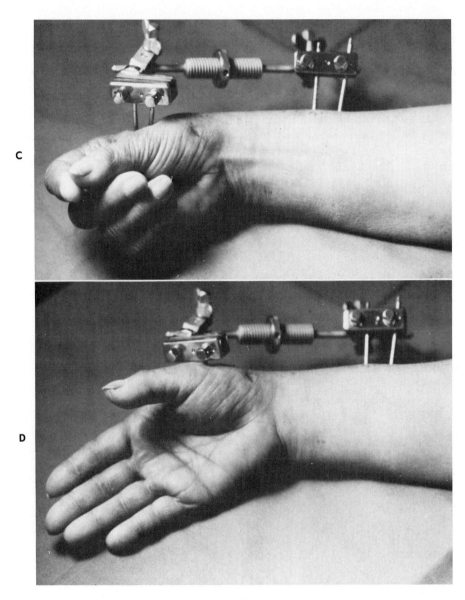

FIG. 10-1, cont'd. C and **D,** A heavy external fixator retained an excellent closed reduction. **E** and **F,** At time of removal of external fixator there was good but not full motion. **G,** Final result shows union and maintenance of radial length. External fixators usually give anatomic result but in some instances there is slow rehabilitation.

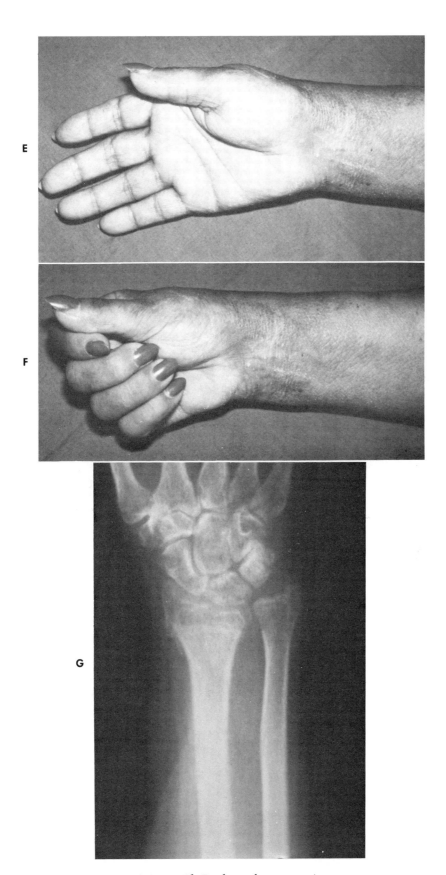

FIG. 10-1, cont'd. For legend see opposite page.

maneuver or the application of the Chinese finger trap traction. They should be placed immediately distal to the flare on the second metacarpal. The pins should be placed transversely through the second metacarpal into the base of the third. Care should be taken that the pin does not exit the shaft of the third metacarpal because of the danger of the winding up of the extensor digitorum communis tendons or their paratenon. The pin size should be comparable to the skeletal size of the patient, and the pin should definitely be threaded. A second pin at 60 to 70 degrees is then drilled into the more distal portion of the second metacarpal from dorsum to volar. Adequate and even generous skin relief should be achieved around these pins. Placing the pins with the hand balled up to a tight fist passively avoids impaling tendons, paratenon, or significant muscle tissue. Also it ensures that full flexion is possible. Placement of the proximal pin should be in either the radius or the ulna. After covering the pin-skin interface with sterile dressings, traction reduction can be achieved. Once the position has been checked radiographically in two planes, a short arm plaster cast is applied incorporating the threaded Steinmann pins.

Immediately before cast application a careful clinical assessment of the distal radial ulnar joint should be carried out in varying degrees of forearm rotation. In general, dorsal subluxation of this joint is most common and is easily aggravated by prolonged pronation in a plaster of Paris cast. The greatest stability is usually achieved with 30 to 45 degrees of supination of the forearm. Likewise, this slightly supinated position allows the patient the greatest chance for use of the hand during immobilization periods and helps to decrease stiffness. These comments about forearm rotation only apply if the proximal pin is placed in the ulna. Rotation is then not possible. If, however, the proximal Steinmann pin is placed in the radius, some forearm rotation will be possible during immobilization, although full rotation will not be achievable. Therefore some thought should be given to the position of greatest stability

of the distal radioulnar joint. Volar subluxation of this joint is far less common than dorsal and usually does not affect rotation to the same extent as dorsal instability. The diagnosis of the subluxation, volarly or dorsally, is not easily made radiographically, especially when there is an associated distal radial fracture, but it usually can be detected quite easily if searched for clinically. The position of forearm rotation should be the position of greatest stability for this joint.

With the popularity of external fixators in the treatment of comminuted open or closed fractures of the pelvis and long bones, their application to fractures of the distal radius was inevitable. The original Roger Anderson half pin set as well as other light external fixators have appeared. In general, the results with the use of external fixation have been very good. Anatomically, the results are superior in most series to other closed-reduction maneuvers. However, great attention to the details of pin care and rehabilitation are necessary. In general, joint stiffness both of the fingers and the wrist are greater with the static traction methods. The rehabilitation period is likewise somewhat longer because of the stiffness as compared with the more functionally treated series of patients.[1,2,9]

The technique of pin placement with external fixators, however, varies from the pin-and-plaster technique. The external pins of the threaded type are usually 2.5 mm in diameter. Two should be placed in the second metacarpal and two in the distal radius. The pins in both instances should converge at an angle of about 60 degrees to each other. This adds considerably to the stability. In addition, both sets of pins should be inserted halfway between straight dorsal and straight lateral, or about 45 degrees to the frontal planes. Following the covering of the pins with a sterile dressing, traction is applied again and reduction obtained. The external portion of the fixator is applied, and then an ulnar plaster splint is put on to prevent excessive ulnar deviation of the wrist.

It may be that because of osteoporosis this treatment modality, as well as the use of pins and plaster, is open to some questions. Usually an adequate reduction can be maintained, but stiffness of the finger, wrist, elbow, and shoulder are more frequently seen in the elderly than in younger patients. According to Jakob and Fernandez,[9] this tendency to stiffness is accentuated by delayed fixation for loss of reduction following closed manipulation and cast application.

Adequacy of reduction is generally in the eyes of the beholder, especially in Colles' fracture. There are, however, some guidelines that should be kept in mind when looking at a film of reduction in a typical patient. The major deformities that one is attempting to overcome in this fracture reduction are shortening and dorsal angulation. Of the two, shortening is the more important functionally and cosmetically. Is it possible to maintain length with other than external pin fixation or internal fixation? The answer is "Yes, sometimes." In the typical fracture even though there may be considerable comminution, the comminution is largely dorsal. The volar cortex of both the proximal and distal fragments is usually intact or relatively so. However, the distal fragment has, because of the dorsal comminution, translated dorsally, and shortening results. If after a reduction attempt the dorsal angulation is restored to normal, shortening will still be present unless the volar cortices of the two fragments are reduced anatomically or very nearly so. Only by restoring the volar cortex anatomy can shortening be prevented. This is the real hallmark of a good reduction and is necessary even if retention of the reduction is by an external fixator, pins and plaster, or plaster of Paris cast. In many cases of the fracture slipping in the cast or loss of reduction there was really no volar reduction initially.

The other functional and cosmetic deformity in the fracture is persisting radial deviation of the distal fragment. One might say that this is shortening, but that would not be accurate. This does not equal shortening, but rather it is angulation radially of the distal fragment. This deformity is far more damaging than simple shortening

without angulation. Equal shortening, even with moderate dorsal tilt, can be managed by some type of ulnar shortening procedure. Radial angulation, however, does not respond to this relatively simple surgery but rather requires an osteotomy of the radius to realign the hand or the forearm. The presence of this deformity is frequently missed because of inadequate radiographs taken of the fracture site when determining the initial reduction adequacy. Enough of the proximal radius must be seen so that this deformity is appreciated on the initial reduction films. With simple radial shortening, the Darrach distal ulnar excision or the creation of a distal ulnar nonunion will improve wrist motion as well as forearm rotation.[3,6]

Fracture dislocations with a significant persisting interarticular component following closed reductions require more aggressive treatment than has usually been accorded to them in the elderly. These fractures in younger patients bring out the entire orthopaedic armamentarium from screws to buttress plates and bone grafts. There is a great tendency, however, to undertreat all fractures in the elderly with the exception of fractures of the upper end of the femur. This is justified by saying that the bone stock is poor, that comminution is great, or that the functional requirements of the patient are low. All of these may or may not be true, but it is difficult for both the patient and the physician to accept a severe cosmetic deformity with functional loss. I feel that one should attempt to restore as closely as possible the interarticular anatomy of fractures of Smith type 3 even if this requires plate, screws, and bone grafts.

In general, osteotomy of distal radial fractures that have healed with deformity fall outside the scope of treatment of fractures in the elderly. Osteotomy for intra-articular or extra-articular distal radial fractures is usually reserved for young patients with high functional demands. However, an occasional patient will be adamant about anything to improve appearance and function. It must be remembered that at least 70% of the normal range of wrist motion should be present before osteotomy is considered. Certainly full range of motion of the fingers, elbow, and shoulder must be added to this. Stiffness is such a major problem in these patients that all attempts should be made to secure and maintain an adequate reduction of the initial fracture.

Complications

These fractures are a hallmark of old age and although the fracture may heal in 6 to 8 weeks, the patient may require up to 1 year for total rehabilitation of the extremity even without complications. Carpal tunnel syndrome, acute or superimposed on an already present situation, may be the condition that triggers a dystrophic pattern in the extremity. Many patients in this age group will have had electrical evidence of median nerve compression at the wrist before the fracture. Their symptoms, however, may have been so minimal or intermittent that they were blamed on "arthritis" or "poor circulation." Older patients expect both of these conditions and so physicians are not particularly concerned about their symptoms. The fracture, however, may trigger a painful condition of median nerve compression. The usual testing methods of physical diagnosis may show no two-point discrimination and thenar atrophy. These are obviously signs of a long-standing problem. The electromyogram (EMG) and nerve conduction tests will show an old carpal tunnel syndrome with marked slowing of median nerve conduction and fibrillation potentials in the abductor pollicis brevis. Compression of the nerve exists and the patient will not move the fingers well in the cast. The patient complains of considerable pain in the cast. In these situations must something be done in order to save hand function? I think that the liberal use of stellate ganglion blocks and carpal tunnel release are useful in improving the use of the limb. Usually I try several stellate ganglion blocks, especially if there is a considerable increase in the skin temperature of the hand and fingers with the blocks. If there is little long-lasting relief after several blocks, carpal tunnel release should be performed early following fracture and reduction.

Before all this is done or even contemplated, the position of the wrist should be evaluated. Severe wrist flexion in a circular cast, splint, sugar-tongs, or external fixator may bring on or accentuate a carpal tunnel syndrome. At the least it will be painful and may trigger a dystrophic picture. Simply having greater wrist extension in the external device may reduce pain and improve finger motion. In addition to being painful, wrist flexion past 30 degrees is probably not needed in order to maintain fracture reduction. Wrist flexion of greater than 30 degrees makes full finger flexion difficult. Flexion of the wrist greater than 45 degrees, if continued until fracture union, may result in a rather rigid wrist flexion contracture that further compromises function.

Following wrist evaluation, swelling of the hand should be assessed. Swelling of the dorsum of the hand and fingers may mirror the conditions within the fibro-osseous carpal tunnel. Elevation of the wrist above heart level almost continuously will reduce swelling and improve finger motion. Elevation in older patients presents a problem, but it must be constantly stressed that loss of dorsal edema will improve finger motion in addition to reducing median nerve compression. Only active finger range-of-motion exercises and elevation will reduce edema and for all practical purposes all early edema will respond to these two modalities. These two modalities, however, are difficult for many patients to carry out. Patients often believe that they are not to move or should be unable to move their fingers with a fracture and a cast. Explanations that this is not the case will need to be repeated.

In addition to a loss of wrist motion following an intra-articular distal radial fracture, two other joints usually lose some motion. The most common is the shoulder. Immobilization of the wrist and/or elbow is also usually followed by secondary immobilization of the shoulder in a position of internal rotation. A sling used to support the arm fosters internal rotation because the arm naturally rests across the abdomen and lower chest. If slings are used, the arm should be removed several times each day for external rotation and flexion exercises to the shoulder. The development of shoulder stiffness makes rehabilitation of the entire extremity difficult after the fracture and in addition sets up a painful condition in the shoulder when one tries to increase the range of shoulder motion. The other joints that may become stiff following this fracture are the metacarpophalangeal joints of the fingers. Swelling with wrist flexion reduces the patient's ability to flex these joints fully. More distal joint motion or interphalangeal joint motion may be free and easy, but the metacarpophalangeal joint of the finger must be looked at constantly for full flexion. If swelling is controlled and distal joint motion is fair, then a cast or splint extension should be added to push the metacarpophalangel joint into flexion. This extension can only be added if the distal palmar crease area is free of external encumbrances. With this freedom, dorsal pressure from the cast, splint, or even rubber band loops will improve metacarpophalangeal joint flexion. Once this joint flexion is achieved, full finger range of motion will soon follow.

Thus, in conclusion, the most frequent complications of Colles' fracture may not be related to the fracture geographically at all. The stiff shoulder with metacarpophalangeal joint stiffness, the wrist flexion contracture, and the carpal tunnel syndrome all compromise the overall result. Great attention to detail in managing these patients will avoid a poor functional result.

HAND INJURIES IN THE ELDERLY

The subject of hand injuries involves so many different injuries that whether one is talking about all ages or just older patients, the possibilities are vast. In general, however, certain fractures are not seen in elderly patients. Basilar fracture dislocations of either the thumb or ulnar border digits are examples of fractures that are unusual in this age group. Likewise, the fifth metacarpal neck fracture so common in young men is rarely seen in the elderly. Certainly any type of fracture, open or closed and with or without tendon injury, is possible if one adds work activities or machinery to the usual activities of daily living.

With the exception of injuries resulting from work or machinery, most hand fractures in the elderly age group occur as a result of falls, and consequently they are usually bending fractures with some comminution. Union does not seem to be a problem in hand fractures, just as with fractures in this age group in other parts of the body. Fracture geography and the quality of bone for maintenance of internal fixation may compromise a final anatomic result, but union will not be a problem in most of the cases.

With all of these generalities, what makes hand fractures in the elderly a topic unto itself? One word—stiffness. Nonarticular finger fractures in patients over the age of 60 are likely to result in only about 40% of normal motion in the digit as compared to the undamaged finger.[22] This is without significant degenerative joint disease in the joints adjacent to the fracture. Stiffness may occur not just in the obviously damaged parts, but also in the adjacent undamaged digits. Not using portions of the hand for only a few days may result in considerable loss of motion. These subclinically arthritic patients not only lose motion quickly but also they do not regain motion rapidly. Considerable discomfort is encountered in attempting to regain this lost motion. Adjacent joints in the hand and also more proximal joints will stiffen during treatment for hand fractures. In addition, it should be remembered that loss of elbow and especially shoulder motion are common accompaniments of more distal injuries in older patients and in some younger ones as well. The elbow, forearm, and shoulder should be put through their full range of motion several times each day in order to prevent this stiffness.

Another problem that perpetuates or invites stiffness is swelling. Swelling is a normal accompaniment of injury, but its presence does not mean it is good, and therefore swelling must be dealt with. Early swelling limits motion because of its space-occupying nature; late swelling with its protein-rich fluid may glue tendons and ligaments to bone, thereby further limiting motion. Swelling can be reduced only by elevation and by active motion of the digits. Both should be instituted as soon as possible. Elevation should be carried out as soon as the fracture is recognized and should be continued until the hand has regained tissue equilibrium and motion is improving. It has been said that elevation must not be continuous, but instead should be intermittent. However, in spite of all sorts of instructions, patients will lower their injured hands below the level of the heart several times each hour for special activities. So even with a desire to institute a continuous elevation program, one really achieves only intermittent elevation. The dependency of the damaged part when it is below the level of the heart usually signals the need for elevation by causing discomfort. However, elevation must be strict; slings should be avoided. Slings place the extremity in a nonuseful position, encourage no hand use, and likewise encourage loss of elbow and shoulder motion. In addition, elevation is not achieved. Elevation must be above heart level and this is difficult to maintain because it requires active muscle control. Resting the elbow on the arm of a chair when sitting will rest the muscles around the shoulder and elbow. Joint symptoms at the elbow and shoulder may occur during this period of elevation and they should be treated by active motion as a method of relieving the static holding of the arm and forearm. This again encourages total motion of all proximal joints.

What about motion? When should it be instituted? Usually, in younger patients motion started by 3 to 4 weeks following the fracture results in achieving function of the joint at a 70% to 80% level.[22] I think that waiting this long in older patients will add significantly to the stiffness problem. Certainly, if open reduction and internal fixation are utilized, the surgeon seeks to protect the anatomic reduction and therefore there is a tendency to hold off on early or immediate motion. Because of this, there is a place for closed-fracture treatment in the hand along with the institution of mo-

tion within a few days of reduction. Note that not all hand fractures can be treated in this way; however, there is a place for closed treatment and I believe that in nonarticular fractures it should be used initially. Surgery on a fracture adds to the injury and in certain cases violates undamaged structures in order to gain surgical exposure. If the part cannot be moved immediately, the stage is set for tendon adherence with further limitation of motion. Fixation failures are common in older patients because of the poor quality of bone stock to support the fixation devices as well as the high degree of comminution in many of these fractures.

Closed treatment method in proximal phalangeal fractures

Nonarticular phalangeal fractures can be called a no-man's land fracture.[23] Just as the injury of flexor tendons over the proximal phalanx was called by Sterling Bunnell the no-man's land tendon injury, these fractures are also special. Both the fracture and the tendon injury are difficult problems. I feel that reduction and retention of these fractures can be achieved by closed means.

The usual deformity of nonarticular phalangeal fractures is related to the intrinsic extensor tendon system and results in dorsal angulation and/or displacement of the distal fragment. Angulation or rotation may be present, but reduction is achieved by flexing the distal fragment toward the palm until one can palpate the loss of the dorsal dished-out deformity over the proximal phalanx. When this disappears completely, the fracture is reduced in the lateral or sagittal plane.[16] A plaster of Paris cast is applied with the wrist at about 30 degrees of dorsiflexion. A dorsal block extension is added to this cast, maintaining the same amount of finger flexion that resulted in the reduction initially. This is usually 70 degrees or more through the metacarpophalangeal joints. This extension block extends to all fingers, not just to fractured digits. With all metacarpophalangeal joints close to full flexion, there is convergence of all digits toward the scaphoid tuberosity. Then if all fingers are closed simultaneously through the proximal interphalangeal joints, the rotation and angulation problems can be appreciated and reduced if necessary. Rotation and angulatory problems are resolved by adjacent digits splinting the fractured finger.

How can one at this time determine radiographically an adequate reduction? Obviously a lateral x-ray film of the damaged digit is important for seeing the adequacy of the reduction. A plain film through a plaster of Paris cast with superimposed adjacent digits will not be useful. I use linear tomograms to determine radiographically the adequacy of reduction. A complete set of tomograms is not necessary. The x-ray technician needs only to measure the distance from the cassette to the finger in question with a ruler and to make the cuts at that distance. This will blur out the cast and other digits and show on a lateral tomogram whether or not the fracture is reduced. If dorsal angulation persists, additional flexion of the distal fragment can be carried out by adding felt to the dorsal extension block.

Once the reduction is satisfactory, motion is instituted. The metacarpophalangeal joints are already all in full or nearly full flexion. This is the safe position for these joints. The motion instituted is proximal interphalangeal flexion and extension. The patient should be encouraged to gain full flexion as soon as possible. Most patients with encouragement are able to do this within a few days; however, there is usually an extensor lag of 30 degrees or so. Generally the joint should be extended several times a day using the opposite hand so that the lag will not become a contracture. In certain cases a light sling with rubber bands can be added to the cast to maintain full extension passively. This, however, should not be done until full flexion of the proximal interphalangeal and distal interphalangeal joints is achieved. The patient should be seen frequently during the first few days in order to supervise motion and to check to see if the proximal interphalangeal joint extension can be achieved passively as well as actively. Union of this fracture functionally is usually achieved in 3 to 4 weeks. At that time the cast can be removed and the metacarpophalangeal joints are allowed to move into extension, and the wrist is free to gain motion. The patient may be left with a slight extensor lag of the proximal interphalangeal joint of the fractured digit but should have full flexion of all joints in the finger. There should be no angulatory or rotational deformity. I have been using this method for unstable proximal interphalangeal fractures for approximately 3 years and have found it to give predictable results in fractures that can be reduced closed.[15] If reduction cannot be achieved, then some thought should be given to open reduction and internal fixation.[14,17-19,21] Even following open reduction and internal fixation, stability is increased considerably by use of the cast described. More severe injuries to the digits may result in amputation to speed hand recovery (Fig. 10-2).

Postoperative rehabilitation is made easier by asking the patient to move only the distal joint of the finger during rehabilitation. External support aids in the maintenance of the reduction during motion.

As the injury site moves more distally in the digits, concerns regarding joint stiffness diminish somewhat. It must be remembered that approximately 80% to 85% of digital function resides in the metacarpophalangeal and proximal interphalangeal joints. So if proximal joint motion can be maintained in the presence of more distal joint injury, a satisfactory finger should result. In the more distal injuries, of bone, joint, soft tissue, or all three, the primary aim must be maintenance of proximal joint motion and the secondary aim is to deal with the actual injury (Fig. 10-3). Again there is the recurring problem of stiffness.

In the case of fingertip injuries, crushings, or actual amputations, I avoid sophisticated techniques of wound cover and closure. Instead, using a digital block or better yet a metacarpal block, I perform primary wound care. I avoid the digital rubber band tourniquet and instead use a pneumatic tourniquet well padded in the upper arm. All patients can tolerate 10 to 20 minutes of ischemic time, especially if the arm is well exsanguinated with an elastic bandage

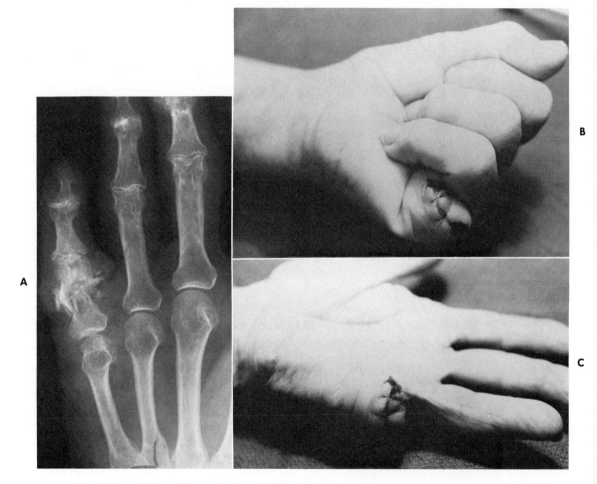

Fig. 10-2. A, X-ray films of 75-year-old woman with highly comminuted fracture of proximal phalanx secondary to gunshot wound. Initial treatment consisted of wound exploration and debridement. After consultation with family and patient following initial surgery, amputation was selected as best treatment option. **B** and **C,** Total hospitalization was 3 days. Note that there was no loss of motion, even in early period. Motion was begun 3 days following injury.

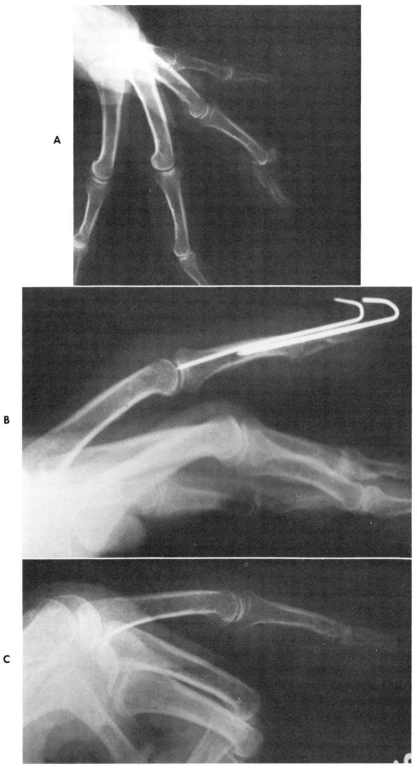

FIG. 10-3. A, X-ray film of 69-year-old woman with open crush injury of distal interphalangeal joint. **B** and **C,** Treatment consisted of debridement and primary arthrodesis. Longer of two K wires was subsequently backed out. *Continued.*

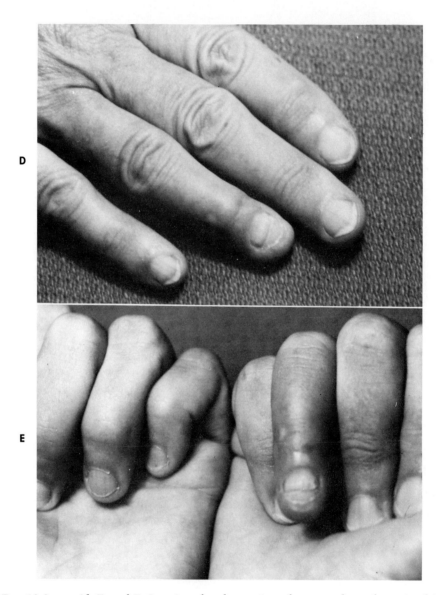

FIG. 10-3, cont'd. D and **E,** In spite of early motion, there was loss of proximal interphalangeal joint motion.

before tourniquet elevation. Pressures of 100 mm Hg over the systolic blood pressure are usually adequate and make local pressure on the arm less of a problem. The tourniquet is not elevated until the anesthesia is complete in the digit. At this time wound debridement, nail excision, or bony shortening can be carried out. In the case of actual intra-articular crush with damage on both sides of the joint, thought should be given to arthrodesis or at least prolonged intra-articular stabilization. A stable fibrous ankylosis may be a useful alternative to a formal arthrodesis in the presence of moderately severe degenerative joint disease.

Following appropriate initial surgery, what should be done? Following the achievement of hemostasis after tourniquet release, there are several alternatives. In the case of the crushed distal phalanx with an open fracture and nail bed injury, I remove the nail completely. How does one stabilize the digit so that union of the fracture occurs and the sterile nail matrix heals? Since the injury is distal to the lunula or sterile matrix, only distal stabilization is needed and a simple finger cast can be used. Before application of the finger cast, fine mesh gauze that is either dry or highly impregnated with petrolatum is applied to the nail or open wound. The finger cast is applied by using tincture of benzoin or topical adherent to the intact skin and one layer of cast padding while the benzoin solution is still wet. This results in a cast that is adherent to the digit through the cast padding. One-inch plaster is placed over the cast padding. The cast extends from the tip of the digit to the area immediately distal to the proximal interphalangeal joint crease. The cast immobilizes the damaged soft tissues, stabilizes the fracture, and offers protection from further injury to the digit.

In the absence of signs of infection, this cast may be kept in position for 3 weeks. During this time joint motions of metacarpophalangeal and proximal interphalangeal joints of the digit are performed. Normal use of the hand is encouraged.

In the case of distal injuries with exposed

bone, I do not believe that sophisticated coverage techniques should be employed. Y-V plasty, rotation flaps, and cross finger flaps are techniques that are all available. Relatively diminished vascularity and the problem of stiffness will, however, relegate these to use in younger patients. Simple bone shortening and secondary intention wound healing with maintenance of proximal joint motion from the day of injury will give a far better result. The result will be functionally better and cosmetically as good.

Fractures of the thumb including the metacarpal or proximal phalanx pose different problems from these same fractures in the other digits. The basis of thumb motion is not the metacarpophalangeal or interphalangeal joint but the basilar joint. Even with complete absence of metacarpophalangeal or interphalangeal joint motion, a nearly normal thumb for most activities will be possible with a full range of basilar joint motion. Therefore any treatment of fractures about the thumb must concentrate on maintenance of the basilar motion and avoiding contractures of the thumb and the index web space as well as avoiding a supination-extension contracture of this most important digit. Most extra-articular fractures of the thumb can be quite easily treated in a thumb spica cast. Considerable deformity can be accepted in the metacarpal, for instance, if there is no loss of basilar motion. Intra-articular Bennett's fractures of the thumb are unusual in this age group. Likewise, collateral ligament injuries in and around the metacarpophalangeal joint with joint instability problems are usual.

Immobilization of thumb proximal phalangeal or metacarpal shaft fractures is best carried out in a thumb spica cast. The interphalangeal joint may be left out in the case of metacarpal fractures or in fractures of the proximal portion of the proximal phalanx. The cast, however, should be applied with the thumb in full or in normal thumb opposition. The transverse metacarpal arch of the hand should be maintained or even exaggerated. The positioning of the thumb in full opposition avoids the development of a nonfunctional contracture of the most important digit in the hand. Last, but not least, the metacarpophalangeal joint of the thumb should be in slight flexion. Hyperextension of the metacarpophalangeal joint in order to improve the reduction of the fracture, either proximal phalanx or metacarpal, will only result in a persistent hyperextension contracture of the joint. This deformity will persist even after union of the fracture. Hyperextension of the metacarpophalangeal joint will reduce the ability of the thumb to reach the fingers even with a normal basilar joint. Slight flexion of the metacarpophalangeal joint is preferable, almost regardless of the fracture position. In treating fractures of the hand in the elderly, function must come first. Stiffness is a major problem in hand fractures in any age group, but it is much more of a problem in the elderly. If the hand can be positioned into the safe or intrinsic-plus position during fracture healing, stiffness will be reduced and function maintained.

What is the safe or intrinsic-plus position? It is metacarpophalangeal flexion of 70 degrees of all fingers with maintenance or exaggeration of the transverse arch of the hand or its cup. In addition, the proximal interphalangeal joint should be free to move and the thumb should be placed in full opposition. It is not the functional position, but the position from which all function is possible.

Elbow Fractures

Interarticular fractures of the elbow in any age group constitute a difficult treatment problem. To be sure isolated radial head fractures and certain olecranon fractures can be treated with expectations of excellent functional recovery. However, older patients usually do not incur isolated radial head fractures or olecranon fractures that can be internally fixed easily. Instead, the two most common elbow fractures in older patients are the comminuted fracture of the olecranon and the interarticular fracture of the distal humerus. In general, if

these fractures are displaced, open reduction and internal fixation will probably be required to achieve a reduction of the fracture and to maintain that reduction until union occurs. As in other fractures in the elderly, there is a great tendency to accept a reduction that is less than ideal because of the patient's age and activity level. However, it is important to guard against this attitude because we should all remember a mobile painless stable elbow joint is extremely important for useful hand function. The most useful range of motion of the joint is the so-called midrange. Loss of the last 30 to 40 degrees of elbow extension and the last 20 to 30 degrees of flexion results in little functional loss to the patient if normal hand, wrist, and shoulder motion are present. Therefore, when thought is given to a loss of the range of motion, which is usually inevitable in the elderly age group, remember the midrange.

Easily the most devastating elbow fracture in this or any age group is the interarticular distal humeral fracture.[26-28,31] The forearm bones are uninjured, but the distal humerus must be stabilized in order to start early range-of-motion activities to avoid the old problem of stiffness. How can one stabilize the fracture in order to achieve union and also institute early range of motion exercises of the elbow joint? The only reasonable solution is open reduction and internal fixation, but this is more easily said than done since exposure is easily the biggest problem in this fracture.[32] The distal humerus needs to be seen both radially and ulnarly and also on the posterior aspect of the bone.

I feel that the best method of exposure for interarticular distal humeral fractures is the inverted U incision.[25] The radial arm, after passing through the skin and subcutaneous tissue, identifies the triceps muscle-tendon unit laterally and anteriorly. The medial or ulnar limb identifies the ulnar nerve and the medial anterior aspect of the triceps muscle. The plan is to raise a myocutaneous flap utilizing the triceps and overlying skin. The radial (lateral) and ulnar (medial) incisions are continued across the subcutaneous border of the ulna. The triceps tendon attachment to the ulna is identified, both medially and laterally, and an extra-articular osteotomy of the proximal ulna and olecranon is created.[33] Before this, a drill hole may be created from the olecranon into the ulna via the intramedullary route. This may be helpful in the later reattachment of the triceps tendon, which is best managed with a large intramedullary cancellous screw and a tension band wire with a washer. The intramedullary cancellous screw should have a washer proximally in order to protect the triceps tendon portion of the tension band. The intramedullary screw gives alignment, while the washer and tension band avoid displacement of the triceps tendon and the bone of the olecranon. Once exposure of the distal humerus has been achieved by osteotomy of the ulna and proximal retraction of the triceps, the ulnar nerve is freed proximally down the level of the intermuscular septum. No formal ulnar nerve transposition, however, is needed. Traction anteriorly allows complete exposure of the fracture site. Using interfragmentary compression screws with or without washers or malleolar screws gives anatomic reduction fixation of the fragments. If not, small plates may be used medially or laterally. One third tubular plates may be bent to conform to the distal humeral flares. It must be remembered that anatomic reduction must be achieved in order for this fixation to retain the reduction adequately. With elbow flexion the most important plate is the posterior tension band plate and this is more important for fixation of the fracture if screw fixation is inadequate. The triceps osseous tendon unit is reattached utilizing the screw tension technique, as mentioned before, and loose skin closure medially and laterally to complete the procedure (Fig. 10-4). If hemostasis is difficult to obtain before closure, portions of the medial and lateral incisions may be left open for drainage during active motion. This is most important because early motion may result in hematoma formation, which has a tendency to restrict motion. These midaxial incisions

about the elbow heal well by secondary intention during the active range of motion. Immediately postoperatively, the elbow is splinted in nearly full extension for 1 to 2 days. Flexion exercises are then started from 30 degrees working for full flexion. Between exercise periods the elbow is maintained at about 30 degrees in a splint. If portions of the lateral or medial wounds are left open, only light sterile dressings are applied and these are changed several times a day. In the elderly it is necessary to be constantly aware of the problems of a stiff shoulder and so, between supervised elbow exercises while the elbow splint is in position, shoulder motion must be encouraged. The patient should be taught full range-of-motion exercises for the shoulder joint. These, as well as the elbow range-of-motion exercises, are best carried out when the patient is in the supine position. One must remember that early exercises are important. After surgery the elbow and shoulder joints are as close to normal as they are going to be for a long time and the fracture fixation is as good as it is going to be for a long time. Early motion avoids stiffness that comes with waiting. Thus, permitting range-of-motion exercises immediately is even preferable to waiting for a few days. Shoulder exercises should be performed early with the elbow splinted at 30 degrees. This allows a patient to achieve control of the arm from the shoulder and also to concentrate exercises on only one joint at the time.

Older patients require close supervision postoperatively. These exercise programs are uncomfortable and there is a great tendency on the part of the patient to put off that which is not pleasant. In addition to explanations about what is going to be required postoperatively for rehabilitation, daily supervision is important at least initially. This situation is not the same as with the patient with the internally fixed upper femoral fracture who can be sent home with follow-up in 1 month. With intra-articular distal humeral fractures, one is looking not only for union but also for a useful range of elbow motion and a mobile

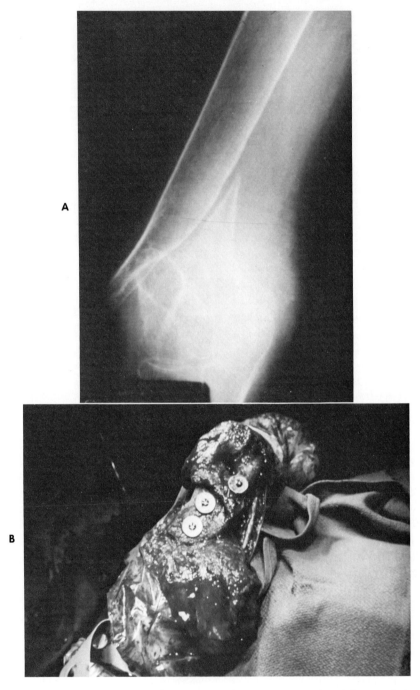

FIG. 10-4. **A,** Sixty-eight-year-old woman with nonunion of distal humeral fracture. Osteoporosis with age and disuse made osseous stabilization difficult. **B** and **C,** Extensive surgical exposure with large bone graft and cancellous screws and washer gave enough stability to begin early motion.

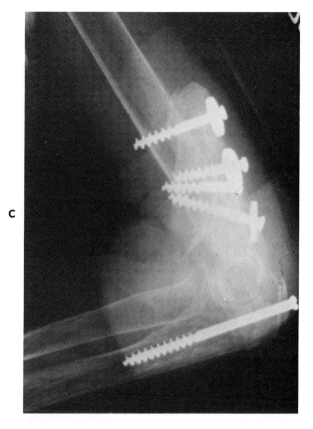

FIG. 10-4, cont'd. For legend see opposite page.

shoulder. These will only be achieved by close supervision in the postoperative rehabilitation process. One should concentrate on the midrange of elbow motion, that is from 30 to 130 degrees (Fig. 10-5).

The comminuted olecranon fracture is another fracture that is seen about the elbow in older patients. Much has been written regarding the advisability of olecranon excision and triceps attachment to the remnants of the proximal ulna.[24] This has had a great deal of appeal, but is also much easier talked about than performed. With bony excision a real length problem exists as far as the triceps tendon is concerned. The periosteum over the olecranon is thin and bringing good tissue from medial and lateral is difficult. In general, the result is a triceps-deficient elbow. The joint is comfortable and moves well into flexion and goes into extension weakly and/or with the aid of gravity. However, before excision is elected, the fracture should be explored to determine whether or not internal fixation of this fracture is possible. A far better functional result can be obtained if solid union of an olecranon fracture can be obtained without postoperative immobilization. If fixation gives enough stability to begin early motion, then the patient would be far better off. If, however, stability cannot be achieved, then excision is preferable. If more than three quarters of the olecranon is involved in the fracture, the patient may have an anterior translation of the elbow. This is a fracture dislocation of the elbow. This is also a potential problem when the entire olecranon is excised with the loss of bony support posteriorly because the brachioradialis, brachialis, and biceps muscles begin to act as translators of the elbow joint not as elbow flexors, making dislocation a possibility. If this is the case, internal fixation of the fracture is a requirement. With high degrees of comminution, partial fixation to provide bony support posteriorly and partial excision of the more proximal portion of the olecranon are indicated.

The entire distal humerus may not be fractured. Instead, the capitellum or lateral condyle may be injured. Usually there is comminution. Also, there is the presence of considerable joint effusion much like that seen with an isolated radial head frac-

ture. In the elderly the management of these two fractures, that is, the radial head fracture and the comminuted capitellum fracture, should be treated considerably differently from in the young. Here the aim is not necessarily a stable joint but one that moves and is comfortable. In the case of the capitellum fracture, attempts at open reduction with internal fixation are difficult. There is usually considerable comminution with attendant osteoporosis. These both

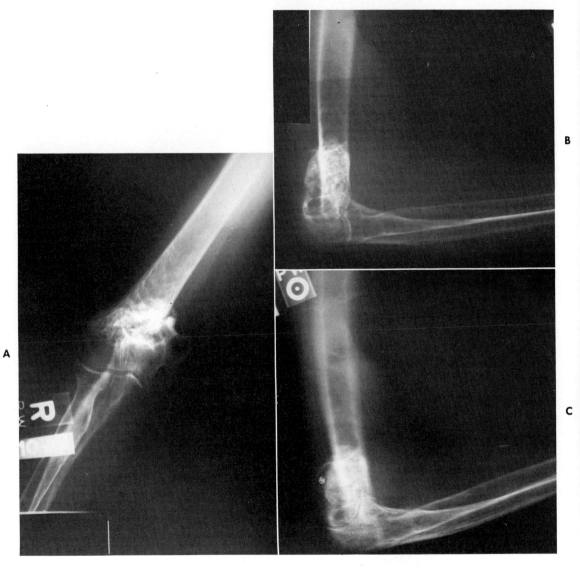

FIG. 10-5. **A** and **B**, Seventy-three-year-old woman with psoriatic arthritis with fracture of distal humerus that has healed with limited flexion. **C**, Latest x-ray film shows possible osseous block anteriorly that is confirmed by tomography. In older patients loss of motion is not entirely from joint stiffness and immobilization.

make fixation of the fracture difficult and even if successful the fixation is usually not stable enough to allow early range-of-motion exercises of the elbow. In this case I believe that excision of the capitellum is indicated. Elbow stability will be diminished, but motion will be nearly normal and the joint will be comfortable. Excision of the capitellum is not necessarily a good idea in younger patients, but I believe that it is a viable alternative in the elderly. Excision avoids elbow immobilization with its resultant stiffness and gives a more comfortable joint.

Radial head fractures are usually a far different problem. Such fractures are not present in any great numbers in elderly patients and when one does occur, the fracture is usually not widely displaced but may be highly comminuted. Here the problem is not the radiohumeral joint so much as the proximal radioulnar joint. In general, patients with radial head fractures treated either operatively or nonoperatively, if there is any loss of motion, lose supination and extension. I feel that most radial head fractures can be treated nonoperatively in the young as well as in the elderly. Younger patients need the stability that the radial head provides even at the expense of losing a few degrees of elbow extension. The decision regarding radial head excision should, I believe, be a clinical decision, not necessarily a radiographic one. I also believe that the elbow joint should be aspirated under sterile conditions within 24 hours of fracture diagnosis.[29] Removal of the blood reduces the effusion so that the patient can move more comfortably. The injection of a small amount of a local anesthetic agent, such as lidocaine (Xylocaine), will nearly eliminate intra-articular pain in the joint. The patient is asked to move the joint actively through its full range of motion. If there is no bony block to motion and no crepitus during a full range of motion including forearm rotation, then closed treatment is preferable. The presence of a bony block or crepitus in the midrange of elbow motion should suggest the need for radial head excision. If closed treatment is used, active motion exercises should be started immediately. Between exercise sessions, which should be 4 times daily, the elbow should be splinted in 30 degrees and full supination. In the splint the shoulder should be moved through its range of motion 4 times daily so that excellent shoulder motion and control can be maintained. Within 7 to 10 days, splinting may be discontinued and light normal use begun during the day. Splinting should be continued at night until the elbow is comfortable and nonreactive.

If an operative procedure is carried out because of bony block, a set of cirumstances that is also seen following excision of the capitellum is encountered. In both situations intra-articular surgery is performed with bony excision. Bleeding must be controlled in order to avoid an effusion of the elbow joint that will be painful and will reduce motion. Bone wax may be used on the cancellous surface of the radial neck or distal humerus to control bone ooze. In addition, leaving the synovium and a portion of the skin open at the conclusion of the surgery will allow the elbow to decompress itself during active motion. If surgery is carried out, immediate range-of-motion exercises should begin the day following surgery. With no fracture present and with control of effusion within the joint, rehabilitation should go fairly easily. The aim of either open or closed treatment is not necessarily an excellent anatomic result but rather a comfortable, mobile elbow joint.

Upper extremity fractures in the elderly require good basic orthopaedic management plus patience and the realization that more time will be required on the part of the physician in order to achieve a satisfactory result. These patients will be grateful for the time and patience.

References
Wrist
1. Cooney, W.P.: External mini-fixators, clinical applications and techniques. In Johnston, R.M., editor: Advances in external fixation, Chicago, 1980, Year Book Medical Publishers.
2. Cooney, W.P., Linscheid, R.L., and Dobyns, J.H.: External pin fixation for unstable colles fracture, J. Bone Joint Surg. **61A:**840-845, 1979.

3. Darrach, W.: Partial excision of lower shaft of the ulna for deformity following colles fracture, Ann. Surg. 57:764-765, 1913.

4. Frykman, G.: Fracture of the distal radius including sequelae, Acta Orthop. Scand. Suppl. **108,** 1967.

5. Gartland, J., and Werley, C.: Evaluation of healed colles fractures, J. Bone Joint Surg. **33A:**895, 1951.

6. Goncalves, D.: Correction of disorders of the distal radio-ulnar joint by artificial pseudoarthrodesis of the ulna, J. Bone Joint Surg. **56B**(3):462, 1974.

7. Green, D.: Pins and plaster treatment of comminuted fractures of the distal end of the radius, J. Bone Joint Surg. **57A:**304, 1975.

8. Griffin, T., and Huster, R.: Rush rod fixation of colles fracture in the elderly, J. Bone Joint Surg. **57A:**1030, 1975.

9. Jakob, R.P., and Fernandez, D.L.: The treatment of wrist fractures with the small A. O. external fixation device. In Uhthoff, H.: Current concepts of external fixation of fractures, Berlin, 1982, Springer-Verlag.

10. Milch, H.: Cuff resection of the ulna for malunited colles fracture, J. Bone Joint Surg. **23:**311-313, 1941.

11. Sarmiento, A.: The brachioradialis as a deforming force in colles fracture, Clin. Orthop. **38:**86, 1965.

12. Sarmiento, A., Pratt, L., Berry, N., and Sinclair, W.: Colles fracture, J. Bone Joint Surg. **57A:**31, 1975.

13. Scheck, M.: Long term follow-up treatment of comminuted fractures of the distal ends of the radius by transfixation with kirschner wires and cast, J. Bone Joint Surg. **44A:**337, 1962.

Hand

14. Brown, P.: The management of phalangeal and metacarpal fractures, Surg. Clin. North Am. **53:** 1393-1437, 1973.

15. Burkhalter, W.: Functional treatment of fractures. In Boswick, J.: Current concepts in hand surgery, Philadelphia, 1983, Lea & Febiger.

16. Coonrad, R.W., and Pohlman, M.H.: Impacted fractures in the proximal portion of the proximal phalanx of the finger, J. Bone Joint Surg. **51A:**1291-1296, 1969.

17. Crawford, G.: Screw fixation for certain fractures of the phalanges and metacarpals, J. Bone Joint Surg. **58A:**487, 1976.

18. Green, D.P., and Andersen, J.R.: Closed reduction and percutaneous pin fixation of fractures phalanges, J. Bone Joint Surg. **55A:**1651-1653, 1973.

19. Lister, G.: Intraosseous wiring of the digital skeleton, J. Hand Surg. **3:**427-435, 1978.

20. Murray, J. and McMurtry, R.: The management of phalangeal fractures, Paper presented at the 36th annual meeting of the American Society for Surgery of the Hand, Las Vegas, Nev., Feb. 1981.

21. Ruedi, T., Burri, C., and Pfeiffer, K.: Stable internal fixation of fractures of the hand, J. Trauma **11:**381-389, 1971.

22. Strickland, J., Steichen, J., Kleinman, W. and Flynn, N.: Factors influencing digital performance after phalangeal fracture. In Strickland, J., and Steichen, J., editors: Difficult problems in hand surgery, St. Louis, 1982, The C.V. Mosby Co.

23. Swanson, A.: Personal communications, 1982.

Elbow

24. Adler, S., Fay, G.F., and MacAuglard, W.R.: Treatment of olecranon fractures. Indications for excision of olecranon fragment and repair of the triceps tendon, J. Trauma **2:**597-602, 1962.

25. Cassebaum, W.H.: Operative treatment of T or Y fractures of the lower end of the humerus, Am. J. Surg. **83:**265-270, 1952.

26. Cassebaum, W.H.: Open reduction of T and Y fractures of the lower end of the humerus, J. Trauma **9:**915-925, 1969.

27. Knight, R.A.: Management of fractures about the elbow in adults, American Academy of Orthopaedic Surgeons Instructional Course, Lecture **14:**123-141, 1957.

28. Miller, W.A.: Comminuted fractures of the distal end of the humerus in the adult, J. Bone Joint Surg. **46A:**644-652, 1964.

29. Quigly, T.B.: Aspiration of the elbow joint in the treatment of fractures of the head of the radius, New Eng. J. Med. **240:**915-916, 1949.

30. Radin, E.L., and Riseborough, E.J.: Fractures of the radial head: A review of 88 cases and analysis of the individuals for excision of the radial head and non-operative treatment, J. Bone Joint Surg. **48A:** 1055-1064, 1966.

31. Riseborough, E.J., and Radin, E.L.: Intracondylar T fractures of the humerus in the adult (a comparison of operative and non-operative treatment in 29 cases), J. Bone Joint Surg. **51A:**130-141, 1969.

32. Van Gorder, G.W.: Surgical approach in supracondylar T fractures of the humerus requiring open reduction, J. Bone Joint Surg. **22:**278-292, 1940.

33. Zagorski, J., Uribe, J., Burkhalter, W.E., and Jennings, J.: Comminuted intra-articular bicondylar fractures of the distal humerus, Paper presented at the 48th annual meeting of the American Academy of Orthopaedic Surgeons, Las Vegas, Nev., Feb. 1981.

SECTION II

Hand Disorders in the Geriatric Patient

Richard R. McCormack, Jr.

Problems of the hand in the elderly population are quite common and they account for a significant percentage of the orthopaedist's practice. The prevalence of osteoarthritis in the general population increases with age; however, symptoms of arthritis in the hand are less likely to bring the patient to the physician than those in other joints. It is the symptoms of osteoarthritis in the large joints that prompt the elderly patient to seek medical attention. Patients with osteoarthritis in the large weight-bearing joints often will give a history of osteoarthritic involvement of the hands as well. In addition, many other afflictions of the hand are seen predominantly in the elderly. These include stenosing tenosynovitis, local nerve compression syndromes (such as carpal tunnel syndrome), and Dupuytren's disease. These and other afflictions although not unique to the elderly population, are seen frequently in this age group and will be discussed in the following section. The clinical presentation, pathophysiology, and essentials of diagnosis, as well as the conservative and operative treatments of each entity will be discussed.

OSTEOARTHRITIS IN THE HAND

Osteoarthritis of the hand is extremely common in the geriatric population. The onset is seen late in the fifth or early in the sixth decade and increases in frequency with age so that it is almost universally present in those over the age of 65.

Osteoarthritis is a disease of the articular cartilage of diarthrodial joints, which is characterized by progressive deterioration of the cartilage followed by joint inflammation and pain leading to eventual stiffness and deformity. Biochemical analysis of osteoarthritic cartilage reveals that the earliest change is an increase in water content followed by a decrease in proteoglycan content.[17] This diminution in proteoglycan content leads to an alteration of the physical properties of articular cartilage resulting in fissuring, fibrillation, and eventual destruction of the articular surface. Proteolytic enzymes and lyzosomal enzymes are thought to play a role in the destruction of articular cartilage in the inflammatory phase of the disease. Prostaglandin synthesis is also noted to be increased. It is unclear whether the inflammatory reaction is primary or secondary; however, it is probably in response to intra-articular debris from fibrillated articular cartilage. Calcium pyrophosphate and bony debris are present as a result of joint destruction. Biochemical changes in the articular cartilage itself are most likely the primary defect in the disease. The term *osteoarthrosis* previously used to denote a lack of inflammatory response is probably not accurate because almost all cases of osteoarthritis, regardless

of the joint involved, show some evidence of inflammation. Interestingly enough, despite the progressive degeneration of the joint cartilage, biochemical marker studies show enhanced synthesis of proteoglycan and collagen during the early stages of osteoarthritis, which is suggestive of an attempt by the body to effect a repair process. However, in most cases, the natural history is one of progressive joint destruction.

The clinical picture of osteoarthritis involving the hand is that of distal interphalangeal joint involvement.[16] The distal interphalangeal joints are probably the most commonly involved joints in osteoarthritis. Localized swellings about the articular margins of these joints, which represent marginal osteophytes, are termed Heberden's nodes (Fig. 10-6). Patients complain primarily of mild stiffness in the joints that is more noticeable on arising in the morning or after periods of rest. Stiffness and discomfort are relieved by activity. Often, warm-up exercises or range-of-motion activities in a basin of warm water improve function.

During the natural history of distal interphalangeal joint arthritis there is often an intense inflammatory phase with local swelling, redness, and effusion about the joint. This inflammatory phase may be followed by a loss of joint stability and progressive deformity with flexion or lateral deviation at the joint. As joint motion continues to decline, pain in the affected joint may diminish. Indeed, in many patients spontaneous ankylosis of the distal interphalangeal joint is the end result.

Involvement of the proximal interphalangeal joints may also be seen, but less commonly. Often proximal interphalangeal joint involvement is seen in the systemic arthritides such as lupus erythematosus, scleroderma, and rheumatoid arthritis. However, when it is seen with osteoarthritis, again juxta-articular osteophytes produce nodes or nodules about the joint, which are referred to as Bouchard's nodes. Involvement of the proximal interphalangeal joints, as with the distal interphalangeal joints, may also go through an inflammatory phase. Though less common, in-

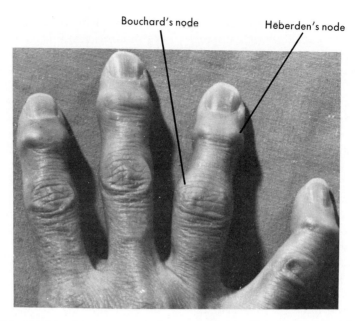

Bouchard's node   Heberden's node

FIG. 10-6. Heberden's nodes are common in osteoarthritis. (From Swanson, A.B.: Flexible implant arthroplasty in the hand and extremities, St. Louis, 1973, The C.V. Mosby Co.)

volvement of a proximal interphalangeal joint is more disabling since full range of motion of this joint is more critical to overall hand function. As with the distal interphalangeal joints, instability, stiffness, and deformity may be the end result.

Metacarpophalangeal joint involvement in osteoarthritis is rare; it is more commonly seen in rheumatoid arthritis. When present, it usually involves the metacarpophalangeal joint of the thumb and index finger.

More common, however, and seen with almost the same frequency as distal interphalangeal joint arthritis, is involvement of the thumb basal joint. This finding is also seen predominantly in women. The symptoms referable to this joint may be found occasionally in women in their third decade. Presentation at this early age is often associated with abnormal laxity of ligamentous structures. Usually, however, involvement begins towards the end of the fifth decade, initially appearing as inflammation and soreness at the base of the thumb, which may radiate up the arm and which is associated with difficulties with functions requiring power pinch and grasp.

Patients will complain of problems opening jars, wringing washcloths, turning keys in locks, and opening car doors with pushbutton latches. Weakness of pinch is universal and is the result not only of inefficient joint mechanics but also of disuse atrophy of the intrinsic muscles of the hand secondary to pain.

The natural history of basal joint arthritis is one of progressive destruction of the carpometacarpal joint of the thumb with subluxation in a dorsal radial direction of the metacarpal on the trapezium. Secondary contracture of the adductor muscle occurs followed by a hyperextension deformity of the metacarpophalangeal joint of the thumb in an effort to get a grip on large objects. With complete subluxation of the basal joint, a "swan neck" deformity of the thumb may exist (Fig. 10-7). In elderly patients with severe basal joint arthrosis and dislocation, symptoms of pain in the basal joint are usually minimal. Although such patients are able to cope with activities of daily living, functions requiring power pinch, as described above, are performed with great difficulty and the patient usually adapts her life-style around this disability.

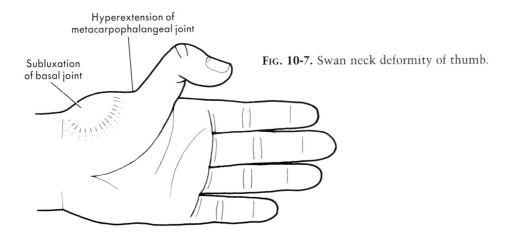

Hyperextension of
metacarpophalangeal joint

Subluxation
of basal joint

FIG. 10-7. Swan neck deformity of thumb.

The radiographic appearance of degenerative arthritis in the joints of the hand is one of a slowly progressive narrowing of the joint space indicating degeneration of articular cartilage. Narrowing is followed by subchondral sclerosis and marginal osteophyte formation with an apparent widening of the joint surface. In later stages, deformity is often present with subluxation and lateral deviation at the interphalangeal joints. In the basal joint, as discussed above, subluxation is frequent. Fragments of hypertrophic spurs with apparent free osteocartilaginous bodies are seen with advanced disease. Occasionally end-stage involvement in the distal interphalangeal joint may result in bony ankylosis.

The treatment of osteoarthritic involvement in the joints of the hand is one of exercises to maintain motion and intrinsic and extrinsic muscle strength. Heat is often beneficial in relieving discomfort and in enabling patients to perform active range-of-motion exercises. Soaks in a basin of warm water or paraffin baths are the most commonly applied modalities.

The main stay of medical therapy is aspirin. It appears to be the most effective, economical, and safe drug for long-term use in this chronic condition. Buffered or enteric-coated preparations minimize gastrointestinal complications. The finding of increased prostaglandin synthesis in the inflammatory phase of osteoarthritis may explain why aspirin is so effective. The nonsteroidal anti-inflammatories are also ef-

fective, their primary advantage being, in some cases, less gastrointestinal irritation and less frequent administration.

The use of systemic corticosteroid preparations is contraindicated in osteoarthritis. However, intra-articular cortisone injections are often helpful in control of the acute inflammatory phase. Such injections, however, should be used with caution. Recent evidence shows that corticosteroids can inhibit proteoglycan synthesis by chondrocytes and that excessive use may actually promote articular destruction.[1]

The use of splints for the resting of symptomatic joints may also be helpful, especially in distal interphalangeal and basal joint involvement. Distal interphalangeal and proximal interphalangeal joints may be splinted using a narrow, foam-backed aluminum splint. Distal interphalangeal joints should be splinted in neutral position. Proximal interphalangeal joints are best immobilized in about 15 degrees of flexion. In no case should immobilization be prolonged because stiffness will ensue. The splints may be removed several times a day for gentle active range-of-motion exercises. The use of a molded Orthoplast thumb immobilization splint for basal joint involvement is usually quite effective during the symptomatic phase of disease.

The surgical treatment of osteoarthritis is tailored to the particular joint involved. The distal interphalangeal joint rarely requires surgery since the arthritis is usually self-limited in this location. As mentioned above, spontaneous ankylosis is often common. However, an indication for surgical treatment of the joint is the presence of a bothersome mucous cyst. A mucous cyst is a synovial outpouching of the distal interphalangeal joint arising in the interval between the extensor tendon and the collateral ligament where the capsule is unsupported. Inflammatory synovitis within the joint accompanied by increased synovial fluid production contributes to the progression of the size of this cystic lesion. It often appears as a small fluid-filled mass dorsally between the distal interphalangeal crease and the nail cuticle. It is often translucent and effaces the skin. It may, on occasion, rupture or become secondarily infected. Extension into the space dorsal to the eponychial fold creates a depression in the germinal matrix resulting in a longi-

tudinal groove in the growing nailplate (Fig. 10-8). Such a finding belies the chronicity of this lesion. Lateral and often oblique roentgenograms of the distal interphalangeal joint will always reveal an osteophytic spur associated with the origin of the cyst.

Surgical treatment is performed through a J-shaped incision (Fig. 10-9). A flap is developed with great care to avoid injury to the underlyng nail germinal matrix. The cyst is traced proximally to the joint line in the interval between the extensor tendon and the collateral ligament. A longitudinally directed ellipse of capsule is then excised in this interval without destabilizing the joint. The offending osteophyte is located and removed with a small rongeur. The wound is closed with interrupted 6-0 plain catgut sutures. Rarely, a skin graft is required if the cyst has effaced a large area of dermis. Postoperatively the digit is splinted in extension for 10 to 14 days after which active motion is initiated. Infected cysts should be dealt with promptly since they are tantamount to septic arthritis. Appropriate antibiotic therapy should be instituted. Of note is the fact that mucous

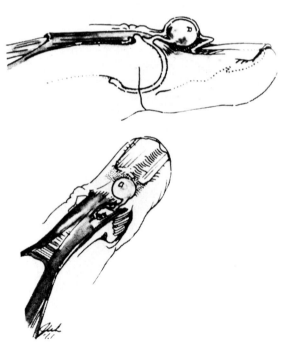

FIG. 10-8. Relationship between mucous cyst and a marginal osteophyte of distal interphalangeal joint. Note that cyst communicates with joint. This thin communication may become pinched off, but at some stage in development it is in direct communication with joint space. Marginal osteophyte produces attrition of extensor tendon expansion with motion. (From Eaton, R.G., et al.: J. Bone Joint Surg. **55A:**570, 1973.)

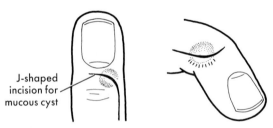

FIG. 10-9. J-shaped incision is preferred for treatment of mucous cyst.

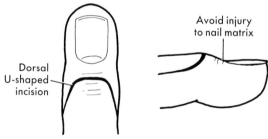

FIG. 10-10. U-shaped incision is used for arthrodesis of distal interphalangeal joint.

cysts are seen in joints that are only moderately involved with cartilage destruction and active motion of the joint is usually preserved.

In those joints that are severely destroyed and in which an unsightly or painful deformity exists, arthrodesis of the joint is the treatment of choice. Fusion can be performed through a dorsal U-shaped incision (Fig. 10-10). The incision is carried straight down to the extensor apparatus, which is incised and reflected with the flap. Collateral ligaments are released and a small burr is used to remove all remaining articular cartilage. Prominent osteophytes are removed to improve the cosmetic appearance of the digit. The alignment of the finger is then restored and fixed with a longitudinal Kirschner wire. The preferred position of arthrodesis in the index finger is at full extension with increasing amounts of flexion in the middle, ring, and small fingers not to exceed about 30 degrees. The extensor tendon is reapproximated with buried 5-0 Mersilene sutures and the skin is closed with 6-0 plain catgut. The joint is protected with a dorsal aluminum splint, leaving the proximal interphalangeal joint free to flex and extend. The Kirschner wire is retained for 8 weeks or until the joint shows radiographic evidence of bony union. The result is a stable, painfree, cosmetically acceptable finger that despite lack of motion, is extremely functional.

Arthritis of the proximal interphalangeal joint is more disabling because the large amount of motion inherent in this joint is required for accommodation in grasping objects of various sizes. Pain and deformity of a proximal interphalangeal joint that is unresponsive to conservative therapy are best treated by arthrodesis. The technique of arthrodesis is as follows: The joint is exposed through a dorsal straight midline or dorsal delta-shaped incision. The central slip is divided longitudinally in its midportion and reflected on either side of the joint. Care is taken not to detach the central slip from the middle phalanx because a significant disruption in the balance of the extensor mechanism will ensue (boutonniere deformity). The collateral ligaments are released

to provide adequate exposure of the joint. A small saw or burr is used to remove cartilage and a thin sliver of subchondral bone from the articular surface of the middle phalanx. A burr is used to remove articular cartilage from the condyles of the proximal phalanx; small portions of the condyles are removed with a fine saw. This cut determines the angle of flexion for the arthrodesis as well as correcting any radial or ulnar malalignment.

Considerable discussion should be made with the patient preoperatively regarding expectations, activities of daily living, and hobbies to determine the best functional compromise with regard to the position of the proximal interphalangeal joints. Basically the more ulnar joints are placed in more flexion. Again the joint is fixed with Kirschner wires; one longitudinal wire and one oblique wire to control rotation are usually sufficient. The closure is performed by reapproximating the extensor tendon with interrupted buried 5-0 Mersilene sutures and the skin is closed with fine nylon or plain 6-0 catgut. As with distal interphalangeal joints, immobilization and internal fixation are maintained for a minimum of 8 weeks or until bony union is perceived on x-ray films.

In cases where preservation of proximal interphalangeal joint function is essential to the patient, implant arthroplasty may be utilized at the expense of some weakness or mild instability. Swanson's technique for silicone implant arthroplasty is followed.[19] A more recently developed prosthesis using an elastomeric rubber hinge with titanium stems, requiring acrylic cement for fixation, has shown some preliminary promise for increased range of motion and stability over the Silastic component.[8] However, the requirements for cement and difficulties associated with revisions for either implant failure or infection must be weighed against these potential advantages.

Degenerative arthritis of the thumb metacarpophalangeal joint is seen less frequently than interphalangeal and thumb basal joint arthritis. If severe, it is best treated by arthrodesis of the joint using a technique similar to that described for the proximal interphalangeal joints of the fingers. However, a portion of the metacarpal condyle is used as a peg bone graft. Arthrodesis of the thumb metacarpophalangeal joint provides excellent stability and function as long as there is preservation of interphalangeal and basal joint motion.

Surgical treatment of basal joint arthritis that has failed to respond to conservative therapy as outlined above may be divided into three basic procedures: (1) excision, (2) arthrodesis, (3) arthroplasty.

Excision involves removal of the trapezium with resection of the metacarpal into the defect left by the trapezium so that it now articulates with the scaphoid. Although stability and pain relief can be achieved with this procedure, relative lengthening of the intrinsic musculature to the thumb by shortening of the bony architecture of the first ray leads to weakness and mild cosmetic deformity that may be unacceptable in many female patients.

Arthrodesis of the metacarpal to the trapezium in a position of 35 to 40 degrees of palmar abduction and 20 degrees of radial abduction (fist position) provides a painfree stable thumb if there is no evidence of scaphotrapezial degeneration.[14] This is a good operation for physically active men for whom power of grip and pinch are more important than fine motor control. However, many patients complain of an inability to bring the thumb ray into the plane of the remainder of the hand, especially when placing the hand on a table or pushing up from a flat surface. These points certainly must be discussed with the patient before arthrodesis is recommended.

In younger or middle-aged patients with isolated metacarpotrapezial arthritis, a fascial interposition arthroplasty with volar oblique ligament reconstruction, as advocated by Glickel, Eaton, and Littler[7] may be helpful. For severe disease involving pantrapezial arthritis and/or moderate to severe subluxation, I prefer excision of the trapezium with trapezium implant arthroplasty using a silicone prosthesis of the Eaton design.[3] Several points in the operative procedure bear special mention. First, care should be taken to avoid superficial branches of the radial nerve that ramify in the operative field and that are particularly prone to traumatic neuroma formation. Second, a slip of the abductor pollicis longus is utilized as an autogenous collagen suture when passed through the tunnel in the prosthesis to enhance stability and prevent dislocation. Meticulous capsular closure and prolonged postoperative immobilization with the Eaton type or the Swanson type of silicone rubber implant minimize the incidence of late dislocation.

The results of trapezium implant arthroplasty have been gratifying with excellent pain relief and good stability with functional motion. Grip and pinch strength return almost to normal levels with a postoperative program of graded exercises. These exercises along with pain relief and increased usage of the hand for daily activities often reverse the preoperative disuse atrophy of the thenar musculature.

RHEUMATOID ARTHRITIS

Although the onset of rheumatoid arthritis and related collagen vascular diseases such as systemic lupus erythematosus and psoriatic arthritis is usually seen in the younger or middle-aged population, the more severe deformities and late sequelae of these problems persist into the geriatric population. The manifestations of these illnesses in the hand are variable, ranging from extremely mild involvement to marked joint destruction and deformity. The older the patient with one of these illnesses is, the more likely the hands are to be involved. In contrast to the situation with osteoarthritis, complaints of stiffness, pain, weakness, and loss of function in the hands may bring the patient to seek medical attention before the involvement of the large weight-bearing joints. Despite marked deformities and functional losses in the hand as a result of rheumatoid arthritis, it is remarkable how these patients are able to cope with the activities of daily living by altering their life-style and the manner in which they use their hands.

It is beyond the scope of this chapter to delve deeply into the pathophysiology of collagen vascular diseases. Suffice it to say that there is an inflammatory response arising within the joint that involves an inappropriate response of the immune system to an antigen that has not yet been characterized but may be related to a previous viral infection. As a result of the intra-articular release of the by-products of immune reactions, such as immune complexes and lyzosomal and proteolytic enzymes, detrimental enzymatic effects are wrought on the articular cartilage. Proteoglycan content is diminished and collagen is degraded and weakened. A synovial proliferation called pannus extends out over articular cartilage, thus cutting it off from its normal synovial nutrition.

The release of proteolytic enzymes such as collagenase from cells involved in these immune reactions in concert with synovitis and synovial effusions weakens the capsular supporting structures, including ligaments, leading to joint instability. In the late phases, subluxation and frank dislocation of the joints as well as pain on any attempted motion result in deformity, loss of strength, and hence function.

In distinction to osteoarthritis, the pattern of joint involvement in the hand in rheumatoid arthritis is primarily one of metacarpophalangeal and proximal interphalangeal involvement. In many cases the wrist also is involved. Indeed, very early signs of rheumatoid disease may be detected in the distal radioulnar joint. The inflammatory process is not confined to the joints alone and may also involve the tenosynovial structures, most commonly in the extensor tendons and on the dorsum of the wrist as well as the flexor tendon synovium both in the fingers and within the carpal tunnel. The invasion of rheumatoid synovium within the substance of flexor and extensor tendons and also the release of enzymatic by-products may lead to tendon rupture.

Capsular instability involving the distal radioulnar joint may result in dorsal subluxation of the distal ulna. The sharp margins of rheumatoid bony erosions at the level of the distal ulna may further contribute to extensor tendon rupture with the exten-

sor digiti quinti, the common extensor of the small finger, and finally the ring finger rupturing sequentially. Rupture of the extensor digiti quinti is often not noticed by the patient, but it is a good sign that rupture of the extensors of the small and ring finger is impending and that surgical intervention is indicated.

The diagnosis of rheumatoid arthritis has usually been established before the patient is seen by the orthopaedist. However, occasionally patients with distal radioulnar joint arthritis, extensor tenosynovitis, or carpal tunnel syndrome will turn out to have rheumatoid arthritis. At this point in their presentation less than 70% will have a positive latex fixation test. The picture of bilaterally symmetrical metacarpophalangeal joint involvement with redness, swelling, active synovitis, stiffness, and loss of motion makes the clinical diagnosis more secure. Patients with lupus and psoriasis tend to have predominantly proximal interphalangeal joint involvement with relative sparing of the metacarpophalangeal joints. These patterns are in contrast to osteoarthritis where the distal interphalangeal joints are involved primarily. Thus, the pattern of joint involvement in the hand can be particularly helpful with regard to the diagnosis. In addition to joint and tendon synovitis, many rheumatoid arthritis patients have atrophy of the intrinsic muscles of the hand, the etiology of which is probably twofold. Many patients with rheumatoid arthritis, when given a careful neurologic and electrodiagnostic examination, are found to have peripheral neuropathy. Denervation of the small muscles of the hand, by virtue of this neuropathy, may result in atrophy. However, more commonly there is an atrophy resulting from disuse because of the pain and instability associated with power grasp and pinch in the rheumatoid hand.

Treatment of rheumatoid arthritis and related collagen vascular diseases is primarily medical and is best left to the direction of the rheumatologist. Suffice it to say that milder cases are usually managed with aspirin or one of the other nonsteroidal anti-inflammatory medications. The use of systemic corticosteroid preparations should be evaluated carefully with respect to the risk:benefit ratio afforded by these drugs because of their powerful anti-inflammatory effect as well as their central nervous system effect on generalized well-being. A rheumatoid arthritis patient once started on these drugs will seldom be able to discontinue them. All of the above medications provide only symptomatic relief. Only the use of gold salts has shown any ability to arrest the progression of the disease. The use of these medications with their potential toxic side effects should be given under the direction of a rheumatologist.

The orthopaedist, working in conjunction with the rheumatologist and an experienced occupational therapist, can help the patient by providing simple exercises to be used judiciously to maintain range of motion and muscle tone and also night resting splints to slow the progressive deformity of ulnar drift. Paraffin baths may also provide symptomatic relief. The surgical treatment of rheumatoid arthritic involvement in the hand is usually limited to severe end-stage deformity and disability with a few exceptions when prophylactic intervention is of extreme benefit. It should be emphasized that the goal of hand surgery in rheumatoid arthritis is primarily to restore function in the form of grasp, pinch, stability, and strength rather than to correct cosmetic deformities. It serves no purpose to the patient to take a hand that may be deformed and unattractive but capable of performing the patient's activities of daily living and converting it to an aesthetically pleasing hand that is unable to perform these vital functions. Preoperatively, the expectations and requirements of the patient should be examined in great detail before deciding which surgical procedure is to be done. An occupational therapist can be extremely helpful by performing a standardized assessment of activities of daily living; however, it is the responsibility of the operating surgeon, armed with the knowledge of the patient's specific requirements, to make the most therapeutic decision regarding surgery.

A multitude of surgical procedures have been developed for the rheumatoid hand. Again, it cannot be emphasized too strongly that the procedure to be performed should be tailored to the requirements of the patient. Those procedures that are somewhat prophylactic in nature involve synovectomy of the extensor tendons in the face of an impending tendon rupture. Those patients with impending tendon rupture often have significant involvement of the intercarpal and radiocarpal joints as well as the distal radioulnar joint; therefore, the procedure of dorsal stabilization as outlined by Straub and Ranawat[11] has been extremely successful as long as volar instability and radiocarpal subluxation have not yet occurred. The procedure involves a complete synovectomy of the extensor tendons with repair or reconstruction of any ruptured tendons. A limited distal ulnar resection with a capsular reconstruction to prevent dorsal subluxation of the ulna and a complete synovectomy of the radiocarpal and intercarpal joints through a dorsal approach with reconstruction of the dorsal capsule using the extensor retinaculum are also performed. Postoperatively patients enjoy a stable wrist with dramatic pain improvement. Although it is expected that they will lose some wrist motion, most patients retain motion within a functional arc of 45 to 60 degrees. Extensor tendon repairs or reconstructions must be immobilized appropriately during the healing period. The postoperative pronation and supination achieved are most gratifying.

For wrists with more severe involvement, including marked destructive changes, carpal collapse, volar subluxation, or dislocation of the carpus on the radius, a formal wrist arthrodesis or a wrist implant arthroplasty should be performed.

The efficacy of synovectomy for metacarpophalangeal joint involvement has not been uniformly established; therefore, surgery at this level is usually reserved for severe deformity with volar-ulnar dislocation of the metacarpophalangeal joints. The technique of Silastic implant arthroplasty as described by Swanson[19] is the most popularly utilized method of metacarpophalangeal reconstruction. Specific attention must be paid to the release of tight ulnar intrinsic tendons to reduce ulnar deforming forces as well as to allow proximal interphalangeal flexion. Swanson stresses reconstruction of a radial collateral ligament, particularly on the index finger, and centralization of the extensor tendons over the axis of metacarpophalangeal flexion with extensor hood reconstructions. Fixed "swan neck" deformities at the proximal interphalangeal joints are best treated by arthrodesis.

Similar surgical reconstructions are available for the thumb involved with rheumatoid arthritis. Some of these are discussed in the section on osteoarthritis. The use of implant arthroplasty at the basal joint with arthrodesis at the metacarpophalangeal joint gives the most reliable results. Where metacarpophalangeal joint motion is required, such as in patients with previously arthrodesed interphalangeal or basal joints, implant arthroplasty of the Silastic or Biomeric types is most effective.

It should also be emphasized that the results achieved with hand surgery in rheumatoid arthritis patients are also to a large extent dependent on the postoperative treatment plan, which in most cases involves a formal program of rehabilitation therapy under the supervision of a hand or occupational therapist.

TENOSYNOVITIS

Tenosynovitis is an inflammation of the synovial sheathed tendons, which is seen commonly in the hand. It begins primarily in the fifth decade but may be seen in older persons especially when it has become chronic. It is seen more commonly in women than in men and may be related temporally to menopause.[10] It is found both in extensor and flexor tendon groups about the hand and wrist in areas where a tendon passes through a fibrous or fibro-osseous tunnel or pulley. The etiology is uncertain. It has been related to repetitive muscle tendon activities and to activities that require forced resistive motions. It is probably most frequently seen in persons performing a

task or motion for which they have not been previously acclimated or conditioned. In addition, in the elderly population tenosynovitis may be related to degenerative or ischemic changes in the tendon.

Patients initially have pain and on occasion locking or clicking referable to the affected tendon system. They often feel that this is the onset of arthritis and are relieved when reassured that this is not an arthritic process. However, tenosynovitis can be associated with rheumatoid arthritis and indeed may be an initial sign of rheumatoid arthritis. Patients often complain of stiffness in the morning that improves gradually with use and exercise. In many cases there is a grating, crepitant sensation or locking, as in trigger finger. There may be evidence of mild inflammation with thickening and swelling along the course of the synovial portion of the tendon sheath and this is associated with mild tenderness. In acute cases, often seen in the younger population, marked swelling, redness, tenderness, and a diminished range of motion can be seen. This may be contrasted to the more chronic appearance of tenosynovitis in the older population. A discussion of specific syndromes now follows.

Trigger finger is probably the most common form of tenosynovitis in the hand. Strictly speaking this is a stenosing flexor tenosynovitis characterized by stiffness and decreased range of motion both in flexion and extension of the involved digit, which is related to synovial inflammation of the flexor tendon sheath in the region of the A-1 pulley. The patient may just have pain and mild stiffness or in full-blown cases there will be locking of the digit. The finger may lock in extension so that the patient is unable to make a full fist or, more characteristically, the finger may lock in flexion and often passive manipulation will be required for regaining extension. The action of locking and passive manipulation to obtain the extended position is quite painful. Palpation will usually reveal crepitation along the course of the flexor sheath at the base of the proximal phalanx and in the palm. Gentle passive flexion and extension of the finger while palpating the volar palm in the region of the A-1 pulley often will reveal tenderness and crepitation.

Pathologic findings show a loss of the normal shiny, glistening quality of the tendon. Instead it is opaque and somewhat yellowed. There is an increase in the volume of tenosynovium present, which instead of being thin and flexible is thickened and adherent especially in the region of the bifurcation of the flexor digitorum superficialis where it is closely related to the profundus. In addition, there is thickening of the metacarpophalangeal (A-1) pulley with some degeneration and scarring seen histologically. Occasionally, small ganglia arise in the interval between the A-1 and A-2 pulleys.

Because of the relationship of the bifurcation of the superficialis tendon, the profundus tendon, and the A-1 pulley, patients who have the inability to make a full fist can often demonstrate the triggering phenomena by taking advantage of differential gliding of the two tendon systems.

The patient is asked first to flex the proximal interphalangeal joint only of the affected finger while holding the remaining fingers in extension (flexor superficialis test). When active flexion of this joint is full, the patient is then asked to make a full tight fist using the profundi. When the patient is then asked to extend the finger slowly, the affected finger will be locked in flexion and may require passive manipulation to regain extension. Such a test clearly localizes the difficulty to the flexor tendon sheath. However, it is important to make sure that the inability to flex or extend the finger fully is not related to an intrinsic joint contracture or to other soft tissue contractures such as Dupuytren's disease. This can be confirmed by demonstrating full passive motion of the joint both in flexion and in extension by relieving the contracture with the metacarpophalangeal joint flexed.

The presenting symptoms, signs, and pathophysiology of the trigger thumb are identical to those of trigger finger except that the thumb is a one-tendon system involving the flexor pollicis longus.

The next most common area of tenosynovitis about the hand and wrist occurs in the extensor system at the fibro-osseous tunnel of the first dorsal compartment. This is known by the eponym of de Quervain's disease and, like trigger finger, it is associated with an inflammation in the region where the abductor pollicis longus and extensor pollicis brevis traverse a fibro-osseous tunnel at the radial styloid. The patient complains of pain localized at the radial styloid, which may radiate proximally into the forearm or distally into the thumb. Symptoms are aggravated by motions that require forced abduction extension of the thumb ray, such as reaching behind the back as to scratch the back or to release a brassiere hook. Patients also are symptomatic with motions that require setting or stabilizing the wrist in radial deviation, such as in lifting a heavy pot or skillet off the stove.

Physical findings include tenderness and swelling in the region of the radial styloid. In acute cases there may be swelling and edema proximal to the first dorsal compartment. In chronic cases, however, there is a firm, hard swelling directly in the area of the first compartment, which is related to fibrosis and thickening of the fibrous portion of the tunnel. There may also be synovial cysts or degeneration of the tunnel so as to produce a ganglion.

Tenosynovitis in the other extensor tendons of the wrist is considerably less common. Occasionally the extensor pollicis longus may be involved in the region where it traverses Lister's tubercle. Inflammation and an attrition rupture of the extensor pollicis longus is a well-described complication of Colles' fracture and is discussed under that heading. Inflammation of the radial wrist extensors and the extensor digitorum communis may occur on an idiopathic basis; however, they are more commonly associated with rheumatoid synovitis. Inflammation of the extensor carpi ulnaris where it traverses its fibro-osseous sheath in relation to the head of the ulna has also been seen. The treatment of tenosynovitis depends on whether the process is an acute or chronic one. Acute involvement, characterized by swelling, edema, redness, or tenderness, is often responsive to immobilization using splints, systemic anti-inflammatory medication (either aspirin or nonsteroidal anti-inflammatory preparations), or injection of corticosteroid preparations into the tendon sheath proper. A combination of all of these modalities may be utilized in severe cases.

The two-syringe technique is preferred as the technique for injection of tendon sheaths. I use two tuberculin-type syringes with 25-gauge ⅜-inch needles. One syringe is filled with 0.5 ml of a local anesthetic, such as 1% lidocaine (Xylocaine) or mepivacaine (Carbocaine), and the second syringe is filled with between 0.5 and 1.0 ml of 4 mg/ml dexamethasone. Dexamethasone is preferred over methylprednisolone acetate for the injection of tendon sheaths because it avoids the deposition of an *insoluble* vehicle within the tendon sheaths, which could cause a late chemical synovitis.

The technique for injection of a trigger finger is as follows: The hand is prepared in a sterile fashion with either a povidone-iodine (Betadine) solution or alcohol. The needle containing the local anesthetic is then introduced into the digital palmar crease in the midline. It is angled obliquely from a distal to proximal direction. The bevel of the needle is kept parallel to the long axis of the tendon. Intrathecal location can be verified by removing the syringe from the needle hub and asking the patient to produce a minimal excursion of the flexor tendon. With this maneuver the needle is observed to toggle slightly. The syringe is then relocated to the hub and is withdrawn very slowly while gentle pressure on the plunger is maintained. The local anesthetic will be found to flow freely into the synovial space and its flow proximal to the A-1 pulley in the palm can be perceived with a palpating finger. Only enough lidocaine is injected to confirm intrathecal location. The syringe is then removed from the hub and the dexamethasone is instilled in a similar fashion. Again confirmation of intrathecal location is made by palpating proximal to the A-1 pulley and by the ease of flow of the solution. A digital flexor tendon sheath will usually not accommodate

more than 1 ml of solution. Difficulty in depressing the plunger indicates that the point of the needle is probably in the tendon and that the needle should be pulled back further. If the needle is pulled back too far and is brought out of the sheath and into the subcutaneous tissue, a local subcutaneous swelling will result and palpation of fluid proximal to the A-1 pulley will not be perceived. Following completion of the injection, the patient is asked to bring the fingers through a full range of motion to distribute the medication throughout the sheath. Because of the increased volume of fluid in the sheath, full motion is often not possible and the patient may have the sensation of fullness in the finger. However, the initial pain should be completely eliminated by the lidocaine injection. If not, the proper location for the injection has not been found.

Although some authors use splints following injection of a trigger finger, I have not found this to be particularly helpful. I encourage active but not strenuous range of motion activities and caution the patient that the locking phenomenon may take several weeks to resolve if indeed the injection is successful. Injection of a trigger thumb is performed in a similar fashion just distal to the metacarpophalangeal pulley using the same precautions as outlined for injection of a trigger finger. Injection of the first dorsal compartment for de Quervain's tenosynovitis again follows the same basic principles as outlined for trigger finger. The injection is placed just distal to the first compartment. The flow of the solution may be perceived proximal to the fibro-osseous tunnel. With de Quervain's disease a lightweight thumb-forearm splint is often helpful in immobilizing the thumb.

CARPAL TUNNEL SYNDROME

Carpal tunnel syndrome may be defined as a compression neuropathy of the median nerve at the wrist where it passes beneath the transverse carpal ligament along with the flexor tendons. Although the syndrome has its onset in middle age, often it is not diagnosed by the physician until considerably later in life at which time the symptoms and signs may be severe. Patients usually come to the physician with complaints of weakness, clumsiness of the hand, paresthesias in the fingers, and numbness in the fingertips. Pain at the wrist extending into the fingers of the hand is often reported. These symptoms may be acute in onset, which is most characteristic of the disease earlier in life. Such acute onset is often associated with pregnancy or the onset of rheumatoid arthritis. In the elderly age group, however, the onset is usually insidious with almost imperceptible changes that are not realized until the disease is well advanced. A frequent complaint is pain and numbness awakening the individual from sleep or on arising in the morning. This may or may not be relieved by shaking the hands. In some cases the pain may radiate proximally into the forearm. The syndrome is found more frequently in women than in men with a ratio of 2:1. Over half of the patients with carpal tunnel syndrome are between the ages of 40 and 60 years.

The etiology of carpal tunnel syndrome is not completely certain. It has been associated with hypothyroidism, diabetes mellitus, acromegaly, and rheumatoid arthritis. It is a common complication following Colles' fracture. In all cases, however, increased pressure within the confined dimensions of the carpal tunnel because of flexor tenosynovitis or hypertrophy of the transverse carpal ligament or alterations in the bony architecture secondary to fracture or dislocation create pressure and relative ischemia of the median nerve at that point. Idiopathic carpal tunnel syndrome is associated with flexor tenosynovitis at the wrist and is seen in a population similar to that for trigger finger. Pathologic changes in the nerve include local ischemia, local fibrosis, and narrowing at the nerve at the level of the transverse carpal ligament with dilatation proximal to that point. A diagnosis can be made in most instances by a history of numbness, tingling, and paresthesias in the digits innervated by the median nerve. The long finger is most commonly cited for complaints. Occasion-

ally pain may be referred to the small finger. Objective findings of decreased pseudomotor activity and fine touch sensibility, however, are limited to the median-innervated digits. Atrophy of the thenar muscles (abductor pollicis brevis and opponens pollicis), which are innervated by the median nerve, are often seen in long-standing, chronic cases. What has been referred to as Tinel's sign is a sensation perceived as paresthesias distally in the median nerve distribution following percussion over the nerve just proximal to the wrist flexion crease. This is a reflection of irritability of the nerve from either a neurapractic or a neurotemetic lesion as a result of compression neuropathy. It is more prominent early in the disease and is often absent in chronic cases.

Phalen's sign, which is the onset of paresthesias in the median distribution within 60 seconds following acute volar flexion of the wrist, is a fairly reliable and specific sign for carpal tunnel syndrome. Other compression neuropathies of the median nerve either at the cervical level or in the forearm (pronator syndrome) must be looked for and ruled out. When any question exists, physical findings can be confirmed by nerve conduction and electromyographic testing. This is especially helpful in discriminating between cervical lesions and more distal compression neuropathies and is done by comparing the distal palmar latency, that is, the sensory latency distal to the transverse carpal ligament with that proximal to the transverse carpal ligament. The diagnosis of surgically correctable carpal tunnel syndrome in patients with peripheral diabetic neuropathy can be made using this technique.[4]

The treatment of carpal tunnel syndrome depends on the stage in which it is diagnosed and the etiologic factors. In cases resulting from an endocrine disturbance, all efforts should be made to rectify that disturbance (such as replacement of thyroid hormone) since in most cases this leads to the resolution of symptoms. In acute, idiopathic cases resting splints that keep the wrist in the extended position and avoid the marked volar flexion attitude often adopted during sleep can be extremely helpful, especially in reducing symptoms at night or on arising in the morning. Oral anti-inflammatory medications including nonsteriodal and short courses of corticosteroid preparations have also been reported as helpful. Recent reports of treatment with pyridoxine (vitamin B_6) have given mixed results.[4] In those cases where thenar atrophy is present or electromyographic studies reveal denervation potentials in the median-innervated intrinsic muscles of the hand, a neurotemetic lesion must be postulated and surgical intervention is indicated. Surgery is also indicated for those individuals who do not respond to the conservative treatments outlined above.

INFECTION

Although as a general rule the hand is relatively resistant to infection, infections do occur in all age groups. The hand is the most frequently injured part of the body and it is surprising that infections are not more common. Although infections do involve all age groups, certain types of infections in the hand occur with increasing frequency in the elderly population. As might be expected, these are often seen with increased frequency in those individuals with a se-

vere debilitating illness or alterations in the immune system because of disease or chemotherapy.

Paronychia is most commonly seen in this group. It is an abscess of the periungual soft tissues on the dorsum of the finger and involves the area adjacent to the lateral nail border and may extend superficially or deep to the germinal matrix. It is almost uniformly a staphylococcal infection and quite commonly results following inoculation after the manipulation of the cuticle at the time of a manicure. Although antibiotics may be helpful in controlling cellulitis and localizing the abscess, the treatment, as with any other abscess, is surgical drainage. Fig. 10-11 shows several methods of making the incision for drainage. I prefer incision 1, which utilizes excision of an ellipse of skin to prevent premature wound closure and obviates the requirements for a drain. Healing following this incision is remarkably cosmetic.

Chronic paronychial infections with fungal or mixed bacterial flora may be encountered in chronically ill or debilitated patients or in patients with altered sensibility in the hand as a result of peripheral nerve or spinal cord injury. In many of these cases, a true abscess cannot be localized. They are also frequently found in people who are continuously immersing their

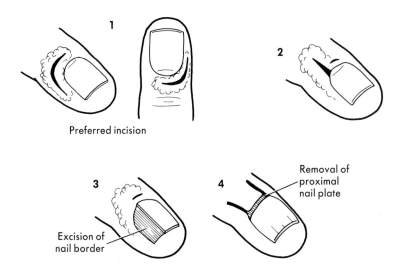

FIG. **10-11.** Incisions for drainage of paronychia.

hands in water, which provides a moist environment for these facultative organisms to reproduce. In these cases, the eponychial fold and cuticle are often found to be receded, thus eliminating the normal barrier to collection of detritus and bacteria in the eponychial fold. I find it most effective to keep the finger dry and uncovered and to apply a clear tincture of iodine solution to the nail fold 2 to 3 times daily. Not only does the iodine kill yeast and fungi, but also the alcohol in the tincture preparation promotes drying of the area. Recalcitrant cases are best treated by the marsupialization method as described for acute paronychia.

A less common but more serious infection of the fingertip involves the volar pulp of the fingertip and is called a felon. The felon is an abscess that arises in the pulp of the fingertip following inoculation by a puncture wound (often from a sewing needle or pin) and it is extremely painful. Pus develops under pressure in the specialized

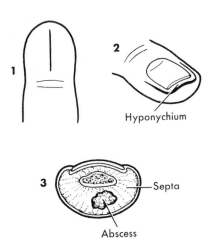

Fig. 10-12. Incisions for surgical treatment of felon.

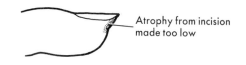

Fig. 10-13. Deformity caused by improperly treated felon.

pulp of the fingertip, which is divided into small compartments by connective tissue septa extending from the terminal phalanx to the skin. For this reason a neglected or improperly treated felon can result in osteomyelitis with erosion of the terminal tuft. The treatment of the felon is surgical. Fig. 10-12 shows the two incisions that I prefer. Incision 1 is used for felons pointing in the midsubstance of the pulp. Incision 2 is used for more diffuse involvement of the entire pulp space. In both cases it is extremely important to release all of the septa to drain the abscess adequately and to prevent persistence of infection. Special care must be taken when making incision 2 so that the transverse limb across the tip of the finger is made at the level of the hyponychium as indicated in the drawing. Incisions made volar to this will result in atrophy of the pulp between the hyponychium and the incision causing marked deformity (Fig. 10-13).

A word should be mentioned about distinguishing herpetic whitlow, a viral infection of the fingertip simulating a felon, from the true felon. Herpetic whitlow is treated nonoperatively. Fluid-filled vesicles characteristic of a herpes viral infection confirm the diagnosis of this condition, which is most commonly seen in dental hygienists. It will resolve spontaneously over a 7- to 10-day course.

True infections of the flexor tendon sheaths are extremely rare and they are almost always secondary to puncture wounds or animal bites. The diagnosis is suspected by the presence of Kanavel's four signs,[9] which are (1) excessive tenderness over the course of the sheath, limited to the sheath; (2) symmetrical enlargement of the whole finger; (3) excruciating pain on extending the finger, most marked at the proximal end; (4) flexion of the finger. The treatment is immediate surgical decompression of the tendon sheath at both the proximal and distal limits with insertion of continuous irrigating catheters. Prompt intervention and adequate drainage is necessary to prevent septic necrosis of the tendon and subsequent rupture.

VASCULAR-RELATED PROBLEMS

Vascular-related problems in upper extremities are rare and they are certainly less common than the problems caused by peripheral vascular disease involving the lower extremities. However, vascular-related problems do occur in certain instances in the upper extremity. One such problem is Raynaud's phenomenon, which is a peripheral vasospastic disease characterized by marked sensitivity to cold, although other stimuli may also trigger the phenomenon. The phenomenon consists of marked blanching of the skin secondary to arteriospasm and cessation of inflow to the affected extremity. This is associated with intense pain and occasionally numbness and tingling, and it may last for several minutes. This initial phase is followed by a second phase consisting of relaxation of the vascular spasm and postischemic reflex hyperemia during which time the extremity appears suffused and erythematous in color. The phenomenon may be limited to single digits or it may involve the entire hand. Exposure to cold is the most common inciting factor. Such minor exposures as removing frozen food from the freezer may bring on this reaction. It is often associated with systemic diseases such as systemic lupus erythematosus, scleroderma, and collagen vascular disease. There is also an idiopathic variety.

The sequelae of repeated episodes of ischemia of the fingertips include decreased sensitivity as a result of ischemic nerve damage. In some cases, where ischemia is prolonged, necrosis of the fingertip resulting in dry gangrene may ensue. In less severe cases, chronic changes in the fingernail and pulp atrophy may occur.

Treatment is aimed at prevention of exposure to cold stimuli. Patients are advised to wear mittens rather than gloves and to be particularly careful in handling of frozen foods. Peripheral vasodilators, including a recent medication, nifedipine, have been shown to be helpful in some cases. Surgical sympathectomy has been advocated by others. Usually, a good response to a local anesthetic blockade at the wrist is indicative of a good response to sympathectomy. Although the classic approach has been to perform a central sympathectomy with a section at the level of the superior cervical ganglion, more recently Flatt[5] has described a digital sympathectomy that is performed in the palm. It involves a microdissection of the adventitia of the common digital arteries to the involved fingers both proximal and distal to the level of bifurcation into the proper volar digital arteries. Initial results with this technique have been promising with an increase in fingertip temperature and healing of trophic ulcers. The long-term benefit remains to be seen.

Volkmann's ischemic contracture is the late sequela of a compartment syndrome in the forearm of the upper extremity. Although this entity is more common following supracondylar fractures in children, it does exist in the geriatric population and is most often related to prolonged compression of the arm or forearm in patients who have been lying on the arm as a result of a drug overdose or cerebrovascular accident. Other causes of the syndrome can be an intravenous infusion that infiltrates deep to the antebrachial fascia or postoperative or postfracture swelling within the confines of a tight circular plaster dressing. In each case, an increase in the pressure within the confined fascial space of the forearm is created, which tends to collapse thin-walled veins and thus obstruct the venous outflow. As a result of venous outflow obstruction and persistent arterial inflow, additional edema within the compartment ensues until the tissue pressure exceeds that of the mean arterial pressure. At such a time the flow of oxygenated blood to the contents of the compartment, including muscle and nerve, is compromised and permanent ischemic damage follows.[18] Experimental studies have determined that irreversible changes take place after 8 hours of ischemia that lead to infarction of muscle. Infarcted, edematous muscle is slowly replaced by fibrous tissue leading to a scarred contracture of the flexor groups in the forearm and the characteristic posture of the affected extremity (Fig. 10-14).

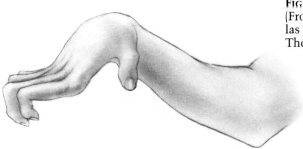

FIG. 10-14. Volkmann's ischemic contracture. (From Goldstein, L.A., and Dickerson, R.C.: Atlas of orthopaedic surgery, ed. 2, St. Louis, 1981, The C.V. Mosby Co.)

The treatment of compartment syndrome in the upper extremity in the elderly is first one of early recognition. The index of suspicion for this syndrome should be high for any patient who has a history of lying dependent on the extremity for a long period of time. The primary symptom is pain that is out of proportion to what should be expected for that patient. Unfortunately, patients with drug overdoses or global cerebrovascular accidents are unable to give an adequate history. However, in such patients the hand will be noted to be maintained in a position of flexion both at the wrist and at the fingers. The forearm is usually swollen and may be tense. Attempts at passive extension of the fingers are met with resistance and guarding, which may produce pain or withdrawal in the semiconscious patient. Pulselessness and pallor in the affected extremity are late findings. One should not wait for the occurrence of these findings to initiate treatment. Paresthesias in the distribution of the nerves running through the affected compartment may also be present as well as loss of sensation. Again, these are relatively late findings.

The treatment of impending Volkmann's ischemia is surgical. Recent authors have suggested the use of intracompartmental pressure readings using various types of catheters.[15] The finding of pressures greater than 30 mm of mercury or 20 mm over the diastolic blood pressure have been advocated as guidelines to determine when to decompress surgically the compartment.[20] Decompression involves a fasciotomy performed through an incision from the medial epicondyle to the carpal tunnel at the wrist.

The deep antebrachial fascia is incised the length of the wound. The muscles within the compartment are also explored and epimysiotomies are also performed, if necessary, to relieve pressure on individual muscle bellies. Before decompression, the muscle bellies appear pale and somewhat tan in color. After decompression, assuming that it has been done before the onset of irreversible changes, a return of normal color to the muscle with active bleeding will be noted. In addition, there will be marked edema in the muscle so that the wound cannot be closed. Attempts should not be made to try to close this wound; rather it should be left open. Protruding muscle may be covered either with a nonadherent dressing or with a split-thickness, meshed skin graft. Secondary closure of the wound or contracture of the split graft may be utilized to bring the skin edges together. Postoperative rehabilitation following early detection and closed treatment will ensure a remarkable functional recovery. It is beyond the scope of this chapter to discuss the treatment of those cases that have gone on to complete ischemic necrosis of the muscle. The reader is referred to a text on reconstructive hand surgery for this purpose.

One additional new problem seen commonly in those in the geriatric age group who are receiving systemic chemotherapy for malignant tumors is the extravasation of antineoplastic agents into the soft tissues during intravenous administration. The most notorious offender is doxorubicin. The toxic effects of this agent will rapidly lead to a full-thickness necrosis of the overlying skin with a marked delay in wound-healing ability and the ability of the bed to accept skin grafts. This has been related to the discovery that insoluble crystals of doxorubicin remain in the subcutaneous tissues and inhibit wound healing. The treatment for infiltration of this agent is a prompt surgical incision of the area of infiltration with full irrigation of the wounds. An ultraviolet (Wood's) lamp may be utilized to aid in the detection of crystals in the subcutaneous tissue.[2,13]

SPASTIC HEMIPLEGIA

Spastic hemiplegia is unfortunately an all too common residual of a cerebrovascular accident or a mass lesion in the central nervous system in the elderly patient. Proper management of this complication remains one of early prevention. Cerebral deficits involving upper motor neuron lesions initially leave the patient with a flaccid paralysis. However, this is invariably followed over a variable period of time by gradually increasing spasticity as a consequence of the release of cortical inhibitory control over the spinal cord anterior horn cells. The degree of deficit is directly related to the amount of cortex involved since the cortical representation for a given extremity increases as one goes distally in the extremity. It is statistically more likely that the distal functions comprised of multiple muscle tendon units and fine control, including the intrinsic musculature of the hand, will be more severely affected than the proximal functions. Fine motor function is also severely impaired, leaving the patient only with gross function in the affected extremity.

The characteristic posture of the patient with the spastic hemiparesis is one of adduction of the shoulder with slight internal rotation. The elbow is held in a flexed position. The forearm is pronated and the wrist flexed. Fingers are held in a clenched fist position and the thumb is adducted into the palm.

The most important therapeutic intervention for the musculoskeletal system in these unfortunate patients is the institution of early intervention. The physical and occupational therapists should encourage active and passive range-of-motion exercises, instruct in sensory reeducation, and fabricate resting splints to maintain the hand and wrist in a functional position. Regardless of the prognosis for recovery, splinting is important to prevent the occurrence of fixed joint deformities that are not only aesthetically unpleasing but also may interfere with the hygiene of the patient.

REFLEX SYMPATHETIC DYSTROPHY

Reflex sympathetic dystrophy, also known as Sudeck's atrophy or causalgia, is a vasomotor dysfunction in the upper extremity that is characterized by pain, swelling, discoloration, and stiffness in the hand and forearm. It is most commonly seen after trauma to the extremity; however, the trauma may be of a trivial nature. It is most commonly seen following Colles' fracture in the elderly age group; it may also be seen after a minor hand surgery such as trigger finger release or carpal tunnel release.

Reflex sympathetic dystrophy should be suspected in patients who have pain out of proportion to the inciting trauma. They often complain of a burning sensation with painful paresthesias to light touch. These begin first as localized phenomena that then become generalized to the entire upper extremity. There are often swelling, stiffness, brawny edema, and loss of the normal skin wrinkles. The skin may appear shiny. This is followed in the late stages by fibrosis of the subcutaneous tissues as well as of the pericapsular structures, which results in joint stiffness. There may be discoloration in the extremity and changes in sudomotor activity. Late stages also reveal osteoporosis on x-ray films and atrophy of normal subcutaneous fat. Lankford[12] has described three stages in the progression of reflex sympathetic dystrophy. The first stage occurs between 1 and 3 months after the onset of the inciting incident. The patient is noted to have pain and edema that diminishes with elevation. There is often periarticular redness around the metacarpophalangeal and proximal interphalangeal joints. There is increased sweating noted on the palm, and the skin is cool to the touch. Motion is diminished because of the pain, and there is the beginning of demineralization on radiographs.

Stage 2 may begin as early as 3 months but is usually seen 9 to 12 months after the inciting incident. This is a period of maximum pain in the extremity, and the pain is especially aggravated by motion. There is brawny edema that does not diminish despite adequate elevation. The rubor seen in the extremity in stage 1 is replaced by pallor and cyanosis. Sweating gives way to dryness of the skin with increased stiffness of the skin and subcutaneous tissue. Periarticular thickening and atrophy of the skin and subcutaneous tissues diminish the range of motion of the joint. Increased bone demineralization and osteoporosis are also seen.

Stage 3 may occur several months to years following the inciting incident. By this time pain has decreased somewhat as has the edema, which is replaced by fibrosis especially around joint capsular structures. Atrophy of the skin and subcutaneous tissues is well established. There is usually a loss of the normal flexion creases. The skin is dry and cool and there is marked stiffness and pain with any attempted passive motion. Osteoporosis is well established.

Involvement of the hand may also lead to problems in the ipsilateral shoulder with adhesive capsulitis and decreased motion. This has been referred to as the shoulder-hand syndrome and is more prominent in women than in men.

The precise etiology of reflex sympathetic dystrophy is unknown. It is thought that there may be a "short circuit" within the central or peripheral nervous system that sets up a spontaneous reflex sympathetic arc. There appear to be three requirements for the disease: (1) an inciting, painful episode; (2) a diathesis or predisposition; (3) the establishment of an abnormal sympathetic reflex.

The primary criteria for diagnosis are pain, swelling, stiffness, and discoloration.

Secondary criteria include osseous demineralization, pseudomotor changes, changes in skin temperature, trophic skin changes, vasomotor instability, and palmar fibrosis.

The treatment of reflex sympathetic dystrophy depends on early recognition of the problem. As discussed above, it should be considered whenever a patient's pain and concern for the extremity is out of proportion to the injury received. Sympathetic stellate ganglion blocks with local anesthetics are occasionally helpful in the early stages. Phenoxybenzamine (Dibenzyline), an alpha receptor blocker, in dosages of 10 mg 1 to 4 times daily, has also been shown to be helpful.[6] Most important, however, is the removal of any current painful stimuli, the most common of which is probably a cast that is too tight. The presence of a neuroma resulting from a minor superficial laceration may be an inciting stimulus. Mood-modifying drugs such as amitriptyline (Elavil) are also sometimes helpful. It is important to disrupt the vicious cycle by eliminating any painful stimuli.

The therapy for the affected extremity is also particularly important to maintain tone and range of motion and to prevent atrophy and demineralization. Therapists, however, should be instructed to use extreme caution and not to inflict any pain on the patient as this will only promote the abnormal reflex. Passive motion should be avoided except when performed by the patient himself. Active exercises and massage are the mainstay of treatment modalities. Local heat is often helpful in increasing active motion. However, whirlpools, which may cause dependent edema, are to be avoided.

Only cases that are detected and treated early have a good prognosis. Unfortunately, most cases are detected well into the second stage of the disease and these usually require a protracted course of therapy and pharmacologic intervention often lasting more than 18 months. In severe cases some patients may be left with a completely functionless extremity.

References

1. Behraus, F., Shepard N., and Mitchell, N.: Alteration of rabbit articular cartilage by intra-articular injections of glucocorticoids, J. Bone Joint Surg. **57A:**70-76, 1975.
2. Cohen, F.J., Manganaro, J., and Bezozo, R.C.: Identification of involved tissue during surgical treatment of doxorubicin-induced extravasation necrosis, J. Hand. Surg. **8:**43-45, 1983.
3. Eaton, R.G.: Replacement of the trapezium for arthritis of the basal articulations, J. Bone Joint Surg. **61A:**76-82, 1979.
4. Ellis, J.M., et al.: Response of vitamin B6 deficiency and the carpal tunnel syndrome to pyridoxine, Proc. Nat. Acad. Sci. **79**(23):7494-7498, 1982.
5. Flatt, A.W.: Digital artery sympathectomy, J. Hand Surg. **5:**550-556, 1980.
6. Fowler, F.D., and Moser, M.: Use of hexamethonium and dibenzyline in diagnosis and treatment of causalgia, JAMA **1611:**1051-1053, 1956.
7. Glickel, S.Z., Eaton, R.G., and Littler, J.W.: Ligamentous reconstruction with interposition arthroplasty for arthritis of the carpometacarpal joint of the hand, Presented at the American Society for Surgery of the Hand 38th Annual Meeting, Anaheim, California, March 9, 1983.
8. Heiple, K.G., Lacey S.H., and Idziknowski, C.: Preliminary experience with the biomeric finger joint prosthesis, Presented at the American Society for Surgery of the Hand 39th Annual Meeting, Atlanta, Feb. 8, 1984.
9. Kanavel, A.B.: Infections of the hand, Philadelphia, 1933, Lea & Febiger, p. 364.
10. Kelsey, J.L.: Epidemiology of musculoskeletal disorders, New York, 1982, Oxford University Press, p. 172.
11. Kulich, R.G., DeFiore, J.C., Straub, L.S., and Ranawat, C.S.: Long term results of dorsal stabilization in the rheumatoid wrist, J. Hand Surg. **6:**272-280, 1981.
12. Lankford, L.L.: Reflex sympathetic dystrophy. In Green, D., ed.: Operative hand surgery, New York, 1982, Churchill Livingstone, p. 539.
13. Linder, R.M., Upton, J., and Osteen, R.: Management of extensive doxorubicin hydrochloride extravasation injuries, J. Hand Surg. **8:**32-38, 1983.
14. Littler, J.W.: The hand and upper extremity. In Converse, J.M., ed. Reconstructive plastic surgery, Vol. 6, Philadelphia, 1977, W.B. Saunders Co., p. 3115.
15. Mubarak, S.J., et. al.: The wick catheter technique for measurement of intramuscular pressure, J. Bone Joint Surg., **58A:**1016-1020, 1976.
16. Rodin, E.L., Parker, H.G., and Paul, I.L: Pattern of degenerative arthritis: preferential involvement of distal finger joints, Lancet **1:**377-379, 1971.
17. Rodnan, G.P., Schumacher, H.R., and Zvaifler, N.J., eds.: Primer on the rheumatic diseases, ed. 8, Atlanta, 1983, Arthritis Foundation, p. 105.
18. Sarokhan, A.J., and Eaton, R.G.: Volkman's ischemia, J. Hand Surg. **8:**806-809, 1983.
19. Swanson, A.B.: Flexible implant resection arthroplasty in the hand and extremities, St. Louis, 1973, The C.V. Mosby Co., pp. 160-170.
20. Whitesides, T.E., Haney, T.C., Morimoto, K., and Hirada, H.: Tissue pressure measurements as a determinant for the need of fasciotomy, Clin. Orthop. **113:**43-51, 1975.

chapter 11
THE LUMBAR SPINE

Thomas P. Sculco

The spine is a common site of severe disability in the geriatric patient. As in other areas of the musculoskeletal system in the elderly, afflictions of the spine are superimposed on biologic changes occurring as part of the aging process. Diseases that affect the locomotor system in general also produce dysfunction in the spine, and in the lumbar area degenerative problems predominate. Disorders of the cervical spine and metabolic disorders, particularly osteoporosis, that commonly affect the spine have been discussed in other areas of this text.

It is a frequent complaint of many geriatric patients that they experience pain in the low back, which limits their activity and function and which is not uncommonly ascribed to "old age." The treating physician may view these complaints as trivial, but to the patients the pain may be interfering with their continued ability to function in an independent fashion. Along with spondylosis as a source of low back or radicular pain in these patients, neoplastic and infective disorders may be hidden and overlooked by the casual examination.

In this chapter primary consideration will be given to the evaluation and treatment of those conditions that affect the lumbar spine in the geriatric patient; particular attention will be directed to the entity of spinal stenosis and its treatment.

ANATOMY

The low back must be considered as a complex mechanism with important contributions to its function from many areas.

Although the physician strives for a specific diagnosis and anatomic area of dysfunction, the low back rarely, when awry, has a single unit out of focus because the vertebrae, intervertebral discs, apophyseal joints, and paraspinal ligamentous and muscular supports are closely integrated. Along with these structures the neural elements that are encased and protected by these stabiliz-

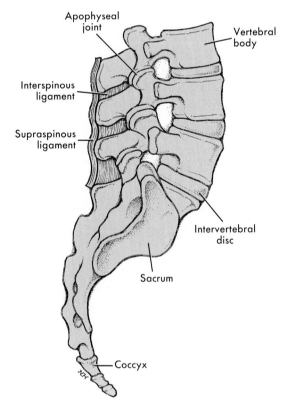

FIG. 11-1. Anatomic sketch of lumbar spine demonstrating elements in complex: apophyseal joints, intervertebral discs, vertebrae, ligament, and muscle.

ers are also vulnerable to damage when pathologic states exist. Although separate anatomic areas can be discussed, it is important for the physician to realize that a continuum of aging and pathology are present in this entire integrated area. (Fig. 11-1).

The vertebrae in the lumbar area undergo morphologic changes with aging.[10] Osteoporosis, although more commonly considered to affect the thoracic spine, is present in the lumbar area and compression may occur with concomitant widening and loss of vertebral height. Marked sclerosis may be seen at the verterbral end plates as a reactive change to stresses created by severe degeneration of the intervertebral discs.

Alterations in alignment may be seen in the aging spine in the anteroposterior, mediolateral, or rotational planes. Scoliosis, with at times severe lateral subluxation of vertebral bodies, can be the result of progression of an adolescent curve or, probably more frequently, it may be secondary to combined osteoporosis and degenerative apophyseal joint disease (Fig. 11-2). Degenerative spondylolisthesis, completely unrelated to isthmic defects, can also be a predominant feature in patients with advanced spondylosis.

Osteophytic bone can develop about the perimeter of the vertebra and alter its configuration. In the most advanced form complete anterior and/or posterior ankylosis may occur with formal ossification of the anterior and posterior longitudinal ligaments.

Apophyseal joints

The apophyseal joints because of their diarthrodial nature undergo changes not dissimilar to those of other weight-bearing joints. The specific changes related to the aging process and those associated with the common forms of degenerative joint disease in the elderly population are difficult to differentiate and probably are coexistent. Most often joint alteration is noted in the lower lumbar segments, L3-4, L4-5, and L5-S1. However, changes may be seen throughout the lumbar spine with advanced aging.

The earliest change noted in the apophyseal joint in the aging spine is the presence of a synovitis that is secondary to the continual rotational and axial stresses on these joints. Early changes are seen in the hyaline cartilage of these joints with evidence of thinning and exposure of subchondral bone. The capsular investment of the joint becomes involved in this process and initially laxity occurs that may lead to subluxation of these joints in some patients. Eventually, as the joint continues to demonstrate evidence of damage, a futile attempt is made by the biologic system to repair the joint and this leads to the evolution of subperiosteal osteophytes. In more advanced situations enlargement of the joint takes place secondary to both

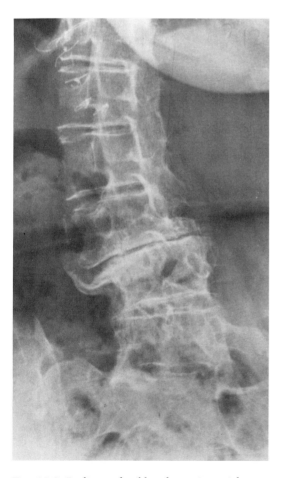

FIG. 11-2. Radiograph of lumbar spine with scoliosis with degenerative spondylosis and lateral subluxation of vertebral bodies.

these osteophytes and the severe pericapsular fibrosis.[19,10]

In those patients with apophyseal joint damage instability may occur and forward, lateral, or rotational displacement can result. The patient with severe degenerative spondylosis and forward displacement may manifest a compromise of neural structures and a spinal stenosis aggravated by further narrowing of the canal by the degenerative spondylolisthesis. Another common series of changes includes progressive osteophyte formation, fibrosis, and ankylosis. A biologic fusion occurs in this latter group of patients that in many cases results in marked improvement in their symptoms.

Intervertebral discs

The three-joint complex popularized by Farfan[11] includes both apophyseal joints and the intervertebral disc, and dysfunctions in these areas are closely linked. The intervertebral discs reside between adjoining vertebrae and provide a hydraulic buffer for the spine. The constituents of the disc have now been well documented and consist of an avascular fibrocartilaginous matrix that is filled with interstitial fluid, proteoglycans, glycoproteins, and noncollagenous proteins. Morphologic and histochemical changes are known to occur in the intervertebral disc as aging progresses.[20] Coventry[6] in 1945 described the progressive changes seen by decade in the cartilaginous end plate, annulus fibrosus, and nucleus pulposus. In the sixth and seventh decades advanced destructive and degenerative alterations are noted in the hyaline cartilage present in the end plate. The observation is made that degenerative changes occur in the annulus with tears being present in its posterior segment and large, longitudinal tears and clefts are described throughout the discs. Along with these tears complete loss of structure of the nucleus takes place with evidence of severe desiccation.

Kirkady-Willis[19] has demonstrated a spectrum of damage to the disc that begins with circumferential tears in the annulus. These are most probably secondary to trau-

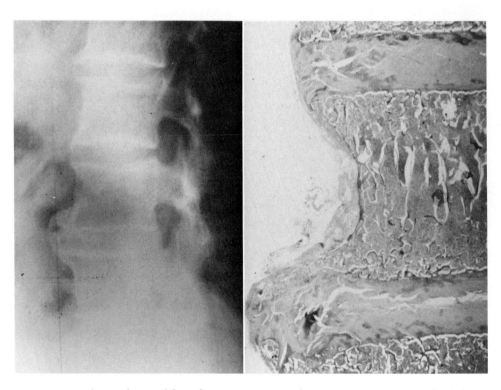

Fig. 11-3. Radiographic and histologic preparation demonstrating intervertebral disc degeneration with traction spurs and osteophytes.

ma to the disc from repeated shear or other stresses during activities of daily living. These circumferential tears tend to extend into the nucleus pulposus with time and produce more confluent radial tears involving a larger cross section of the disc. With further extension of these tears, complete internal disruption of the intervertebral disc can occur. Maceration of the disc as it occurs tends to lead to loss of the height of the disc and much of its stabilizing characteristics.

As this evolution in the structure of the disc is progressing, concomitant biochemical changes of note can be demonstrated. The proteoglycan content diminishes as does the water content and this further alters the turgor and buffering capacity of the disc. The water content of the interstitial fluid varies with age, being 88% at birth and 65% in adulthood, and this content continues to decrease with age.[22] Further changes noted with age include a fall in the total sulphate ester present in the disc with a relative increase in the keratan-sulfate: chondroitin-sulphate ratio, an increase in glycoproteins, an increase in fibrillation and precipitation of collagen, an increase in noncollagenous proteins, and an increase in the beta protein fraction.[22] The morphologic and biochemical changes noted in the disc with aging may also be related to changes in permeability of the disc, which has been demonstrated to occur. This, however, may be primary or secondary to the changing nature of the disc with age.[5]

Fibrosis of the disc ensues and resorption of disc material follows. As the disc becomes severely narrowed and macerated, osteophytes are produced along the margins of the vertebral bodies, more anteriorly than posteriorly. Some of these osteophytes may be under the anterior longitudinal ligament and these are called *traction spurs*. Sclerosis of the vertebral end plates occurs with eventual ankylosis noted in the more advanced conditions (Fig. 11-3).

Soft tissue stabilizers

In the complex integration of all elements of the lumbar spinal unit, the stabilizing soft tissues play a particularly im-

portant role in the geriatric patient. Degenerative changes are commonly present in intervertebral discs and apophyseal joints, and secondary changes are present in the vertebrae in elderly individuals. In these patients there is an associated loss of tone and bulk of abdominal and spinal extensor musculature. Yet, reliance on the abdominal and spinal extensor musculature remains considerable for maintenance of posture and reduction of day-to-day overloading of the spinal elements.

Stability is provided in a static fashion by much of the ligamentous structures of the spine. The supraspinous and interspinous ligaments provide needed stability to the posterior elements of the spinal column. The ligamentum flavum links laminae but also extends to the apophyseal joint and becomes confluent with the medial joint capsule. The anterior and posterior longitudinal ligaments are stout bands acting as bindings front and back for the vertebral bodies themselves (Fig. 11-4). The iliolumbar ligament may play an important role in preventing spondylolisthesis at the lumbosacral level in patients with degenerative spondylosis. This theory has been advanced by Fitzgerald and Newman,[13] who feel that this stabilizer, which is acting primarily between the last lumbar vertebra and the sacrum, maintains the relationship of these structures. This contributes to the documented increased incidence of degenerative spondylolisthesis at the L4-5 level.

The large paraspinal muscles insert from level to level, traversing from occiput to sacrum and providing an interwoven and hardy support to the spine. Because of their individual interconnections at each level yet integrated action as a lengthy unit, the muscles function as a series of box cars. That is, each unit and contiguous units can effect local dynamic responses from the spine but the entire network also is affected in a domino manner. This reinforces the importance of their strength and coordinated functioning and explains the concept of referred pain and muscle spasm when a local pathologic phenomenon occurs. The protective role of these muscles is dem-

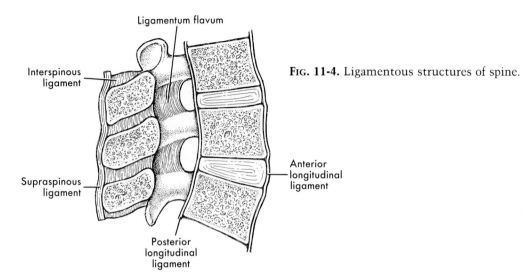

FIG. 11-4. Ligamentous structures of spine.

onstrated by the development of a reversal of lordosis and a list, which is seen in painful lumbar disorders. Severe spasm tends to limit motion at the involved segment and unload to an extent the forces across the painful area. The abdominal and pelvic musculature is equally important, and the spine can be considered to be suspended with anterior and posterior guy supports that have the dynamic function of regulating posture and bending and loading activities of the spine.

SPINAL STENOSIS

Clinical syndromes related to the aging and degenerative processes that involve the intervertebral discs, apophyseal joints, and stabilizing ligaments and other soft tissues are common in the geriatric patient. In general, specific clinical syndromes are characterized by involvement of the entire lumbosacral complex rather than by specific dysfunctions of one anatomic element or another. For example, low back pain with radicular symptoms in the elderly patient may be produced by an isolated herniation of an intervertebral disc with secondary nerve root compromise; however, far more commonly these symptoms are produced by a combination of entrapment of the nerve root by both an intervertebral disc and an arthritic facet joint. The entity of spinal stenosis, first described by Verbiest[28]

in 1954, has now been identified as a common source of lumbosacral dysfunction in geriatric patients. In his initial discussion of this entity, Verbiest demonstrated the pathologic findings in seven patients; he identified in them narrowing of the neural canal primarily from encroachment from the articular processes.

A more formal classification of spinal stenosis has been developed and is given in the box on p. 179.[2] Classically, stenosis implies narrowing, and in caring for a patient with spinal stenosis the treating physician must think of the neural canal in all dimensions and of those adjacent structures that may encroach upon the neural elements within this canal.

Clinical presentation

Patients with the classical symptoms of spinal stenosis manifest increasing pain usually bilaterally arising from the buttocks and traveling down the posterior aspects of the thighs into both calves. This pain is aggravated by standing or walking in most patients and may be confused with the intermittent claudication of vascular insufficiency. Most patients will describe the pain as burning in nature and requiring that they stop and rest and then resume walking as the pain recedes. Most patients will note an improvement in their symptoms if they lean forward, flexing the spine, and resting in this bent-forward position.

SPINAL STENOSIS CLASSIFICATIONS

I. Congenital-developmental stenosis
   A. Idiopathic
   B. Achondroplastic
II. Acquired stenosis
   A. Degenerative
      1. Central portion of spinal canal
      2. Peripheral portion of canal, lateral recesses, and nerve root canals
      3. Degenerative spondylolisthesis
   B. Combined: any possible combination of congenital/developmental stenosis, degenerative stenosis, and herniations of the nucleus pulposus
   C. Spondylolisthetic-spondylolytic
   D. Iatrogenic
      1. Postlaminectomy
      2. Postfusion (anterior and posterior)
      3. Postchemonucleolysis
   E. Posttraumatic, late changes
   F. Miscellaneous
      1. Paget's disease
      2. Fluorosis

Patients will generally give a history of long-standing and recurrent low back pain with progressive referred pain into the extremities. However, it is important to note that although pain is usually bilateral, it may be unilateral and have many of the characteristics of discogenic sciatica. In contrast to discogenic pain, though, sitting is often comfortable and it relieves symptoms in patients with spinal stenosis.

In association with their pain patients generally describe numbness and on occasion weakness in their lower extremities that comes on as they proceed with their walking. The weakness and the pain may be limiting factors in their gait patterns. On careful questioning patients with severe symptoms of neurogenic claudication secondary to spinal stenosis may describe urinary symptoms of retention or on occasion incontinence, indicating more severe compression of the cauda equina itself. Therefore, urinary symptoms should be evaluated carefully and not be considered only in relation to prostatism in the male or bladder relaxation in the female.

Physical examination

The patient usually stands with the spine in the flexed or straightened position and there is marked reversal of normal lumbar lordosis. The stoop test as described by Dyck[8] is generally positive in these patients and is performed by having the patient walk a specific distance until the onset of the leg pain. The patient is then asked to flex forward and if there is relief of the pain and then the pain is again aggravated by extension of the spine, the test is positive and consistent with spinal stenosis. Examination of the spine itself demonstrates significant limitation of spinal mobility secondary to the arthritic involvement of the lumbosacral facet complexes. Lumbar scoliosis may be present. There may be significant paravertebral muscle spasm and a list may be noted in some patients. The Lasegue test is often negative in these patients although hamstring tightness may be present. Direct spinal tenderness is present but not severe. Specific neurologic impairment in the lower extremities is usually completely absent. In some patients patchy areas of loss of sensation without good dermatomal localization are present. Motor changes may be subtle and again without specific nerve root localization. Reflexes in both lower extremities are generally depressed or absent in these patients. The nature of the neurologic abnormalities is consistent with a broadened area of cauda equina compression with multiple levels of mild but true dysfunction.

Radiographic evaluation

Anteroposterior, lateral, and oblique radiographs of the lumbosacral spine demonstrate advanced changes involving both the anterior and the posterior spinal structures. There is noted in most patients severe narrowing of the intervertebral disc spaces with marked sclerosis of the vertebral end plates. Osteophytes are commonly present anteriorly, with frank lipping and ankylosis in severe cases (Fig. 11-5). There are marked osteophytic changes noted with irregularity and enlargement of the apophyseal joints. Posteriorly, these facet joints can become bulbous and quite close to the midline. In some patients lumbar scoliosis with lateral subluxation of the vertebral bodies may be noted in the lumbar area.[9] A spondylolisthesis, most commonly occurring at the L4-5 level, may also be present (Fig. 11-6).

Computed tomography (CT) is a useful adjunct to routine radiographs in these patients. It provides specific localization of the areas of encroachment and the degree of stenosis. The scan is also particularly useful in defining the lateral recesses beneath the apophyseal joints, which are the exit areas for the nerve roots. In spinal stenosis with involvement of the lateral recess a "sombrero" configuration replaces the normal trifoil appearance of the neural canal in the lumbar area (Fig. 11-7). Both apophyseal joint and disc impingement in the lateral recess can be noted on the CT scan.

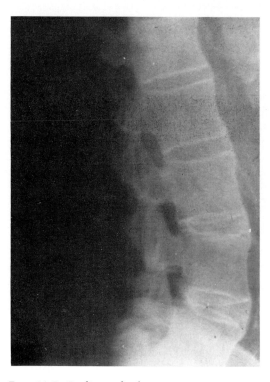

FIG. 11-5. Radiograph demonstrating anterior vertebral ankylosis.

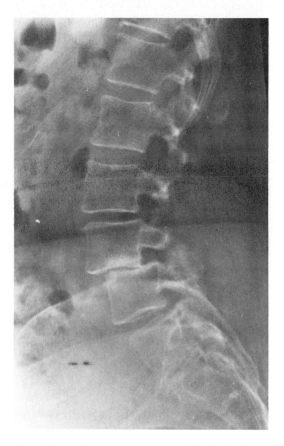

FIG. 11-6. Degenerative spondylolisthesis at L4-5.

In severe cases of spinal stenosis a "pagoda" appearance develops in the neural canal as the superior articular processes become elongated and form a pseudolamina beneath the existing lamina (Fig. 11-8).

Metrizamide myelography further defines the soft tissue encroachment on the diameter of the neural canal. The myelogram provides useful information on the extent of disc impingment as well as on the extent of encroachment from the ligamentum flavum and pericapsular soft tissues arising from the anterior portion of the facet joint. It is not uncommon in patients with

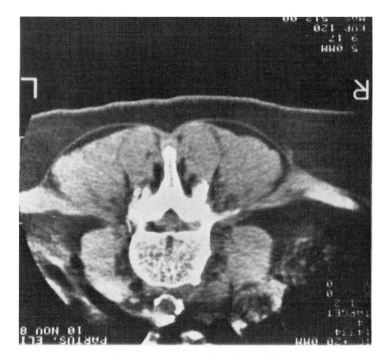

FIG. 11-7. Lumbosacral CT scan demonstrating "sombrero" sign.

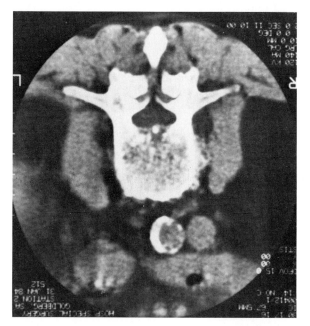

FIG. 11-8. Lumbosacral CT scan demonstrating "pagoda" sign.

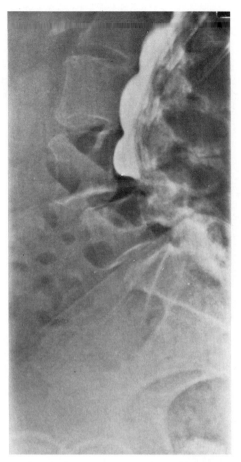

Fig. 11-9. Myelogram showing complete block in patient with spinal stenosis at level of spondylolisthesis.

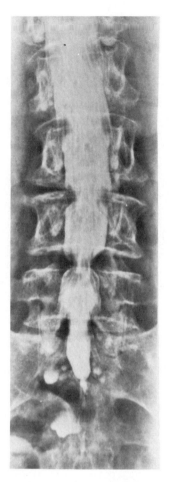

Fig. 11-10. Myelogram showing "waisting" appearance produced by hypertrophic facets.

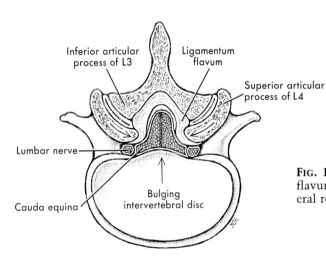

Fig. 11-11. Schematic drawing of ligamentum flavum and pericapsular synovitis narrowing lateral recess.

severe spinal stenosis to have complete blockage of flow at a particular level, most commonly L4-5 (Fig. 11-9). A characteristic waisting (Fig. 11-10) of the dye column is seen in patients with multiple level spinal stenosis predominantly from the apophyseal arthritis as the enlarged and medially protuberant facet impinges on the dura and its contents. Combining the metrizamide myelography with a CT study provides an extremely accurate picture of both the bony and the soft tissue elements contributing to the patient's spinal stenosis.

Pathophysiology

Despite attempts at classification of lumbar spinal stenosis, great controversy persists as to the factors that contribute to the pathologic state. There remains debate as to whether spinal stenosis results from purely degenerative stenosis and its concomitant arthritic involvement of the apophyseal joints or whether an element of pre-existing developmental narrowing is present in these patients.[25,29] Spinal stenosis can be considered to be primarily of the (1) central type, in patients with marked hypertrophy of the laminae, or (2) lateral recess type, where encroachment is in the area of the neural foramen and is secondary to apophyseal joint hypertrophy and further crowding by the degenerative disc anteriorly and ligamentum flavum medially. More accurately, however, the central and lateral types of stenosis are present in a combined fashion in the symptomatic patient and pure central stenosis is rare.

The neural canal becomes narrowed anteriorly by degenerative changes within the disc, posterior weakening of the annulus fibrosus and longitudinal ligament. This produces the common midline multiple level bulging defects noted on myelography in patients over 40. Lipson and Muir[20] have demonstrated osteophyte formation arising from the innermost fibers of the annulus, which are undergoing a metaplasia into frank osteophyes as chronic disc degeneration and herniation occur. This posterior ostephyte development further narrows the spinal canal.

The posterior and lateral recess areas of the neural canal become compromised primarily by hypertrophic facet changes. This pathologic process evolves through a spectrum in which initially there is a localized synovitis within the facet joint, laxity of the capsular structures about the facet joint, and with time progressive articular cartilage damage and osteophyte formation. In the lumbar apophyseal joints the inferior articular process becomes quite hypertrophic, and marked medial prominence of the facet joint is apparent as a result of the posterior and medial enlargement of this inferior articular process. The laminae tend to become thicker and to take on a more perpendicular orientation as the facet joint deforms medially. The ligamentum flavum also assumes a perpendicular direction to the midline as it travels beneath the lamina which is in this more perpendicular position. The ligamentum flavum also thickens in its cross-sectional area as spinal canal narrowing increases, and it crowds the lateral recess because it is forced to take a sharp angulation to pass beneath the facet joint. The lateral recess is compromised not only by the hypertrophic and osteophytic apophyseal joint but also by the lateral portion of the ligamentum flavum and periarticular fibrosis and synovial hypertrophy that occur and extend into the lateral recess around the nerve root (Fig. 11-11). The superior articular process lies directly posterior to the nerve root and its formamen, and this may further compromise the exit pathway of the nerve root. In addition, in patients in whom a degenerative spondylolisthesis occurs, the nerve root is tethered and compressed by the pedicle and is forced to assume a very angular exit around the pedicle into the tightened foramen. In patients in whom a lumbar scoliosis is present, rotation of the lumbar vertebrae produces further abnormalities in the pathway of the nerve root.

In summary, a spectrum of pathologic changes occurs in spinal stenosis both in the soft tissues and in the bony structures about the central lumbar neural canal and the nerve root foramina, producing the clinical manifestations of this entrapment in the geriatric patient. Lateral-recess narrowing at the site of the foramen is aggravated by posterior bulging of the degenerative disc as well as by anterior compromise from the hypertrophic and arthritic facet joint with further narrowing being produced by the ligamentum flavum and pericapsular synovitis and fibrosis occurring about the facet joint. In cases where anteroposterior or lateral malalignment of the lumbar spine is present, aggravation of the nerve root exit pathway is more marked. Wiltse et al.[32] have described compression of the spinal nerve lateral to the pedicle and beyond by degenerative changes lateral to the facet and compression of the spinal nerve between the transverse process of the fifth lumbar vertebra and the ala of the sacrum.

The cause of neurogenic claudication in patients with spinal stenosis has not been well documented. Breig[4] has demonstrated that when the spine moves from flexion to extension the lumbar canal shortens by 2.2 mm and that nerve tissue within the canal is also shortened. He also noted that the intervertebral foramen is narrowed in extension and that there is a slight increase in the protrusion of the posterior aspect of the intervertebral discs at all levels with extension of the spine. This may well explain the increase in symptoms with spinal extension in patients with spinal stenosis. The actual claudication pain that patients perceive is probably on a vascular basis[3] and represents ischemia to the perineurium as traction along the nerve root occurs during ambulation. The nerve root is already severely compromised as it passes through its narrowed foramen, and further tension on the root probably produces a secondary loss of blood supply to the nerve itself and claudication symptoms result.

Degenerative spondylolisthesis

In approximately 15% of patients with spinal stenosis a degenerative type of spondylolisthesis is noted. This takes place primarily at the L4-5 level and plays a significant role in increasing the narrowing of the neural canal in these patients. Junghanns[17] in 1930 first described degenerative spondylolisthesis. Newman and Stone[23] attributed the spondylolisthesis to the development of instability as a result of degeneration of the supraspinous and interspinous ligaments, which leads to a resultant increase in mobility at the L4-5 level.[1] As the inferior articular process develops marked osteoarthritic changes, it slips forward and below the superior articular process of L5. In doing this, the L5 nerve root and at times the cauda equina come under significant compression. The obliquity of the facet joint at the L4-5 level is also implicated as playing a role in degenerative spondylolisthesis. The orientation is oblique to the transverse plane while the facet joints at the L5-S1 level are not and they tend to be more stable. Newman[23] followed the progression of spondylolisthesis prospectively and found approximately a 2 mm progression in the spondylolisthesis after 4 years. Newman states that it is rare for the vertebral body to slip more than one quarter of the diameter of the adjoining vertebral body.

Treatment

Patients with severe signs and symptoms of spinal stenosis rarely improve on a conservative regimen. However, those with milder symptoms often feel better with symptomatic treatment.

Exercise program. These patients, generally because of inactivity, develop marked weakening of the paraspinal and abdominal musculature. A Williams exercise program, designed to exercise these muscle groups isometrically, tends to provide transient relief to some patients. In a small number of patients the exercises may aggravate the underlying pain and they should be discontinued if this occurs. Swimming and a stationery bicycle also are beneficial to the patient with stenosis. Because of the flexed position when the bicycle is used, symptoms are generally not exacerbated. The overhand crawl stroke is recommended because it promotes flexion of the spine in the water.

In association with these exercises the patient should be instructed in proper body mechanics concerning the care of the back.

The patient should avoid lifting, heavy gardening, and activities that require repetitive walking or stair climbing.

Medications. Nonsteroidal medications as a rule are not helpful in the treatment of significant spinal stenosis. Occasionally phenylbutazone or indomethacin given for short periods may provide temporary relief to these patients, but oral cortisone has not been beneficial. More commonly, these medications are poorly tolerated by geriatric patients and care should be exercised and proper discussion of their gastric and other side effects must be given to the patient before prescribing these medications. Analgesics and muscle relaxants are generally of little benefit to patients with spinal stenosis since pain is not present at rest.

Epidural injections. The injection of epidural dexamethasone has been helpful in approximately 60% of patients with spinal stenosis in a current series at The Hospital for Special Surgery. Those patients who improved tended to be the lesser affected. The medication is administered on a weekly basis for 2 or 3 injections and patients who respond to this method of treatment may note improvement in their symptoms for up to 3 to 6 months. Recurrence of pain is common, however, and response to repeat injections has not been as successful as when given intially.

Lumbosacral supports. The use of a lumbosacral support generally relieves back pain if it is of significance, but such supports do not diminish the pain and symptoms from the patient's neurogenic claudication. The warm-and-form type of lumbosacral corset is preferred for the geriatric patient in that it has a Velcro anterior closure that is easy for the geriatric patient to use. It incorporates a molded plastic insert that in some patients is uncomfortable and can be removed. More formal lumbosacral braces of the Knight spinal and the Hoke types are generally poorly tolerated by elderly patients and compliance is poor.

Operative treatment. The goal of the surgeon in the treatment of spinal stenosis is to return the patient to a level of function that allows walking with comfort and daily activities. In patients in whom pain is severe and disabling and in whom all conservative measures have failed, surgical decompression should be considered. The surgeon must decompress the lateral recess area where the primary pathology exists and which is responsible for the patient's radicular symptoms. Decompressions that are limited to the laminae have yielded poor results in most patients and should always be combined with proper lateral recess decompression. It is rare in the geriatric patient that discectomy without adequate decompression will relieve the symptoms of spinal stenosis. In fact, discectomy in patients with spinal stenosis should be performed only when disc herniation is massive and decompression of the lateral recess and neural foramen is incomplete without it.

Technique of surgery

Since these patients tend to have associated medical problems, a careful preoperative evaluation by an internist is requisite before surgery. The operative procedure itself can be prolonged and perioperative monitoring is important to the care of these patients. A urinary catheter is inserted preoperatively and an arterial line for blood gas determinations should be utilized if the patient has pulmonary insufficiency. The patient is placed in the prone position, generally on bolsters or on a frame that leaves the abdomen free from pressure. The blood loss during these procedures can be extensive and therefore ample blood replacement should be available. The use of a Cell-Saver is recommended if available for recirculation of shed blood from the operating field.

After positioning of the patient, a midline lumbar incision is made and the paraspinal musculature is reflected subperiosteally from the spinous processes, laminae, and facet joints. Careful packing is performed above and below the operative site to prevent continued oozing of blood into the operative field. Localization of the involved vertebral levels is then confirmed and, if necessary, an intraoperative lateral radiograph should be taken. The spinous processes are removed and a Leksell rongeur is used to remove laminae first centrally and then extending laterally toward the apophyseal joints. Initial decompression should be done away from the level of a complete block should one be present. The more severe areas can generally be approached from above or below from a site of lesser stenosis. It will be noted in these patients that the facet joints tend to be

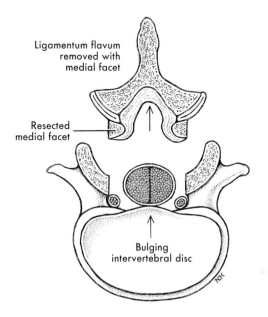

FIG. 11-12. Resection of medial facet for proper decompression of lateral recess.

quite bulbous and close to the midline. As lamina is removed, the ligamentum flavum will be oriented perpendicularly and it will extend laterally beneath the facet joint, thus crowding the lateral recess. This extension should be excised as the laminae are removed. Once the dura has been identified, care should be taken to prevent trauma to it and to avoid epidural bleeding. In these patients epidural fat is usually absent and therefore great care should be taken in protecting the dura as bone is resected further. After removal of the lamina, further dissection is extended laterally. The pars interarticularis can be resected with a rongeur and the inferior facet can be removed. One will then visualize the nerve root, which is passing beneath the superior articular process exiting through the foramen. In patients with severe stenosis, it is necessary to remove the medial border of the superior articular facet to free the nerve root properly as it exits toward the foramen (Fig. 11-12). If necessary, further lateral decompression should be extended into the foramen and beyond until the nerve root can be followed easily with a retractor and until it is noted to be free of compression. In cases of degenerative spondylolisthesis or severe stenosis, the pedicle in part may

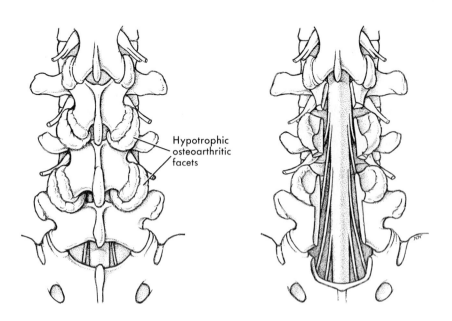

FIG. 11-13. Schematic demonstrating decompression after performed.

have to be removed to relieve pressure on the lateral portion of the nerve root as it passes around this structure. Considerable fibrotic debris will be noted in the lateral recess and it should be excised. Most of this arises from the facet joint and it is formed of pericapsular fibrosis and synovial tissue. This dissection should continue on both sides if involvement is bilateral and the surgeon should decompress as many levels as is necessary to relieve the extent of the stenosis properly (Fig. 11-13). The preoperative CT scan and myelogram are useful in determining the extent of the stenosis, but evaluation at the surgical field is most important.

As the procedure progresses, the dura will become quite dilated and pulsatile activity generally returns to the dura at the completion of the decompression. Fat is excised from the subcutaneous area and is placed over the exposed dura before closure. In patients in the geriatric age group spinal fusion has not been performed in addition to the decompression despite the fact that the extent of the decompression usually involves the facet joints. Progression of spondylolisthesis is also uncommon in geriatric patients who have undergone significant decompression without associated spinal fusion.

Results of operative treatment

Multiple studies report good to excellent results in the range of 55% to 80%.[15,21,24,26,32] The reason for the unsatisfactory results has generally been attributed to failure to decompress adequately either in extent or in number of affected levels. If multiple-level laminectomy has been necessary, patients may be relieved of their radicular pain but back pain may be a problem. This has not been attributed, however, to spinal instability after these laminectomies, although these patients do feel better with a lumbosacral corset.

Although the majority of patients note significant relief of their pain after decompression, persistent radicular symptoms may be present in a small number. These are patients with a chronic history of severe neurogenic claudication with ob-

jective neurologic loss preoperatively. Neural damage may be irreversible in these patients because of prolonged nerve root and cauda equina compression and ischemia. The surgeon may be able to improve somewhat the pain patterns in these patients but return to normal function is doubtful. It is a clinical impression that patients with peripheral vascular disease do less well after decompression. This may also be related to nerve root ischemia as the source of neurogenic claudication.

Although degenerative disease of the intervertebral discs and apophyseal joints is the most common cause of low back pain in elderly patients, in the differential diagnosis the physician must also consider spinal infection, tumor involvement in the spine, and bone collapse secondary to osteoporosis. These conditions may be overlooked and, particularly in those patients with infection or a tumor in the spine, diagnosis may be quite delayed. If routine evaluation and treatment methods are not working, it is important to persist by using more specialized radiographic studies or invasive procedures when the suspicion is present that a more ominous problem may underlie the patient's symptoms.

SPINAL INFECTION

Infections that involve the spine most commonly spread via the hematogeneous route. Their incidence is quite high in patients in the fifth, sixth, and seventh decades and those vertebrae around the thoracolumbar junction and the upper lumbar spine tend to be the most commonly involved.[7,27] Garcia and Grantham[14] found that over two thirds of those affected had involvement in the lumbar spine.

Clinical features

Patients with infections of the lumbar spine may have features of a chronic illness rather than of acute infection. Most patients describe a general feeling of malaise, weight loss, and anorexia. Fever may occur during an acute exacerbation or with bacteremia but tends to be absent or low grade. The pain with spinal infection is persistent with any activity and also persists into the night, resembling the pain found in patients with malignant spine disease. Neurologic signs are infrequent and occur only in severe and widespread infection with secondary meningitis from direct extension of the infection from the vertebral body into the peridural areas.

On examination patients will demonstrate marked paravertebral spasm with reversal of their lordosis. Direct percussion or deep palpation over the affected vertebral level elicits pain in most cases. In those patients with severe pain any range of motion of the lumbar spine is avoided by the patient. Patients will also tend to keep the hip flexed to relax the iliopsoas and will have severe discomfort if the hip is forceably extended. Neurologic deficits are uncommon but should be carefully tested since, if present, they are indicative of advanced and more severe infection.

Patients who are diabetics, alcoholics, or drug abusers may have a greater risk for developing spinal infections.

Pathophysiology

It is debated whether the hematogeneous spread of the infection occurs by the arterial or venous route.[30] The venous drainage from the pelvic area is retrograde through a series of valveless veins and when intra-abdominal pressure is increased, blood is conducted into the venous sinusoids in the cancellous portion of the vertebral body. This may help to explain the high incidence of lumbar spine infections seen in patients after genitourinary instrumentation or surgery or with infections in the urinary tract. Those patients with pelvic or colonic surgery or infection are also at greater risk for developing spinal infections.

The organism most commonly cultured from the infected site is *Staphylococcus aureus.* This organism accounts for from 80% to 90% of these infections. Less frequently, *Escherichia coli, Pseudomonas aeruginosa,* and *Salmonella* are recovered from the infected vertebra or disc space.

The infection develops from the hematogeneous spread first in the vertebral body itself. From there by direct extension the intervertebral disc becomes secondarily infected. It is rare that extension travels to involve the pedicle or the posterior elements except with tuberculous spondylitis. Bone destruction progresses if the infection remains untreated, and severe erosion and eventually changes in alignment of the spine can occur. Most commonly, the vertebral end plates become damaged along with the underlying vertebral body. With narrowing and damage to the disc space, further collapse of the anterior structures ensues and a kyphotic deformity can result. This is associated with instability and often intractable pain.

Laboratory and radiographic data

Serologic tests may be remarkably normal. The leukocyte count may be mildly elevated, but in low-grade chronic infections it is usually unremarkable. Blood cultures unless performed during a febrile episode tend to be negative. The most useful test is the erythrocyte sedimentation rate, which is elevated in most infected patients. It may be markedly elevated in some patients, but a level of 50 is quite common and this should alert the physician to the presence of something other than just degenerative spondylosis.

Plain radiographs of the spine taken early in the infection (weeks 2 to 4) will usually demonstrate paravertebral shadows consistent with an abscess or edema. The intervertebral disc space will also be narrowed early in the disease (Fig. 11-14). The infection progresses, bone changes occur with localized areas of lysis within the vertebral body and destruction of bone in the area of the end plate. The more severe changes with vertebral collapse tend to be seen later in the disease if it remains untreated for several months.

A bone scan will be quite positive in the area of infection and this is the best diagnostic tool for identifying possible infection before radiographic changes occur. The use of CT scans may be helpful in determining more accurately the extent of vertebral involvement as well as the magnitude of the paravertebral abscess. Tomograms further reinforce the information obtained from plain radiographs, CT scans and bone scans. In patients with neurologic involvement metrizamide myelography is recommended preferably with CT scans to define the level of the involvement and the extent of intraneural compression.

Definitive diagnosis is made by recovery of pathologic material from the area of infection. This can usually be done with a Craig needle biopsy under fluoroscopic control. In patients in whom this is not possible, open biopsy should be performed.

Treatment

The treatment for hematogenous infections of the spine is a combination of bed rest and intravenous antibiotics. With microbiologic identification of the infecting organism and its sensitivity, adequate antibiotic coverage can be administered and this should be continued for a period of 4 to 6 weeks. The criteria for cessation of antibiotic coverage are (1) clinical improvement of the patient, (2) return of the sedimentation rate to a normal range, and (3) radiographic improvement, particularly reduction in paravertebral soft tissue mass and the halting of further bone destruction.

Immobilization initially implies bed rest and this is indicated since most of these patients are in significant pain when they are ambulatory. However, in the geriatric patient the concomitant multisystem problems of bed rest must be taken into consideration. A synthetic lightweight jacket or a properly molded polyethelene jacket may be used. These should be worn by the patient until evidence of resolution of the infection is noted on radiographs and until the patient is able to function unsupported without pain. Some type of jacket or corset

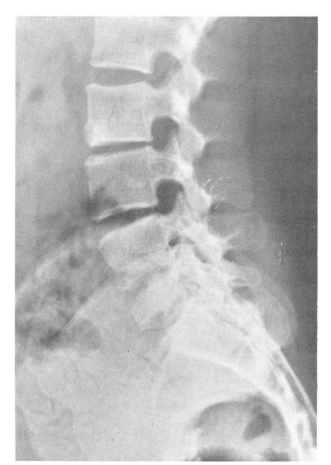

FIG. 11-14. Radiograph demonstrating progression in disc space infection and secondary vertebral body changes.

may be required for a period of up to 6 months.

The patients should be placed on a Williams flexion exercise program early in the course to maintain some tone in abdominal and paraspinal muscles.

Surgical treatment is indicated in the patient who remains quite ill because of a large paravertebral abscess that is not responding to antibiotic therapy. Decompression of the abscess and the disc space can be performed through a costotransversectomy or an anterolateral approach. Necrotic and infected bone can be removed at this time as well. In patients with neurologic involvement decompression should be performed anteriorly and fusion can also be performed.

Most patients on a proper regimen of antibiotic therapy and immobilization will go on to spontaneous fusion across the infected disc space with improvement in symptoms and resolution of infection. The mainstay of treatment is early recognition and aggressive pursuit of the pathogen followed by an adequate course of antibiotic coverage and supportive measures to the infected spine.

Tuberculous spondylitis

Tuberculous infection of the spine is quite uncommon in North America at this time. Its clinical manifestation is similar to that of pyogenic infections of the spine and the diagnosis is made by the recovery of the organism from the site of infection by biopsy, usually of the closed type. Of note is the fact that unlike other bacterial infections of the spine tuberculous infections usually infect not only the disc space but also very commonly the posterior elements of the spine and pedicles. Neurologic damage and severe kyphosis (gibbus deformity) may be seen in the advanced cases. Treatment is with prolonged antituberculous therapy (1 to 2 years), immobilization, and bed rest. Patients who do not respond or who demonstrate neurologic deficits should have anteriorly decompression and fusion.[12]

SPINAL TUMORS

Neoplastic involvement in the geriatric spine is almost always metastatic. Primary multicentric tumors such as multiple myeloma or lymphoma may involve the spine, but more commonly the primary source resides in another area. Those tumors that most frequently spread to bone include lung, kidney, breast, prostate, thyroid, and gastrointestinal tumors.

Clinical presentation

The pain from malignant infiltration of the spine has an unremitting character despite symptomatic treatment. Patients will describe a chronic backache that can become quite intense and that increases nocturnally. Unlike the case with degenerative conditions of the spine, these patients often cannot relieve their pain except with strong analgesics.

Radicular symptoms are rare unless nerve root or intradural spread occurs. Neurologic deficits are likewise rare if the tumor remains localized to the bone. Local tenderness to palpation or percussion is present. Obvious spinal deformity secondary to vertebral destruction is uncommon. Muscle spasm may be quite marked.

Routine radiographs may be negative for obvious morphologic changes in the vertebral body or posterior elements. In more advanced cases tumor may produce areas of bone destruction and collapse, which are most commonly seen in the vertebral body (Fig. 11-15), although pedicle and posterior elements may also be affected. A bone scan is useful for identifying malignant involvement in patients with negative routine radiographs. In patients with radicular symptoms or neurologic abnormalities myelography and CT scans are necessary to demonstrate the areas and extent of spinal cord or nerve root compression.

In patients in whom a primary focus of tumor has not been identified, a thorough oncologic evaluation should be performed. The orthopaedic surgeon should work closely with an oncologist in the care of these patients. If the diagnosis remains unclear, a Craig needle biopsy of the affected area can be performed percutaneously using local anesthesia with fluoroscopic control.

Treatment

Treatment varies depending upon the tumor type, extent of disease, and neurologic involvement. In the early stages radiation therapy with or without chemotherapy is useful in controlling pain from these sites. These patients require considerable support during this period and a team approach by orthopaedist and oncologist is important. Local support, such as the warm-and-form corset, may provide relief and is recommended. Analgesics should be given according to need.

In patients with progressive collapse of vertebral bone with instability and intractable pain despite treatment, surgical stabilization should be considered. This is also true in patients who have progressive neurologic deficits. Anterior decompression is recommended with resection of affected bone and replacement by methylmethacrylate reinforced by fixation rods or screws. In patients who primarily have instability secondary to bone collapse Harrington rod instrumentation augmented with methylmethacrylate can be used. (Fig. 11-16).[16]

The goal of treatment in the geriatric patient with malignant spread to the spine is to provide pain relief and allow continuation of function. Treatment of the primary focus of the tumor is requisite. Close cooperation between the oncologist, orthopaedic surgeon, and of course the patient must be present from the initial phases of treatment. This will be a difficult period for the patient and the family and all methods for assisting the patient should be made available.

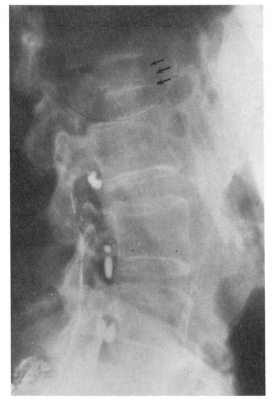

FIG. 11-15. Radiograph of metastatic tumor involvement of vertebral body.

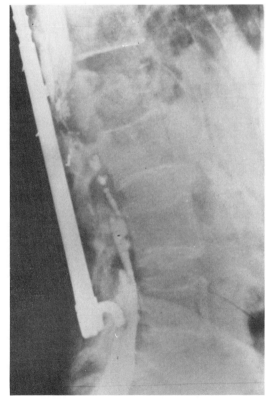

FIG. 11-16. Radiograph demonstrating use of Harrington rods and methylmethacrylate to stabilize pathologic fracture of lumbar vertebra.

References

1. Allbrook, D.: Movements of the lumbar spinal column, J. Bone Joint Surg. **39B:**339-347, 1957.

2. Arnoldi, C.C., et al.: Lumbar spinal stenosis and nerve root entrapment syndrome, Clin. Orthop. **115:**4-5, 1976.

3. Blau, J.N., and Logge, V.: Intermittent claudication of the cauda equina, *Lancet*, **1:**1081-1086, 1961.

4. Breig, A. Biomechanics of the central nervous system, Stockholm, 1964, Almqvist and Wiksell.

5. Brown, M.D., and Tsaltas, T.: Studies in the permeability of the intervertebral disc during skeletal maturation, Spine, **1:**250-244, 1976.

6. Coventry, M.B., Ghormley, R.K., and Kernohan, J.W.: The intervertebral disc: its microscopic anatomy and pathology, J. Bone Joint Surg. **27:**233-247, 1945.

7. Digby, J., and Kersley, J.: Pyogenic non-tuberculous spinal infections, J. Bone Joint Surg. **61B:**47-55, 1979.

8. Dyck, P.: The stoop-test in lumbar entrapment radiculopathy, Spine **4:**89-92, 1979.

9. Epstein, J., Epstein, B., and Jones, M.: Symptomatic lumbar scoliosis with degenerative changes in the elderly, Spine **4:**542-547, 1979.

10. Ericksen, M.F.: Aging in the lumbar spine, *Am. J. Phys. Anthropol.* **48:**241-246, 1978.

11. Farfan, H.F.: Biomechanics of the lumbar spine. Kirhady-Eillis, W.H., editor: Managing low back pain, London, 1983, Churchill-Livingstone.

12. Fifth report of the Medical Research Council: a five-year assessment of controlled trials of in-patient and out-patient treatment and of plaster-of-paris jackets for tuberculosis of the spine in children on standard chemotherapy, J. Bone Joint Surg. **58B:**399-411, 1976.

13. Fitzgerald, J.A.W. and Newman, P.H.: Degenerative spondylolisthesis, J. Bone Joint Surg. **58B:**184-192, 1976.

14. Garcia, A., and Grantham, A.: Hematogenous pyogenic vertebral osteomyelitis, J. Bone Joint Surg. **42:**429-436, 1960.

15. Getty, C.J.M.: Lumbar spinal stenosis, J. Bone Joint Surg. **62B:**481-485, 1980.

16. Harrington, K.: The use of methylmethacrylate for vertebral body replacement and anterior stabilization of pathological fracture-dislocation of the spine due to metastatic malignant disease, J. Bone Joint Surg. **63A:**36-46, 1981.

17. Junghanns, H.: Spondylolisthesen Ohne Spalt Im Zwischengelenkstück, Arch. Orthop. Unfallchir. **29:**118, 1930.

18. Kirkady-Willis, W.H.: Managing low back pain, New York, 1983, Churchill-Livingstone.

19. Kirkady-Willis, W.H., Wedge, J.H., Yong-Hing, M.B., and Reilly, J.: Pathology and pathogenesis of lumbar spondylosis and stenosis, Spine **3:**319-328, 1978.

20. Lipson, A., and Muir, H.: Vertebral osteophyte formation in experimental disc degeneration, Arthritis Rheum. **23:**319-324, 1980.

21. McKinley, L.M., and Davis, G.: The narrow lumbar spinal canal or lumbar spinal stenosis, Clin. Orthop. **114:**319-325, 1976.

22. Naylor, A.: Intervertebral disc prolapse and degeneration, Spine **1:**108-114, 1976.

23. Newman, P.H., and Stone, K.H.: The etiology of spondylolisthesis, J. Bone Joint Surg. **45B:**39-59, 1963.

24. Paine, K.W.E.: Results of decompression for lumbar spinal stenosis, Clin. Orthop. **115:**96-100, 1976.

25. Postacchini, F., Pezzeri, G., Montanaro, A., and Natali, G.: Computerized tomography in lumbar stenosis, J. Bone Joint Surg. **62B:**78-82, 1980.

26. Rosomoff, H.: Neural arch resection for lumbar spinal stenosis, Clin. Orthop. **154:**83-89, 1981.

27. Ross, P., and Fleming, J.: Vertebral body osteomyelitis, Clin. Orthop. **118:**190-196, 1976.

28. Verbiest, H.: A radicular syndrome from developmental narrowing of the lumbar vertebral canal, J. Bone Joint Surg. **36B:**230-237, 1954.

29. Verbiest, H.: Results of surgical treatment of idiopathic developmental stenosis of the lumbar vertebral canal: a review of twenty-seven years experience, J. Bone Joint Surg. **59B:**181-188, 1977.

30. Wiley, A.M., and Trueta, J.: The vascular anatomy of the spine and its relationship to pyogenic vertebral osteomyelitis, J. Bone Joint Surg. **51B:**796-809, 1959.

31. Wiltse, L.L., Kirkady-Willis, W.H., and McIvor, C.W.: The treatment of spinal stenosis, Clin. Orthop. **115:**83-91, 1976.

32. Wiltse, L.L., et al.: Alar transverse process impingement of the L5 spinal nerve (the far-out syndrome), Spine. (In press.)

chapter 12
THE LOWER EXTREMITY

Thomas P. Sculco

The recurrent theme throughout this text, the need to maintain function in the elderly patient, becomes crucial in the treatment of afflictions of the lower extremity. For when ambulation becomes impossible and these patients are confined to a wheelchair or to a bed-to-chair existence their entire level of function generally deteriorates quite rapidly. This is true not only of their physiologic well-being but also in their interactions with their environment. Because of their need to rely on friends, family, or assistance through social services, the geriatric patient often loses the will to be independent. It has been reiterated time and again that failure to maintain walking ability brings on, as a rule, a rapid demise.

In a discussion of musculoskeletal conditions that affect the lower extremity, it is important to emphasize that manifestations in the limb may be produced locally or as a referred condition. That is, a patient may complain of pain on weight bearing and the treating physician must discern if this is caused by a dysfunction of the hip or knee joint or if it is referred pain from osteoarthritis of the lumbosacral spine with sciatica. The need to approach these patients carefully with a thoughtful history and a comprehensive physical examination is of great importance in not being misled as to the patient's underlying pathologic problem.

In this chapter I will focus primarily on degenerative problems of the weight-bearing joints of the lower extremity, particularly the hip and knee, and provide a treatment plan that is reasonable for these conditions. Again, it should be emphasized that neurologic disease as well as peripheral vascular disease may influence the patient's ability to walk and these must be considered in the physician's differential diagnosis and treatment plan in approaching patients with lower extremity dysfunctions.

THE PATIENT WITH PAIN ON WEIGHT BEARING

One of the most difficult diagnostic problems is the geriatric patient who complains of pain on weight bearing. Such pain is particularly disabling and will rapidly bring the patient to the physician for treatment. The treating physician must define more clearly the nature of the pain and its pattern. The pain of neurogenic claudication tends to be aggravated during walking but generally not until the patient has walked some distance. As a rule, neurogenic claudication does not produce pain in the initial weight-bearing process. On the other hand, patients with osteoarthritis of the hip or knee will manifest pain rapidly as they change position from a seated to an upright position or as soon as weight bearing ensues. The pain associated with peripheral vascular disease also tends to be quite dramatic after a certain period of walking has taken place. Inflammatory conditions about the hip and knee, namely greater trochanteric bursitis or pes anserine bursitis, tend to be aggravated with weight bearing but are often with the patient even when the limb is at rest. Along with osteoarthritis such pains may be increased in severity during the night. Pain is also elicited when pressure is applied to them locally.

The duration of symptoms is also helpful information since a more progressive disease process may be described when the patient's symptoms have been gradually increasing in severity and not relenting. With a more acute presentation of pain the treating physician must look to an inflammatory problem as being the underlying source of the patient's complaint. This is particularly true of gouty arthritis, which can occur precipitously and without history of insult. Pain that tends to be constant without remission may be indicative of a malignant process within the bone.

The localization of the pain also bears great importance in providing insight as to its cause. Dysfunction of the hip joint tends to produce pain referred to the groin, anterior thigh, and medial knee area. Pathology localized to the knee joint tends to produce pain in the area of the knee itself with some referred component to the distal aspect of the thigh and proximal aspect of the lower leg. Ankle problems tend to produce pain that is diffuse about the ankle joint and that is, as a rule, more anterior than posterior with a medial and a lateral component. Vascular claudication tends to involve the calf and the pain is of a cramping nature. Neurogenic claudication, on the other hand, tends to produce pain that radiates generally in a bilateral fashion from the buttocks down both lower extremities posteriorly.

It is also important to question the patient as to his response to various medications. If the symptoms are markedly better with anti-inflammatory medications, it lends support to the idea that the problem results from either degenerative joint disease or localized bursitis or tendinitis. Should the pain be responsive only to stronger analgesics, the physician must be more concerned about a possible underlying pathologic process within the bone itself. Severe episodes of sciatica secondary to lumbosacral osteoarthritis can also produce severe pain requiring strong analgesics for relief.

Physical examination

Probably the most important aspect of the physical examination in terms of differentiating the source of the patient's problem is an evaluation of the gait. Fine alterations in weight bearing as well as a specific pattern of limp consistent for hip or knee disease may be noted. Weakness in the lower extremity can be observed from the patient's gait, and it becomes especially apparent on watching the patient arise from a seated position or climb stairs. In general, if the hip is severely involved, the patient will demonstrate an abductor lurch or an antalgic gait. If there is significant loss of motion, the gait will be shuffling; the pelvis will be rotated in a compensatory fashion. If the leg has been shortened, the shoulder will sag on the affected side as weight bearing takes place. The deformed knee in weight bearing will demonstrate lateral or medial shifts away from the side of the deformity. Patients who have referred pain from the lumbar area when they walk tend to describe radiation of the pain from their lower extremity into the paraspinal area.

An evaluation of the active and passive range of motion of the joints of the lower extremity will provide useful information in further defining the patient's underlying problem. Careful evaluation should be given to hip, knee, and ankle motion as well as to muscle power in the lower extremity. Leg lengths should be measured. In patients with spinal stenosis the physical findings will differ from patients with acute sciatica on a discogenic basis. Straight leg raising is often negative and the only findings may be paraspinal muscle spasm and significant limitation of spinal motion. The peripheral pulses should be evaluated and a careful neurologic examination of the lower extremities should be performed. It is important to measure the circumferences of the calf and thigh during the physical examination and to compare them to the contralateral, less symptomatic side. Localized areas of tenderness or swelling should be documented along with an effusion within the joint.

Radiographic evaluation

The physician, having taken a thorough history and performed a careful physical examination, will use radiographs to provide further information for arriving at a working diagnosis. It must be remembered, however, that many geriatric patients will have degenerative joint disease involving multiple areas and this can make interpretation of radiographs difficult. Patients will often have degenerative changes in the facet joints of the lumbosacral spine with disc-space narrowing along with arthritic changes in the hip, knee, and ankle. Therefore, the radiographs must be evaluated with a firm conceptualization of the patient's probable diagnosis, and they should be used to confirm the degree of objective involvement. More elaborate radiographic studies, such as CT scans, are useful in difficult diagnostic problems, particularly those involving an overlap with the lumbosacral spine and spinal stenosis. Arthrography can be useful in defining pathology in the knee joint but because of the high incidence of degenerative meniscal tears, it rarely provides more information in the geriatric patient than do the plain radiographs.

Additional laboratory information

If doubt persists as to the exact diagnosis, further serologic testing can be performed. This includes the erythrocyte sedementation rate, latex fixation test, and uric acid measurements as preliminary screening studies. If joint destruction is suspected to be on a neuropathic basis, a VDRL test should be performed as well as a 2-hour postprandial glucose determination if there is no history of diabetes. More specific immunologic studies including HLA-27 antigen, immunoelectrophoresis, and complement levels can be obtained but whether this should be done is best left to the judgment of the consulting rheumatologist.

In patients with a joint effusion (particularly in the knee or ankle joint) an arthro-

---

DIFFERENTIAL DIAGNOSIS OF LOWER EXTREMITY PAIN

I. Degenerative
  A. Osteoarthritis, primary or secondary
II. Metabolic
  A. Osteoporosis, osteomalacia
  B. Paget's disease
  C. Gout, pseudogout
III. Neoplastic
  A. Primary
  B. Metastatic
IV. Inflammatory
  A. Rheumatoid arthritis
  B. Soft tissue
    1. Bursitis
    2. Tendinitis
    3. Myositis
  C. Polymyalgia rheumatica
V. Infections
  A. Septic arthritis
  B. Osteomyelitis
  C. Tuberculosis

VI. Fracture
  A. Stress
  B. Traumatic
  C. Pathologic
VII. Referred
  A. Spine
  B. Visceral
VIII. Other
  A. Vascular insufficiency, peripheral or central
  B. Neurovascular disease
    1. Peripheral neuropathy with neuropathic joint
    2. Spinal cord diseases (e.g., amyotrophic lateral sclerosis, multiple sclerosis)
    3. Stroke

centesis can be performed. Fluid removed can be evaluated for culture, cell count, latex fixation, complement levels, and crystalline presence.

• • •

The differential diagnosis when a proper history and physical examination is completed will usually be quite narrow. The radiographic and other objective laboratory information will further define the problem. The material in the box on p. 195 gives a brief synopsis of the major categories of diseases that affect lower extremity function. These disease categories are discussed in separate sections of the text. Degenerative joint disease as it affects the lower extremities and its nonsurgical and surgical treatment will now be covered in detail. Inflammatory problems of the soft tissues will also be reviewed.

Emphasis should be on the careful collection of clinical data and the development of a treatment plan that is carefully constructed to meet the needs and concerns of the geriatric patient.

DEGENERATIVE JOINT DISEASE (OSTEOARTHRITIS)

Osteoarthritis affecting the weight-bearing joints of the lower extremity remains the most disabling affliction in geriatric patients. Controversy persists as to whether the alterations in articular cartilage in osteoarthritis are an inevitable result of an aging skeleton or a valid pathologic process. It has been demonstrated that changes occur in osteoarthritis both in the chondrocyte and in the matrix constituents of hyaline cartilage. Chondrocytes in early osteoarthritic articular cartilage demonstrate mitotic activity and metabolic activity not seen in normal cartilage. Desiccation is also noted in the matrix of degenerative cartilage. Proteoglycans are altered both in chain length and in constituent ratio. Reparative attempts by the chondrocytes produce much of the osteophytic bone and debris seen about the arthritic joint.[7] Radin, Paul, and Rose[13] have advanced the theory

that much of the articular cartilage damage is secondary to microfracture in subchondral bone with resultant sclerosis and bony condensation in the area. Impact loading of surface hyaline cartilage is thereby increased leading to degeneration and osteoarthritis.

Although significant involvement of lower extremity joints tends to be limited to one or two joints, a more generalized manifestation of osteoarthritis can be observed throughout the synovial joint system. Typically, articular damage is usually found affecting a particular portion of the entire joint surface (Fig. 12-1). In contrast, in the more inflammatory type of osteoarthritis, generalized joint damage occurs and the pattern may be quite similar to rheumatoid arthritis (Fig. 12-2). As articular cartilage damage progresses, irregularity develops in the cartilage surface with fissuring and fibrillation. Reactive changes in subchondral

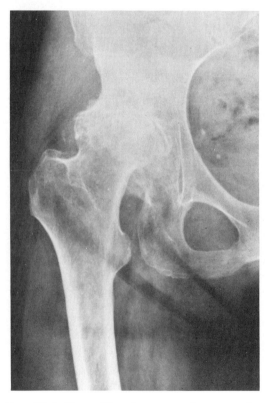

FIG. 12-1. X-ray film demonstrating superolateral involvement of hip joint with osteoarthritis.

bone become more marked with areas of sclerosis and cyst formation (Fig. 12-3). Continued proliferation of osteophytic bone produces further joint incongruity with resultant deformity. Secondary soft tissue changes occur in response to the damage in the joint, and contractures take place with further limitation of joint motion. Along with progressive destruction of the joint surfaces, deformity or subluxation, and periarticular soft tissue contractures, there is a decrease in power as a result of disuse.

Clinical presentation

Pain tends to be most marked on weight bearing and may also be quite pronounced at night. Patients will tend to avoid ambulation and such activities as stair climbing where loads on the affected joints will be significant and repetitive. Pain is relieved by rest and by unloading the joint

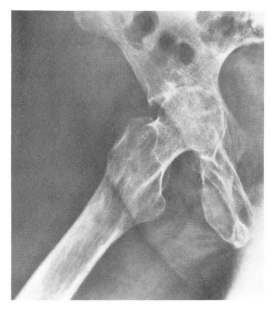

FIG. 12-2. Radiograph of generalized damage to joint surface in inflammatory osteoarthritis of hip.

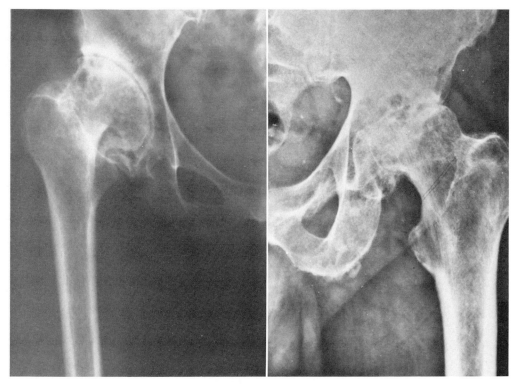

FIG. 12-3. Radiographs demonstrating marked cystic and sclerotic changes in bone in osteoarthritic hip joints.

with assistive devices, such as a cane or crutches.

Range of motion will become limited as the degenerative joint disease progresses. This is caused by the incongruity of the joint surfaces and also by the concomitant soft tissue contracture about the joint. Rotation of the hip is rapidly lost with flexion and abduction becoming more limited later in the course of the disease. External rotation-flexion deformities are particularly common in advanced degenerative hip disease, this being the resting position of the limb that is most comfortable for the patient. As a weight-bearing joint becomes more damaged, compensatory gait patterns develop. In the hip this may be manifested by an abductor lurch or quick step off pattern. As range of motion is lost, a shuffling component to the gait develops. As flexion deformity advances, a crouch may be assumed in standing and walking. Patients with knee osteoarthritis develop an antalgic component to their gait with rapid unloading of the affected leg. Joint instability and deformity are noted during the stance phase of gait. Gross medial and lateral shifts can be seen in ambulation toward the opposite side from the deformity.

In the knee joint flexion contracture develops early. This can be attributed to the knee being more comfortable in the flexed position, to the increased capacity of the knee joint to accommodate effusions in the flexed position, and to spasm in the hamstring tendons. Varus or valgus deformities alone are common in the arthritic knee joint and may be seen in combination with flexion and rotational deformity. In most patients soft tissue contracture is present on the concave side of the deformity (varus—medial, valgus—lateral, flexion—posterior) with laxity of soft tissue on the convex side of the deformity (Fig. 12-4). Motion is lost in flexion as knee joint damage progresses. In the ankle similar loss of motion is noted in both dorsiflexion and plantar flexion.

Pain, loss of motion, and deformity lead to increasing immobility in these geriatric patients and associated muscle weakness develops. Patients will describe a progressive decrease in their activity from community ambulation to being homebound in more severe cases. Atrophy of thigh and calf musculature will be discernible on observation. In the terminal stage ankylosis of an arthritic joint may occur and the geriatric patient may become nonambulatory.

Nonsurgical treatment

Treatment should be directed to the problem areas and their manifestations. In order to promote rehabilitation of the affected joint, pain relief is essential. Nonsteroidal anti-inflammatory medications are used extensively to reduce the synovitis present in the arthritic joint. The mechanism of action is unclear but probably works through the reduction in prostaglandin synthesis. Aspirin in anti-inflammatory levels (greater than 3 g/day) is the time-

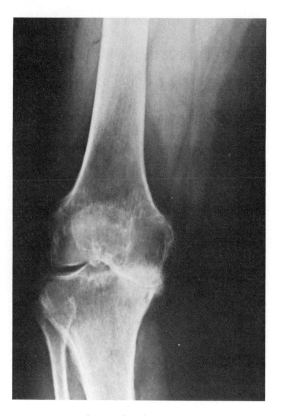

FIG. 12-4. Radiograph of varus deformity. Soft tissue is contracted on concave side of deformity and elongated on convex side of deformity.

proven drug of choice but compliance at these levels is a problem. Indomethacin, 100 to 150 mg/day, in my experience continues to be the most effective of the non-steroidal anti-inflammatory medications. Patients will respond variably to this category of medication, and if one medication is not working another may. Ibuprofen (Motrin), 1800 to 2400 mg/day, and naproxen (Naprosyn), 500 to 750 mg/day, are also particularly useful. The treating physician must inform these geriatric patients of the myriad of side effects from this group of medications. All have gastrointestinal side effects and aside from dyspepsia may produce gastrointestinal hemorrhage. Many will produce alterations in bowel function and at times alterations in cerebral function. The geriatric patient who tolerates these medications may be helped significantly with pain relief and is able to improve his functional level.

Analgesic medications can be used but with caution. Many idiosyncratic reactions to these medicines are noted in the geriatric group. Propoxyphene (Darvocet N-100) is generally safe and effective in these patients and only rarely is stronger analgesia needed.

Muscle relaxants are generally not effective in these patients.

Local injection. Intra-articular corticosteroids are not recommended for osteoarthritis of the hip. Fluoroscopy is needed to confirm the localization of the needle within the hip joint. Also, damage to associated structures can occur during this procedure if it is performed without radiographic control. The knee and ankle joints, being more peripheral and therefore accessible, can be injected safely. If the inflammatory component manifested by the degree of synovial hypertrophy and effusion is significant, relief can last up to 3 to 4 months with intra-articular injections. Absolute sterility must be maintained when injecting intra-articular steroids because the occurrence of infection within a joint may eliminate the possibility of future total joint arthroplasty in these patients. Dexamethasone, 40 to 80 mg, is administered and this can be re-peated at regular intervals in patients benefiting from these treatments. The usual response is a gradually decreasing effect from these injections until they are minimally effective. Patients with severe mechanical dysfunction of the knee or ankle joint secondary to their osteoarthritis are not generally improved. Repeated local steroid injections at short intervals may promote cartilage destruction and this is not recommended.

Rest. The involved joint or joints may be rested by lessening load carriage across these painful areas. This can be achieved by weight-relieving devices such as canes or crutches or periods of non-weight-bearing. It is important in the geriatric patient to maintain mobility and function and strict extended periods of bed rest should be avoided. Bracing for the arthritic knee is occasionally helpful. It must be appreciated by the physician that no static support can effectively counteract the magnitude of forces to the knee joint without significantly limiting knee motion. Bulky knee braces are also not well tolerated by the geriatric patient. The ankle joint lends itself to the use of orthoses to put the inflamed joint to rest. Polypropyline posterior braces with Velcro straps can be fabricated and fitted within the shoe (Fig. 12-5). Immobilization of the ankle is useful, but it must be remembered that stiffness and permanent loss of joint motion may result.

It should be emphasized to the patient that weight reduction represents significant unloading of the arthritic joint and is extremely beneficial.

Exercises. It is often paradoxical to patients when both rest to the affected joint and exercises are prescribed concomitantly. Because of the loss of strength and muscle bulk accompanying the disuse of the muscles about an inflamed joint, exercises are crucial to maintain range of motion and some degree of tonicity in these muscles. These are best done isometrically or without putting the joint through the painful arc of motion. The use of weights to increase resistance is not recommended in the geriatric patient since this can further

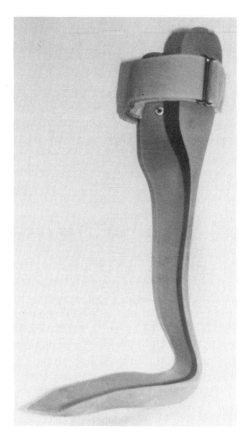

FIG. 12-5. Polypropylene brace to limit ankle motion.

aggravate the joint inflammation. Anti-gravity exercises can be performed in increasing repetitions. The patient may cause pain from an arthritic lumbar spine or associated areas if exercises, particularly straight leg raising, are too stressful.

Swimming is often an excellent way to promote range-of-motion and strengthening exercises because of its buoyant environment. Walking and the use of a stationary bicycle may also be beneficial to the geriatric patient. Passive range-of-motion exercises and supervised active exercises by a physical therapist should be encouraged in patients unable to do exercises on their own. Contractures should be prevented. Modalities such as ultrasound and diathermy also provide transient relief.

Surgical treatment

Surgery should be considered in geriatric patients who demonstrate progressive loss of ambulatory capacity secondary to pain and alteration of joint function. The goals of the treatment plan are to relieve pain and to restore function and independence. The decision to recommend surgery must also be based on the patient's general medical health. In addition, the surgeon must consider the patient's mental status and ability to participate in the postoperative therapeutic plan.

Debridement. The removal of degenerative debris from a joint has generally been performed in the knee joint and rarely in the hip and ankle. Open debridement procedures for an arthritic joint are designed primarily to remove mechanical impediments to joint function. Loose bodies, osteophytes, joint debris, and degenerated menisci have been removed in the knee joint as part of the procedure. Subchondral bone has been drilled where denuded of cartilage in an attempt to promote regeneration of fibrocartilage. Good results have been transient particularly in the older patient. Knee stiffness and prolonged convalescence after open debridement procedures have been common and these are generally disabling to the geriatric patient. Although morbidity is less, arthroscopic debridement has still met with limited success. Long-term follow-up data for these patients are not currently available. Geriatric patients with an element of crystalline synovitis do notice improvement because of the copious lavage at the time of arthroscopy, but the relief has been short term, lasting 3 to 6 months.

Osteotomy. The pattern of osteoarthritis is commonly focal and this is true particularly in the hip and knee. In the hip joint mild forms of hip dysplasia may result in superolateral involvement in the femoral head and corresponding acetabular surface. In the knee joint osteoarthritic involvement is commonly more severe in the medial or lateral compartment of the knee. Associated with tibiofemoral involvement or by itself, the patellofemoral joint may demonstrate degenerative changes.

Intertrochanteric or subtrochanteric osteotomy can be used to shift the load to more spared areas of the hip joint. Preoperative radiographs should be taken with the hip in abduction and adduction to determine maximum improvement in the contact between the femoral head and the acetabular surface. Sparing of the anterior aspect of the femoral head in many osteoarthritic hips has led to an attempt to extend the femoral head by osteotomy, bringing the anterior portion of the head into the hip joint. Fixation of osteotomy has been by blade plate devices, which ensure compression and allow early weight bearing and hip range-of-motion exercises. Results from osteotomy[3,6,14] have been good in the short term with 60% to 75% of patients improved up to 5 years after surgery. The results, however, tend to deteriorate further with time. Weisl[22] reports that only about 25% of patients had a lasting good result in a review of 757 intertrochanteric osteotomies. The procedure remains the preferred one for younger patients with focal hip disease.

Experience with osteotomy about the knee has yielded similar results of increasing failures with time.[4,21] Some authors have advocated combining tibial osteotomy with open joint debridement, but experience with the procedure has been mixed and knee stiffness may result.[11] It is recommended that for varus deformities a laterally based wedge be removed from the proximal tibia above the insertion of the patella tendon (Fig. 12-6). The proximal tibiofibular syndesmosis may be released with an osteotome or periosteal elevator and resection of the proximal fibula is usually not necessary. Internal fixation is also not used at the osteotomy site because these devices may act to prevent coaptation at the osteotomy surfaces during weight bearing. If no fixation is used, it is essential that the cylindar cast applied be snug and well fitted. Synthetic materials that are lightweight are used for casting. It is recommended that the cast remain on for a period of 7 to 8 weeks. Range of motion returns 4 to 6 weeks after cast removal (Fig. 12-7).

For lateral compartment involvement femoral osteotomy is recommended. A blade plate or other fixation method may be used to allow early knee motion (Fig. 12-8). Nonunion may occur in this procedure and healing is slow. Weight bearing remains protected for 2 to 3 months pending healing. Osteotomies remain an important procedure for localized degenerative joint disease in the younger patient or the active older patient.

Excision arthroplasty. Patellectomy remains the chief example of lower extremity excision arthroplasty. Although for isolated patellofemoral osteoarthritis it may be considered, in the geriatric patient results are mixed and persistent weakness of the quadriceps mechanism can occur with an extension lag to the knee. The patient may complain of difficulty on arising from a seated position or on climbing and descending stairs. Tendomalacia can also occur in the area of the patellectomy from contact

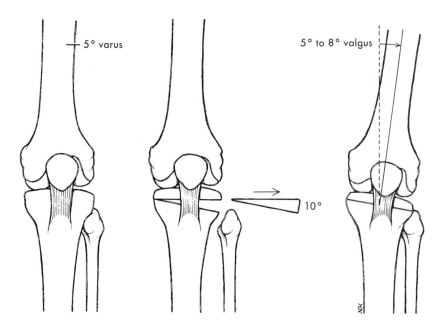

Fig. 12-6. High tibial osteotomy with laterally based wedge.

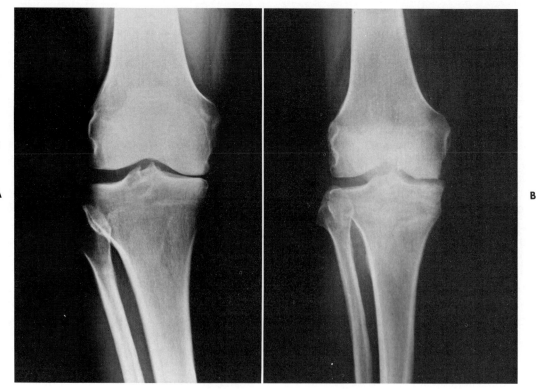

Fig. 12-7. A, Radiographs of patient with high tibial osteotomy for varus deformity. B, Radiograph after 5 years.

of the tendon against the anterior femoral condyle.

In the geriatric patient there is usually involvement of the tibiofemoral compartment and therefore total knee replacement is more frequently recommended. Results of total knee replacement in patients with previous patellectomy have not been as good as in patients undergoing primary total knee replacement.[12] In most geriatric patients total joint arthroplasty has become the procedure of choice because of its rapid recovery and high percentage of predictable good results.

Total joint replacement

The greatest advance in the treatment of degenerative arthritic afflictions of the major weight-bearing joints of the lower extremity has been the evolution of total joint replacement. This has been particularly important in returning the geriatric patient to a high level of ambulatory function as well as in maintaining independence in his daily existence. The techniques used involve the replacement of arthritic surfaces by metals and high-density polyethylene implants that are lubricated by synovial fluid from remaining synovial cells. The technologic advances in the past 15 years have been directed toward improving the biomechanical features of these implants as well as the materials used in their fabrication. In addition, technical advances have been made in lessening the incidence of mechanical failure of these implants as a result of poor fixation of the implant to the bone by the methylmethacrylate. The problem of infection, present in any operative procedure, is particularly catastrophic in patients undergoing prosthetic joint replacement because as a rule infection cannot be eradicated without removal of implant material and bone cement.

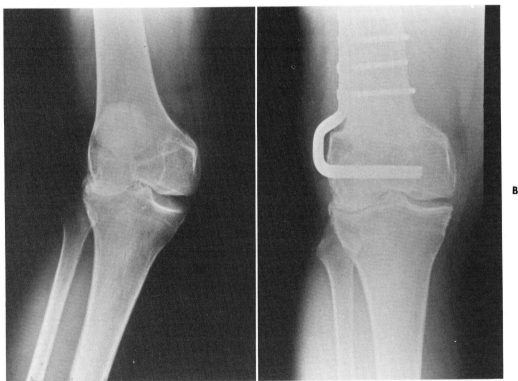

FIG. 12-8. **A,** Radiograph of osteoarthritis of lateral compartment of knee treated by valgus osteotomy and internal fixation. **B,** Radiograph after 3 years.

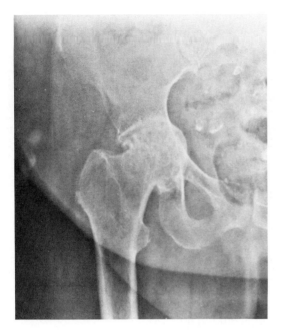

FIG. 12-9. Radiograph of protrusio deformity in patient with erosive osteoarthritis.

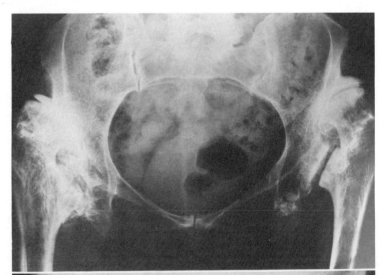

FIG. 12-10. Marked true acetabular deformity in congential hip dysplasia treated by custom total hip replacement.

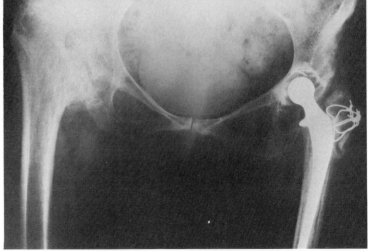

The elderly patient presents specific problems in implant arthroplasty. These include the potential medical complications that are attendant to any major surgical procedure in the geriatric patient. In addition, osteoporosis with bone loss may influence the surgical approach to implant arthroplasty and require methods to augment deficient bone. In patients with advanced deformities, particularly about the knee, custom implants or the use of bone-grafting procedures may be necessary to augment these defects and correct bone deficiencies. Untoward anesthetic reactions may influence the patient's general medical status or cerebration to the point where the patient is unable to participate in the postoperative rehabilitation. The geriatric patient is also prone to urinary retention and secondary infection or infection in other areas that may seed the prosthetic joint, leading to deep infection about the prosthetic implants.

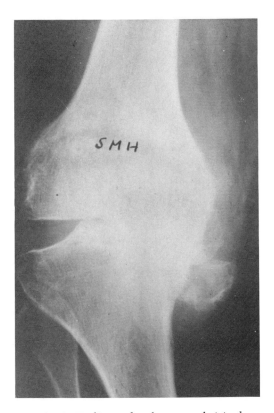

FIG. 12-11. Radiograph of osteoarthritic knee with severe bone defect on tibial plateau.

Bone deficiency in joint replacement. Bone deficiency in the geriatric patient may result from osteoporosis or from progressive bone destruction caused by abnormal loads being transmitted to one aspect of the arthritic joint. This is commonly seen in the hip in the osteoporotic patient who develops a protrusio deformity, which is most commonly seen in patients with Paget's disease or in patients with severe osteoporosis and an erosive or inflammatory-type of osteoarthritis (Fig. 12-9). Protrusio deformities are also common in patients with rheumatoid arthritis. In the osteoarthritic hip in a patient with previous hip dysplasia there may be significant bone loss in the true acetabulum (Fig. 12-10). Bone loss can be significant over the superior shelf of the acetabulum with secondary flattening of the femoral head. In the knee joint varus or valgus malalignment may result in the progressive loss of bone over the medial or lateral tibial plateau (Fig. 12-11). Corresponding bone loss may occur in the knee joint over the distal femur, but this is far less common.

In the hip, bone grafting techniques are employed to improve the position of the prosthetic implant.

Protrusio deformity. In the patient who has penetration of the iliopectineal line by the femoral head a protrusio deformity exists. As a rule, when this evolves over a period of time, the acetabular floor is intact although it is generally weakened. Complete bone deficiency at the base of the acetabulum is unusual.

These patients may present difficulties in the dislocation of the femoral head from the acetabulum if approached without trochanteric osteotomy. If ankylosis of the femoral head exists, it may be necessary to transect the femoral neck in the subcapital area to rotate the femur externally and to remove it from the mouth of the acetabulum. (Fig. 12-12, *A*). The femoral osteotomy can then be modified by a second cut in the area that previous measurements have demonstrated is the correct level for this osteotomy. The remaining femoral head is removed in toto by using curved osteotomes around the femoral head and inner

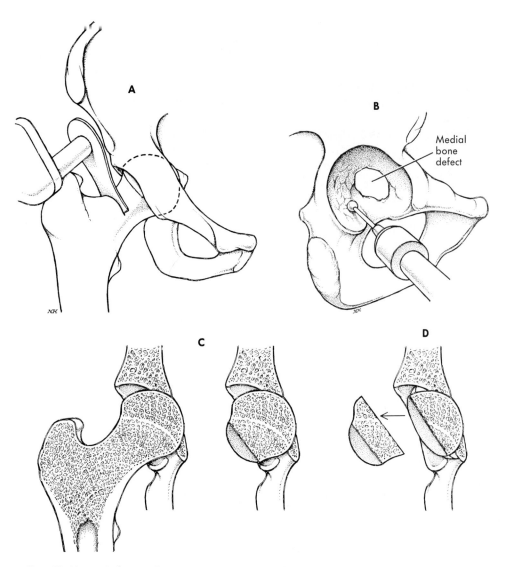

Fig. 12-12. A, Subcapital osteotomy to mobilize femur. **B,** High-speed burr is used to remove debris from floor of acetabulum. **C,** Segment of femoral head is inserted as medial bone graft. **D,** Methylmethacrylate is used as a sealant around the bone graft.

acetabular rim. The base of the acetabulum is often quite sclerotic and a Midas high-speed burr can be used carefully to prepare the mouth of the acetabulum; fibrous debris from the floor of the acetabulum can be gently and safely removed with this instrument (Fig. 12-12, *B*). The femoral head can be decorticated down to cancellous bone and a portion of it inserted into the deepened acetabulum to lateralize the placement of the prosthetic cup. If the femoral head can be dislocated without osteotomy, this decortication is best done be-

fore removal of the femoral head by transection of the femoral neck. Fixation of this bone graft to the floor of the acetabulum is generally not necessary since the femoral head and acetabulum are well mated from being previously coapted (Fig. 12-12, *C*). Methylmethacrylate is used as a sealant around the periphery of this bone graft and it is allowed to harden before insertion of a second batch of methylmethacrylate and the prosthetic cup itself (Figs. 12-12, *D*, and 12-13). If this technique is not used, methylmethacrylate will tend to penetrate be-

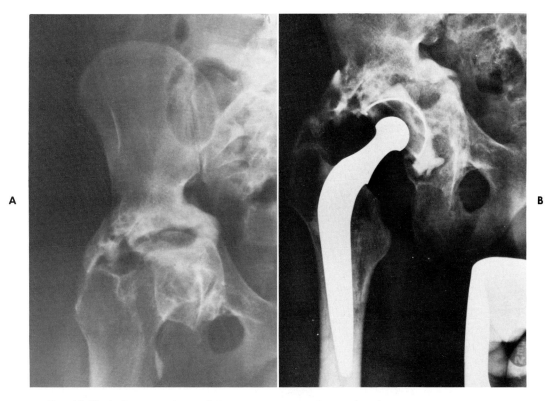

FIG. 12-13. **A,** Preoperative and, **B,** postoperative radiographs of posttraumatic protrusio defect treated with medial bone graft from femoral head.

FIG. 12-14. Use of metal acetabular ring to reinforce deficient medial wall of acetabulum.

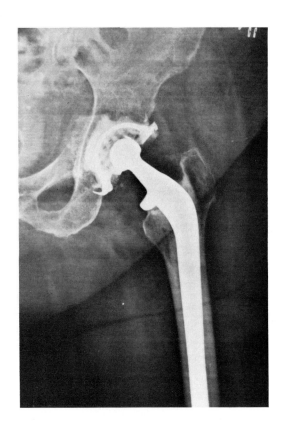

hind the bone graft and this will result in a nonviable piece of bone being situated between two methylmethacrylate layers.

If the floor of the acetabulum is perforated or very weakened, mesh or a Müller ring, which is fixed to the mouth of the acetabulum, may be used (Fig. 12-14).

Superolateral acetabular deficiency. In patients with acetabular deficiency over the superolateral aspect of the acetabulum, bone grafting again can be utilized to fill this defect. Such a deficiency is most commonly encountered in patients with con-

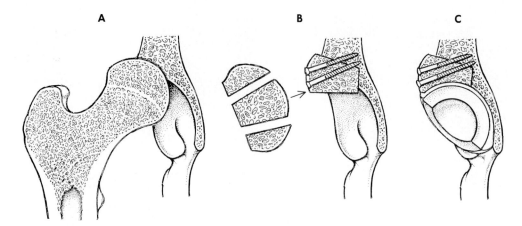

FIG. 12-15. **A,** Acetabulum with superior defect. **B,** Segment of femoral head is used to fill superolateral defect. **C,** Prosthetic acetabulum inserted below bone graft.

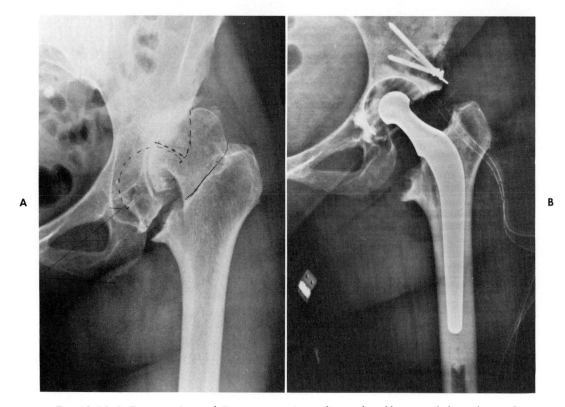

FIG. 12-16. **A,** Preoperative and, **B,** postoperative radiographs of bone graft from femoral head to fill superolateral acetabular defect.

genital dysplasia of the hip in which there has been lateral subluxation of the femoral head with flattening of this segment of the acetabular roof. When reaming has been performed to reposition the prosthetic acetabulum in a more normal position, the surgeon will often be faced with a deficient roof in the superolateral area. Bone grafting may be performed by again decorticating the femoral head and using a Midas or other burr to remove sclerotic bone from this area of the acetabulum. The bone graft is then inserted in the area of bone deficiency and held in position by multiple K wires (Fig. 12-15). Reaming is performed to allow insertion of the prosthetic cup and the reaming can be directly into the bone graft itself. When satisfactory coverage has been obtained, cortical screws may be used to fix the bone graft to the acetabulum. The screws are inserted after the reaming process so that fixation will not be interfered with by the reaming with the screws affixed. Methylmethacrylate is again used to

seal the bone graft surfaces and to prevent intrusion of cement behind the bone graft. A second batch of cement is inserted with the prosthetic cup. Postoperative management for those patients undergoing bone grafting is similar to management after uncomplicated hip replacements. However, if the bone graft is quite large, protected weight bearing should be continued for 3 months postoperatively (Fig. 12-16).

Bone deficiencies in the knee. The knee joint represents a similar problem in patients with advanced varus or valgus deformity. The bone deficit tends to be more on the tibial than femoral side although there may be an element of bone loss on both femur and tibia (Fig. 12-17, *A*).

The knee is exposed as for a routine total knee replacement and the bone is removed, with the distal femoral cut being saved for the later bone grafting (Fig. 12-17, *B*).

The bed of the area of bone deficit is generally very sclerotic and does not lend itself to good coaptation of the bone graft because

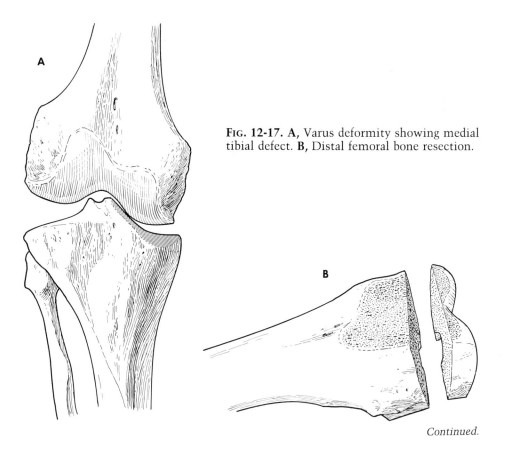

FIG. 12-17. A, Varus deformity showing medial tibial defect. **B,** Distal femoral bone resection.

Continued.

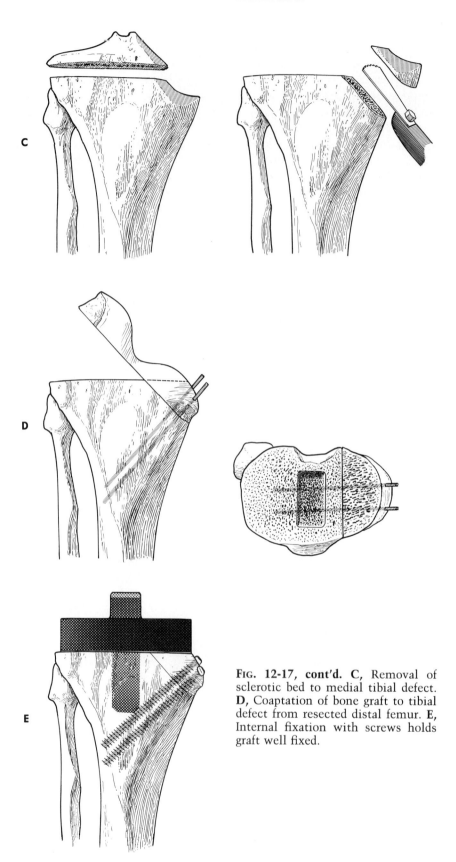

FIG. 12-17, cont'd. C, Removal of sclerotic bed to medial tibial defect. **D,** Coaptation of bone graft to tibial defect from resected distal femur. **E,** Internal fixation with screws holds graft well fixed.

the shape is commonly dished. A technique that I have utilized incorporates excision of this sclerotic area of bone in an oblique fashion to expose areas of cancellous bone below the sclerotic bed of the bone deficit (Fig. 12-17, C). The distal femoral bone can then be apposed to this oblique tibial area and held in position with two K-wires (Fig. 12-17, D). A saw can then remove the segment of femoral condyle that is hanging over the proximal tibia. Two screws are then used to hold the bone graft in position. There should be excellent coaptation of cancellous bone from the graft to the recipient bed (Fig. 12-17, E). The methylmethacrylate sealing technique is again used to prevent penetration of cement beneath the bone graft into its bed and thereby interfere with its ability to be incorporated into the proximal tibia. The tibial component is then inserted directly on this bone graft with a second batch of methylmethacrylate (Fig. 12-18, A and B).

Alternative ways to deal with bone deficits include the use of methylmethacrylate by itself, using screws or mesh embedded in methylmethacrylate, or utilizing a custom-made prosthesis with a metal wedge that fills the area of bone loss (Fig. 12-19). Unsupported methylmethacrylate columns should be avoided for deficits of greater than 0.5 cm because fractures of such columns have occurred with loss of implant position. This is also true for methylmethacrylate reinforced by screws or mesh. The use of a custom implant has been popular at the Hospital for Special Surgery; however, there is difficulty in obtaining these custom implants quickly, and at surgery the fit may not be exact after debridement and preparing the deficit bed. Postoperative management when bone-grafting procedures have been used does not vary from standard postoperative total knee replacement techniques.

Particularly in patients with osteoporo-

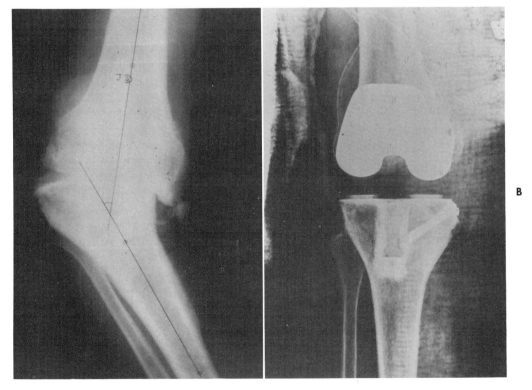

FIG. 12-18. **A,** Preoperative and, **B,** postoperative use of bone graft for deficient tibia.

sis a metal-backed prosthesis should be employed and in the knee the implant should extend to the cortical margin to prevent possible subsidence of the implant into the proximal tibia.

Results. Total joint replacement has led to good results in 85% to 90% of patients.[8,15,18] Relief of pain, improved range of motion, and better function is the rule after total joint replacements. However,

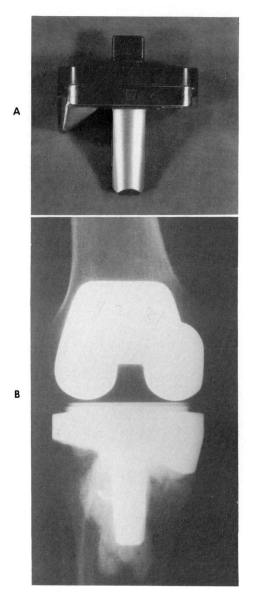

FIG. 12-19. **A,** Custom total knee prosthesis with medial wedge to fill defect in tibia. **B,** Radiograph of custom tibial prosthesis implanted.

complications do occur and their management may be more complicated in the geriatric patient. Prevention is always preferred and therefore careful preoperative and perioperative monitoring is essential in these patients as well as expeditious and accurate surgical technique.

Postoperative management. Geriatric patients after total joint replacement must be mobilized from bed to chair and to an ambulatory status as rapidly as possible. As a rule, after initial incisional pain has subsided, usually 48 hours after surgery, patients are mobilized from bed and are encouraged to ambulate with a physical therapist and external support.

Most patients in the postoperative period are advanced to Lofstrand crutches, although patients after both knee and hip replacement surgery who are quite elderly and have difficulty ambulating with these crutches may be discharged home using either a cane or a walker if they are unable to negotiate ambulation with a cane.

The protocol at the Hospital for Special Surgery is to administer preoperative antibiotics approximately 2 hours before the surgical procedure and to maintain antibiotics intravenously postoperatively for 36 to 48 hours. Penicillinase-resistant penicillins may be used or the cephalosporins.

Thromboembolic complications may occur and in routine venography studies incidence of clot formation in the deep venous system occurs in up to 60% to 84% of patients.[9,10,20] Involvement of the iliofemoral system is significantly less, however, although subclinical pulmonary emboli do occur. Thromboembolic prophylaxis has been debated in the management of patients and currently aspirin, 600 mg orally twice a day, is used in most patients. In those patients with a thromboembolic history or those who are at high risk, such as obese or sedentary patients, warfarin (Coumadin) may be given prophylactically the night of surgery and monitored postoperatively. It has been recommended that the prothrombin time not be elevated beyond 1½ times normal, and this has prevented many of the wound hemorrhagic complications noted in other studies.[16] Should thromboembolism occur, postoperative anticoagulation is continued for 3 to 6 months.

Patients after knee replacement surgery are now being placed in a constant passive motion machine, which has led to the return of knee flexion more quickly and with less pain when the fresh postoperative knee is manipulated by a physical therapist. A recent report by Lynch et al.[10] has demonstrated a reduction in the incidence of deep vein clots when the constant passive motion machine is used and, if available, its use is strongly advocated. Patients should not be discharged home before they have attained 85 to 90 degrees of knee flexion.

Mechanical failures. The problems of wear and breakage of implants have been less than originally surmised. Studies have demonstrated that the polyethylene cup in a total hip replacement in a patient of the geriatric patient's level of activity will last from 30 to 40 years.[2] The problems of breakage that were noted in the femoral component in early total hip designs,[1,5] particularly in men weighing more than 200

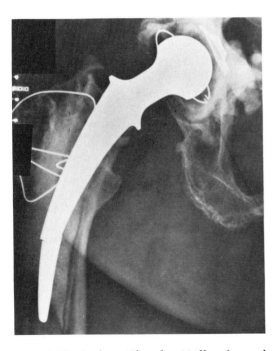

Fig. 12-20. Broken Charnley-Müller femoral component in 240-pound man.

pounds, have been virtually eliminated by the use of super alloy materials and the availability of larger femoral stem sizes (Fig. 12-20).

The main problem that still exists is loss of fixation of the implant to bone by its methylmethacrylate envelope. This occurs variably in the literature and may be completely asymptomatic and solely a radiographic finding. In those patients with symptomatic loosening of an implant, treatment will vary depending on whether the fixation is deficient at the bone-cement interface or the cement-prosthesis interface. More commonly, loosening occurs at the bone-cement interface with fragmentation of the cement and it is necessary to remove this methylmethacrylate as part of the revision procedure (Fig. 12-21). When this occurs, cement-removal instruments and high-speed burrs are necessary so that all methylmethacrylate can be removed and additional methylmethacrylate can then be inserted with reimplantation of the implant. This procedure is often quite tedious and patience is required not to perforate or fracture the bone during the revision procedure. If the cement mantle is intact, the prosthesis can be removed and further cement can be inserted directly into the previous methylmethacrylate column and a new implant is then inserted.

In cases of progressive bone destruction with migration of the implant, it will be necessary to employ bone-grafting techniques to improve the quality of bone into which the revision implant is inserted and, additionally, a custom implant or other metal reinforcement may be necessary to augment these bone deficits. In any revision procedure for mechanical loosening, careful preoperative planning is important to prevent situations in the operating room where the surgeon does not have available the proper cement-removal tools or a variety of implants for dealing with the remaining bone after prosthetic removal. The surgeon should be alert to the possibility that a custom implant may be necessary to deal with excessive bone loss, and this should be fabricated preoperatively by submitting the proper films for use in designing the implant to an implant manufacturer.

Particularly in patients undergoing revision of a total knee replacement, bone loss occurs as the implant loosens in the bone and the surgeon should be prepared to fill these defects with autogenous bone or iliac crest bone at the time of the revision (Fig. 12-22, *A* and *B*).

Dislocations. Dislocation in total hip replacements is reported to occur in up to 5% of cases.[23] The most common cause for in-

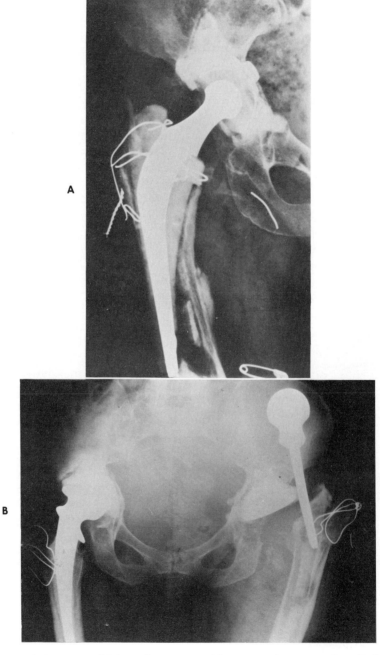

FIG. 12-21. **A,** Loose total hip replacement with cement fragmentation. **B,** Loosening and dislocation of total hip replacement from its methylmethacrylate envelope.

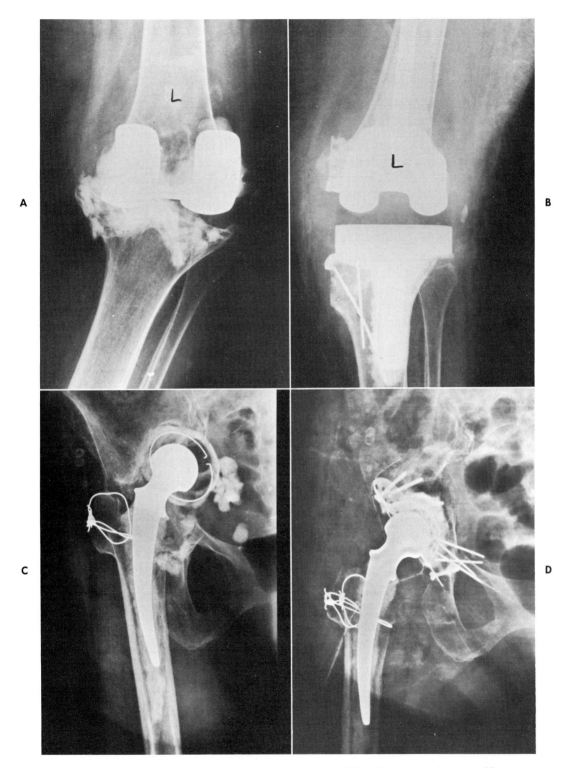

FIG. 12-22. A, Preoperative and, **B,** postoperative x-ray films demonstrating use of bone grafts to augment bone deficit in total knee replacement revision. **C,** Loose acetabular component with massive loss of medial bone support. **D,** Postoperative radiograph demonstrating use of large iliac crest graft to fill acetabulum and metal ring for added support.

stability of the prosthetic components is malposition in their insertion. This is particularly true in insertion of the acetabular or femoral component, which may be retroverted if care is not taken.

If the posterior approach to the hip is used, it is important to have ample visualization of the acetabulum. This requires thorough release about the acetabulum and proximal femur to allow mobilization of the femur anterior to the acetabulum. A curved Hohman retractor may be used over the anterior lip of the acetabulum to hold the femur clear of the acetabular opening (Fig. 12-23).

The insertion of the gluteus maximus into the femur should be released routinely if the posterior approach is utilized, as it allows greater internal rotation and mobilization of the femur without undue tension on the posterior structures.

A capsular closure is recommended in the geriatric patient whose muscle tone may be poor (1) to provide further stability to the prosthesis and (2) to provide another soft tissue layer between the prosthetic components should infection occur.

A technique that I have used in these patients requires identification of the external rotators and using a right-angled narrow Hohman retractor under the abductor superior to the pyriformis tendon. Using electrocautery the external rotators are removed at their insertion into the posterior greater trochanter and elevated off the posterior hip capsule (Fig. 12-24, *A*). A portion of the gluteus minimus can also be incised and released more superiorly. The capsule is then entered, creating a wide-based flap from the posterior wall of the acetabulum (Fig. 12-24, *B*). That is, the capsule is incised along the superior femoral neck and then the capsule is incised superiorly and inferiorly extending posteriorly and diverging as widely as possible. The posterior acetabular retractor is inserted between the labrum and the capsule, and this posterior capsular flap is thereby protected throughout the procedure (Fig. 12-24, *C*).

After completion of the hip replacement, two drill holes are made into the greater trochanter and a suture is placed from inside the capsule through this layer, then through the pyriformis tendon back through the capsule. A similar stitch is performed more inferiorly through the capsule and conjoined tendon (Fig. 12-24, *D*). By having the sutures begin inside the capsule and end in this fashion, the flap is inverted beneath the greater trochanter and the entire posterior aspect of the hip is closed.

In over 500 total hip replacements that utilized this technique, the dislocation rate has been less than 1% and delayed dislocation (after discharge from the hospital) has been extremely rare.

Management of wound complications and infection after total joint replacement. The geriatric patient who develops a wound complication, a superficial or deep wound infection involving the implant itself, is at risk because further, more complicated surgical procedures are often necessary. In those patients with delayed wound healing or persistent culture-negative drainage from the wound or hematoma, local wound treatment should be employed. If a hematoma that is quite extensive develops, it should be evacuated in the operating room

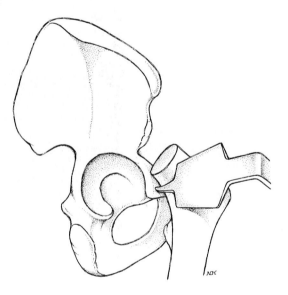

FIG. 12-23. Curved Hohman retractor over anterior rim of acetabulum.

and the wound should be closed primarily. If drainage persists and is culture-negative, sterile dressings must be applied by the surgeon and careful wound care must be continued until the drainage ceases. In the patient with a draining total knee replacement either from hematoma or from seroma, knee flexion in the postoperative period should be postponed until drainage ceases. If drainage persists beyond 5 to 7 days, reexploration of the wound is indicated with closure at that time.

Superficial wound infection. Infections in the immediate postoperative period that do not involve the implant itself may be treated by early debridement of infected tissue and closure with appropriate antibiotics being continued until the wound is healed, usually in 7 to 10 days. In patients with large abscess cavities above the fascia and not involving the implant, the wound may be packed open in the initial period and a secondary would closure can be performed in 7 to 10 days.

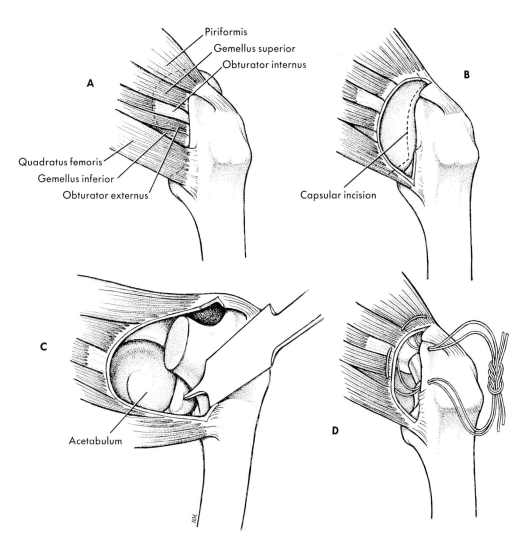

FIG. 12-24. Reconstruction of posterior capsule in total hip replacement. **A,** External hip rotation. **B,** Removal of insertion of external rotator from surface of capsule. **C,** Hohman retractor placed anterior and posterior (not shown) in space between labrum and capsule. **D,** Reattachment of external rotator and capsule to greater trochanter.

Deep wound infection. Deep wound infections (Fig. 12-25) may be classified according to whether or not there is obvious involvement of the implant and its bone-cement interface. As a rule, early deep wound infections involving the prosthetic implants may be treated by thorough debridement and appropriate postoperative antibiotics until the wound is healed and there is no evidence of infection. Generally this would entail a 2 to 3 week course of intravenous antibiotics. Closed tube drainage is generally not utilized because contamination of the arthroplasty may occur with these tubes. However, if an abscess cavity is encountered, closed tube drainage may be used for 48 to 72 hours to irrigate this particular cavity.

In patients with deep wound infections that demonstrate changes in the bone-cement interface, the infection cannot be eradicated without removal of the implants and all the methylmethacrylate (Fig. 12-26). It is emphasized that methylmethacrylate must be removed in toto to prevent reoccurrence of infection and to allow for reimplantation of the implant. Radiographs should be taken in the operating room at the conclusion of the procedure if there is any question as to whether methylmethacrylate is still present in any bony surface. Once all foreign material has been removed, gentamicin-impregnated beads may be used about the pseudarthrosis created to ensure high-level local antibiotic elution. Appropriate intravenous antibiotics are continued 6 weeks postoperatively. More recently, I have been utilizing a Broviac catheter and in some cases discharge from the hospital with administration of antibiotics at home by the patient's family. The implant is then reinserted with antibiotic-impregnated methylmethacrylate (Palacos) after the course of intravenous antibiotics has been completed. Before reoperation, the pseudarthrosis is aspirated and a frozen section and gram stain are performed at the time of the reimplantation procedure to look for evidence of organisms or active acute inflammation. If either is encountered, the reimplantation is not performed at that time. The results at the Hospital for

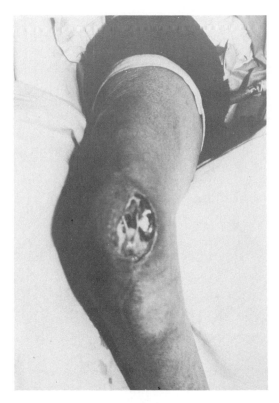

Fig. 12-25. Deep wound infection with major wound slough and prosthesis exposed.

Special Surgery utilizing this protocol have led to a greater than 90% success rate in reimplantation of infected hip replacements without the use of antibiotic-impregnated cement during the reimplantation procedure, although such cement is currently being utilized more frequently. The success rate has been even higher in reimplantation of infected knee implants, approaching 98%, because debridement can be performed more accurately and thoroughly in the knee than in the hip.

Total ankle arthroplasty. Prosthetic replacement of the ankle joint, particularly for osteoarthritis, has not led to nearly the degree of excellent results as prosthetic replacement of the hip and knee joints. In various studies of total ankle replacement, success in the osteoarthritic patient has been only in the 60% to 65% range.[17,19] Failure has been primarily from loosening of the implant or associated pain about the ankle from impingement of the fibulocal-

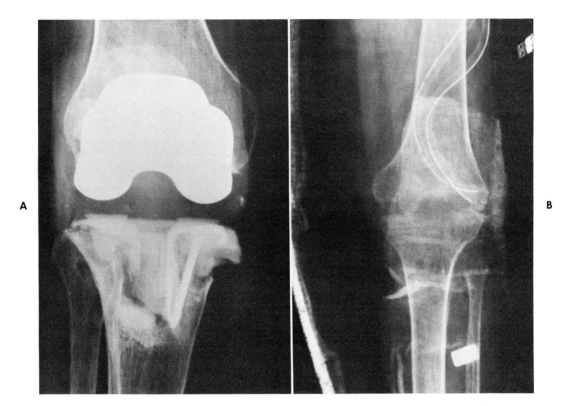

A

B

FIG. 12-26. **A,** Deep infection involving bone-cement interface with loosening of components. **B,** After removal of implant.

caneal area. Range of motion has also been disappointing after arthroplasty in these osteoarthritic patients. Removal of the failed total ankle replacement followed by arthrodesis has been difficult. Shortening is present when the ankle replacement is removed and the bony surfaces do not lend themselves to easy union at the arthrodesis site.

Arthrodesis of the ankle joint also has been problematic particularly in the geriatric patient. Use of external fixation and compression techniques, with or without plaster casting, is cumbersome and greatly limits the geriatric patient's ambulatory capacity. Conservative measures, particularly nonsteroidal antiinflammatory medications, bracing, and protected weight bearing are recommended for ankle arthritis for as long as possible. If all attempts at nonsurgical treatment are not successful, ankle arthrodesis remains the procedure of choice for these patients.

INFLAMMATORY PROBLEMS

Aside from the degenerative process damaging the weight-bearing joints, the most frequent cause of lower extremity pain related to the major weight-bearing areas (the hip, knee, and ankle) is inflammatory involvement of tendons or bursae.

In the hip area the most common involvement occurs around the greater trochanter, where a localized area of tenderness is present and pain is referred proximally and distally about the lateral thigh. Patients will complain of pain when they lie on this involved side and also when they cross their leg, which increases tension across the greater trochanteric soft tissues. Treatment is by local injection of dexamethasone, 40 mg, into the trochanteric area. Oral anti-inflammatory medications usually are inadequate and are not well tolerated by the geriatric gastrointestinal tract. Repeated injections may be necessary in severe and chronic cases.

Localized swelling with tenderness may occur after trauma to the patella area, and prepatellar bursitis may result in significant swelling within the bursa. On occasion this may become infected and require repeated aspiration and antibiotic coverage. In severe cases incision and drainage may be necessary. Pes anserine bursitis can also occur about the knee.

Tendinitis may affect the abductor tendon of the hip, the patellar tendon, or the Achilles tendon, all at their insertions. Treatment is by injection of dexamethasone. On recovery stretching and strengthening exercises are given to these patients.

References

1. Chao, E.Y.S., and Coventry, M.B.: Fracture of the femoral component after total hip replacement: an analysis of 58 cases, J. Bone Joint Surg. **63A:**1078-1094, 1981.
2. Charnley, J., and Halley, D.K.: Rate of wear in total hip replacement, Clin. Orthop. **112:**170-179, 1975.
3. Collert, S., and Gillstrom, P.: Osteotomy in osteoarthritis of the hip, Acta Orthop. Scand. **50:**555-561, 1979.
4. Coventry, M.D.: Upper tibial osteotomy for gonarthrosis, Orthop. Clin. North Am. **10:**191-210, 1979.
5. Galante, J.O.: Current concepts review: causes of fracture of the femoral component in total hip replacement, J. Bone Joint Surg. **62A:**670-673, 1980.
6. Goldie, I., Andersson, G., and Olsson, S.: Long-term follow-up of intertrochanteric osteotomy in osteoarthritis in the hip joint, Clin. Orthop. **93:**265-270, 1973.
7. Howell, D.S., and Moskowitz, R.W.: Introduction: symposium on arthritis. A brief review of research and directions for future investigations, Arthritis Rheum. **20:**96-103, 1977.
8. Insall, J.N., Lachiewicz, P.F., and Burstein, A.H.: The posterior stabilized condylar prosthesis: a modification of the total condylar design: two to four year experience, J. Bone Joint Surg. **64A:**1317-1323, 1982.
9. Lotke, P.A., Ecker, M.L., Alavi, A., and Berkowitz, H..: Indications for the treatment of deep venous thrombosis following total knee replacement, J. Bone Joint Surg. **66A:**202-208, 1984.
10. Lynch, K.A., et al.: Continuous passive motion: a prophylaxis for deep venous thrombosis following total knee replacement, Paper presented at the annual meeting of the American Academy of Orthopaedic Surgeons, Atlanta, Ga., 1984.
11. MacIntosh, D.L., and Welsh, R.P.: Joint debridement: A complement to high tibial osteotomy in the treatment of degenerative arthritis of the knee, J. Bone Joint Surg. **59A:**1094-1097, 1977.
12. Mjos, T., and Premer, R.F.: Total knee arthroplasty after patellectomy, Paper presented at the annual meeting of the American Academy of Orthopaedic Surgeons, Atlanta, Ga., 1984.
13. Radin, E.L., Paul, I.L., and Rose, R.M.: Current concepts of the etiology of idiopathic osteoarthritis, Bull. Hosp. Joint Dis. **38:**117-120, 1977.
14. Salenius, P., Langenskiold, A., and Osterman, K.: Intertrochanteric displacement osteotomy in the treatment of osteoarthritis of the hip, Acta Orthop. Scand. **42:**63-77, 1971.
15. Salvati, E.A., et al.: A ten year follow-up of our first 100 consecutive Charnley total hip replacements, J. Bone Joint Surg. **63A:**753-767, 1981.
16. Salzman, E.W., and Harris, W.H.: Prevention of venous thromboembolism in orthopaedic patients, J. Bone Joint Surg. **58A:**903-913, 1976.
17. Stauffer, R.N.: Total joint arthroplasty: the ankle, Mayo Clin. Proc. **54:**570-575, 1979.
18. Stauffer, R.N.: Ten year follow-up study of total hip replacement, J. Bone Joint Surg. **64A:**983-990, 1982.
19. St. Elmo, N.: Total ankle arthroplasty, J. Bone Joint Surg. **64A:**104-111, 1982.
20. Stulberg, B.N., Insall, J.N., Williams, G.W., and Ghelman, B.: Deep vein thrombosis following total knee replacement, J. Bone Joint Surg. **66A:**194-201, 1984.
21. Vainionpää, S., Läike, E., Kirves, P., and Tiusanen, P.: Tibial osteotomy for osteoarthritis of the knee: a five to ten year follow-up study, J. Bone Joint Surg. **63A:**938-946, 1981.
22. Weisl, H.: Introchanteric osteotomy for osteoarthritis: a long-term follow-up, J. Bone Joint Surg. **62B:**37-42, 1980.
23. Woo, R.Y.G., and Morrey, B.F.: Dislocation after total hip arthroplasty, J. Bone Joint Surg. **64A:**1295-1306, 1982.

chapter 13
THE GERIATRIC FOOT: DISORDERS AND TREATMENT

Alexander Hersh

The Bureau of the Census report in the *New York Times,* May 24, 1981, indicated that there were 25.5 million people over 65 years old, 28% more than in 1970. The large increase in the number of people over 65, which exceeded by far the 11% growth rate of the nation's population as a whole, was caused in large measure by advances in medical science, nutrition, and economic security. The figures also showed 6 million more females than males in the population, mainly because women live longer.

The margin of females over males is a relatively new phenomenon in the nation's history. When the country was developing and immigration was at its height, the influx of single men seeking their fortunes resulted in a predominant number of males. In 1910 there were 106 males for every 100 females. As late as 1940 men still held a slight margin. But in 1950 there were only 98.6 males for every 100 females, and the trend has continued. In 1980 there were 94.4 males for every 100 females. The count conducted in April, 1980, showed 116,472,539 women to 110,032,295 men.

Females were even more dominant in the upper age brackets. In the latest census report there were three women for every two men over the age of 65, and among those over 85, the Census Bureau counted 1,558,293 women and 681,428 men, a margin of more than two to one. Meanwhile the number of persons over 65 doubled from 1950 to 1980 because of increased longevity.

Demographers estimate that 11% of the population is over 65, and the elderly are expected to exceed 20% of the population within 50 years, when the numbers are projected to be 63,000,000. It is well documented that people are living longer, and concurrently, many are "growing younger." Some 70% of the over-65 population report themselves to be in generally good health. Only 5% are in nursing homes. Nevertheless, the elderly do need more than average medical attention to keep them in good health. Foot problems of a wide range are among the most common, along with special footwear needs.

From the early 1900s through the 1960s knowledge and methods in the management and treatment of foot disorders were obtained largely from experience with children and young adults. Now a group of older people whose foot problems are different from those seen in younger patients requires attention.

The limitation of the ability to walk resulting from disorders of the foot in the elderly has an overall deleterious effect on the individual. The enforced immobilization leads to isolation, which can result in depression, boredom, a lack of exercise with the resultant sequellae of diminished muscle tone, muscle atrophy, and osteoporosis of bone itself.

It is essential to maintain mobility in the elderly, to foster communication with others, and to permit these individuals to maintain contact with their environment and to diminish undesirable psychologic aftereffects.

Some comments about the human foot are in order. First, it is unique. Anatomists and anthropologists consider it the single most distinctive feature of the human race. The human is the only creature who can stand and walk upright with a stride. This type of mobility required a whole new architecture, which explains the unique design of the human foot.

The foot is composed of twenty-six bones—28 including the sesamoid bones. It has 107 ligaments, 19 intrinsic muscles, and 13 extrinsic muscles, along with a complex network of blood vessels, nerves, sweat ducts, and 57 separate articulating surfaces. The relationship of the midtarsal bones to the hindfoot and forefoot is analagous to the relationship of the bones or structures in a truss held together with ligaments and, secondarily, by certain tendons in their relationship to these ligamentous structures. The function of this unit is shock absorption by way of a spring-type action. It is this design that allows the foot to bear enormous work loads (1000 or more tons a day), to endure a multiplicity of stresses, and to maintain the upright and balanced position of the body.

The geriatric foot is the product of years of reasonable use or abuse. It also represents the resultant effects of physiologic tissue changes related to the multiplicity of metabolic, circulatory, and environmental factors such as occupation and stresses and the type of shoes or footwear to which the foot has been subjected with the passage of time. The physiologic effects of atrophy of intrinsic musculature results in varying degrees of deformity of the toes.

It is essential to maintain mobility; for many individuals this is the sole form of exercise in maintaining physical fitness. Thus it is essential to foster the ability to function in a useful and interesting manner.

The response of the foot to the changing types of footwear available to the female population in conjunction with the changing patterns of clothing styles has had its effect, over the years, on the feet. Increasing height of heels results in contracture of the

Table 13-1
Age and sex distribution of 100 patients

Age	Male (17)	Female (83)
60-65	8	30
66-70	4	28
71-75	3	12
76-80	2	8
81-85	0	5

posterior elements of the ankle, such as the heel cord and posterior capsular tissues of the ankle joint and hindfoot joints. The height of the toe box has an effect on the position of the toes. The shape of the toe box contours the foot into a triangle, and the thinness of the sole of the shoe increases the shock factors in the foot and diminishes the ability to compensate for them. The major portion of foot disorders are seen in women (Table 13-1).

In order to more objectively evaluate the patterns of geriatric food disorders,, I reviewed a consecutive series of 100 geriatric patients with foot complaints in my office practice. This material forms the basis for the data in Tables 13-1 to 13-4.

It is possible to classify two major types of foot structure that are prone to disorders. One is the flatfoot that has a lowering of the medial longitudinal arch and is associated with varying degrees of pronation, with evidence of thickening of the plantar skin or keratotic areas where there is continual pressure. The other type of foot structure is cavus foot, which is the opposite of flatfoot and presents different types of foot problems. The flat, pronated foot is most often associated with a varying degree of widening or splayfoot, hallux valgus deformity, prominent bunion formation, and associated claw or overlapping toes with a bunionette that is frequently symptomatic. The cavus type of foot often has metatarsalgia associated with prolapsed metatarsal heads and plantar callosities or corns under the metarsal heads. There is also subluxation or dislocation at the metatarsophalangeal joints of the small toes, with claw toe deformity. These are not unlike the deformities seen in the younger age-group of patients, but they are more severe because of the progressive nature of these deformities with the passage of time and the influence of aging factors such as intrinsic muscle atrophy, peripheral vascular problems (for example, varicosities and venous stasis), varying degrees of arterial insufficiency, and nutritional skin changes, which may all modify the problem. The presence of systemic disease is a factor. Conditions such as diabetes and neurologic conditions will all play a part.

The presence of osteoarthritis in various portions of the foot also adds another factor. The foot with rheumatoid arthritis on the other hand, presents a completely different problem.

One type of foot disorder is seen so frequently in the geriatric patient that it almost merits a classification as a distinct entity. The history reveals the long-term presence of flat feet, prominent bunions, and hallux valgus. Yet these patients have managed to get along fairly well with an orthopaedic shoe, with or without a shoe modification or an orthosis. Although shoe fitting has always been a problem, the bunions were painful only when irritated in a closed shoe. With time progressive deformity of the foot is noted: increasing lateral dislocation of the great toe (hallux valgus) and increasing prominence of the bunion, sometimes with an overlying bursa and hammer-toe deformity of toe two, which begins to deviate medially and may overlap or underlap the great toe. In many there is also hammer-toe or claw toe deformity of toes two, three, four, and five, with subluxation of the metatarsophalangeal joint and secondary metatarsal callosities and corns accompanied by increasing pain under the metatarsal heads. In the older agegroup this is often associated with marked atrophy of the metatarsal fat pad.

With the passage of time conservative treatment becomes less and less effective in making the patient comfortable, and the use of orthoses, shoe modifications, and even custom-made shoes eventually offer only minimal relief.

In summary, these patients usually complain of (1) diminishing walking capacity, especially on hard, flat surfaces, (2) inability to obtain comfortable shoes, (3) painful keratoses and corns on the dorsal surface of the small toes, (4) painful bunions, hallux valgus, and overlapping toes, (5) an enlarging bunion bursa that is sometimes infected in some patients, (6) metatarsal callosities and corns, and (7) symptomatic Tailor's bunion or bunionette.

Other conditions present in the forefoot, which are symptomatic and have been noted in the geriatric foot, are stress fractures in the metatarsals, interdigital soft or hard corns, interdigital neuroma (Morton's syndrome), Freiberg's disease (or aseptic necrosis of the second metatarsal head), and arthritic involvement of the metatarsophalangeal joint of the great toe, with limitation of motion and considerable degeneration of the cartilage in this joint and marginal exostoses.

Disorders of the midfoot are usually related to osteoarthritic involvement. Occasionally there is tendonitis, degeneration, and even a tear of the posterior tibial tendon. Disorders of the hindfoot (or calcaneodynia), with pain on the plantar surface of the foot, have localized tenderness in the region of the medial process or tubercle of the calcaneal tuberosity; often there is x-ray evidence of a large calcaneal spur in this area. In the geriatric foot this is often associated with atrophy of the plantar fat pad of the heel. Occasionally, there is retrocalcaneal bursitis and calcific deposits in the tendo achillis at the heel cord insertion.

NONOPERATIVE MANAGEMENT

The nonoperative management of these various foot disorders consists of attempting to fit the patient with a shoe that will provide adequate room for the toes by having an extra depth toe box. The shoe should be a blucher type oxford that will permit lacing to support the foot. The counter should be long to provide medial support. The sole should a fairly thick one, preferably of the synthetic compound type, which acts as a better shock absorber. The shoe may require further modification if the painful area is in the metatarsal region associated with prolapsed metatarsal heads and plantar callosities, such as a long meta-

Table 13-2

Treatment of 100 patients by conservative and surgical methods

Age	Male		Female	
	Nonsurgical	Surgical	Nonsurgical	Surgical
60-65	8	0	15	15
66-70	2	2	21	7
71-75	3	0	7	5
76-80	2	0	7	1
81-85	0	0	5	0
Total	15	2	55	28

Table 13-3

Treatment of various conditions by surgical and nonsurgical procedures

Diagnosis	Number of patients	Treatment	
		Nonsurgical	Surgical
Anterior tibial tendonitis	1	1	0
Bunion	43	25	18
Cavus	10	10	0
Circulation problems	9	9	0
Deformity of toes	48	31	17
Gout	1	0	1
Hallux valgus	43	25	18
Heel pain	11	9	2
Metatarsalgia	4	4	0
Morton's neuroma	18	13	5
Multiple sclerosis	1	1	0
Osteoporosis	3	3	0
Osteoarthritis (hallux rigidus)	12	10	2
Pes planus	14	13	1
Postsurgical status	5	5	0
Posterior tibial tendonitis	4	2	2
Rheumatoid arthritis	4	0	4
Splay foot	12	11	1
Trauma	8	8	0

Table 13-4

Surgical procedures on 30 patients

Type of procedure	Number	Type of procedure	Number
Avulsion of toenail	1	Keller procedure	3
Akin procedure	1	Proximal crescent oste-	11
Silver procedure	1	otomy of first meta-	
Osteoarthritis of ankle	1	tarsal	
(debridement)		Kidner procedure	2
Interdigital neuroma	9	Double-stem Swanson	5
Osteotomy of fifth	4	implant	
metatarsal (chevron		Talonavicular and cal-	1
procedure)		caneocuboid arthro-	
Osteoplasty of fifth	1	desis	
metatarsal		Excision of rheumatoid	1
Mitchell osteotomy	2	nodule	
McBride procedure	1	Hammer-toes	6
		Total	50

tarsal rocker sole. This is frequently highly beneficial. If a separate orthotic insert is constructed, it must be used in properly sized footwear.

The use of a custom-made shoe may be necessary. Such shoes should be fabricated by an orthotist familiar with the technique of taking impressions of the foot and then constructing an appropriate shoe with adequate balancing to relieve pain in the areas that have excessive pressure. Such an orthotic system aims to redistribute plantar foot pressures to achieve foot comfort by way of pressure relief.

When conservative measures no longer help the patient, it is time to consider the surgical approach (Tables 13-2 through 13-4). *Extensive, successful, foot surgery in the elderly is possible.* However, certain criteria must be fulfilled. Although the chronologic age is not a surgical contraindication, the physiologic condition of the patient is most important. It is good health rather than age that matters. The psychologic makeup of the patient is another important factor. The ability to accept realistic goals by a well-motivated patient suggests a good prognosis in those selected for surgery. The question to be answered in the affirmative is, "Can the patient cope with a 2- to 3-month rehabilitation program?"

CRITERIA FOR SURGICAL TREATMENT
General principles

The following factors should be assessed:
1. Medical condition
2. Anesthesia
3. The condition of the skin
4. The peripheral vascular evaluation (venous and arterial)
5. The patient's psychologic outlook

The patient's health status should be verified by a complete medical examination, with evaluation of all medical factors.

Consideration should be given to the type of anesthesia. General anesthesia is desirable if it can be tolerated by the patient. If contraindicated because of a pulmonary condition or other medical contraindications and surgery is a necessity, then the use of spinal anesthesia works very well. The use of regional ankle block or, for small procedures, local digital block is recommended. If, however, the procedure takes an hour or longer, the patient is kept in one position without moving, which is usually uncomfortable.

A positive psychologic approach on the part of the patient is important. The willingness to accept realistic goals should be thoroughly discussed with the patient and family. There should be a full understanding that it is not possible to create a new foot but that a poorly functioning one usually can be improved. Postoperatively it may still be necessary to wear modified shoes, but the fitting should be easier.

Specific principles

Successful reconstructive forefoot surgery demands a thorough analysis of predisposing factors, knowledge of anatomy and anatomic variations, experience with basic documented surgical procedures, and appropriate aftercare. In addition those factors already discussed, as they influence the specific criteria concerning the geriatric foot, must be considered.

Sensory nerves must be protected and the surgery must be meticulously performed. There are more than 100 different types of bunion operations and at least 7 different procedures for hammertoes. The choice of surgery is influenced by factors such as:

Shoe wear

The pronated foot with a hypermobile first metatarsal bone

The cavus foot with prolapsed or plantar flexed metatarsal bones

Neurogenic imbalance

Excessive length or shortening of the first metatarsal bone

Variations in the shape of the head of the first metatarsal bone

Excessive length of toes

Deformities of the lesser toes

Flexion deformities of the distal and proximal interphalangeal joints vary. They may be rigid or flexible, and they may correct passively to neutral position. Fixed flexion deformity of the proximal interphalangeal joint is associated with varying degrees of hyperextension or dorsiflexion at the metatarsophalangeal joint. This results in subluxation or dislocation at this joint, which may be flexible or fixed. These deformities are frequently referred to as hammertoes. The deformity of the distal interphalangeal joint is usually referred to as a mallet toe and that of the proximal interphalangeal joint is a hammertoe. Considerable hyperextension at the metatarsophalangeal joint is referred to as a claw toe. Flexible proximal interphalangeal joint deformities can be corrected by tendon transfer procedures such as transferring the flexor tendon to the dorsal expansion or dorsal tendon.

The treatment of fixed flexion deformities requires bony approaches. Mallet toe is adequately treated by a dorsal transverse elliptic incision over the involved joint with a resection of the distal portion of the middle phalanx. A dorsal mattress suture through the extensor tendon and capsular tissues will hold the distal phalanx in satisfactory alignment. This procedure is indicated in the toe that has developed a plantar keratosis or corn and that is very painful to the patient.

The fixed flexion deformity of the proximal interphalangeal joint is similarly treated with a resection of the distal end of the proximal phalanx if the hyperextension deformity is minimal.

The flexible proximal interphalangeal deformity can be adequately treated with a diaphysectomy of the proximal phalanx. Retrograde pinning is useful in this procedure to maintain alignment. A .045 mm wire is used and kept in place for 3 weeks.

The fixed flexion deformity of the proximal interphalangeal joint associated with more than a minimal degree of hypertension at the metatarsophalangeal joint is best treated by a proximal phalangectomy and either a plantar dermoplasty to fix the toe to the metatarsal skin tissues or syndactyly to the adjacent toe with resection of a portion of the proximal phalanx of the adjacent toe. The surgical approach to the toe, if a proximal phalangectomy alone is done, is made through a plantar incision centered on the plantar surface of the proximal phalanx and adjacent metatarsal skin.

An oval incision is quite adequate for this approach but must be made proximal enough to permit appropriate plantar positioning of the toe postoperatively, thus avoiding dorsal recession of the toe. This prevents dorsal migration of the flail toe.

Deformities of the fifth toe in the elderly are best treated by a modification of the Ruiz-Mora procedure. This is a proximal phalangectomy, extensor tendon tenotomy, and plantar dermoplasty done through a plantar incision, preventing postoperative problems that are common if a less radical approach is used. It is a sound idea to complete a definitive proved procedure that will give a desired end result rather than risk a prolonged type of postoperative management in the elderly.

At times it may be necessary to consider either partial or complete amputation of a digit in the elderly if the digit is the site of a disease process. Amputation of a distal terminal phalanx in a digit with severe involvement works very satisfactorily in a patient with gout.

In certain cases, for example, an elderly patient with a marked hallux valgus and dislocated and hyperextended second toe overlapping, the great toe becomes a potential source of irritation and possible infection in a closed shoe. These patients may also profit from an amputation of the second toe and accept the other deformities if they are not disabling.

Surgical treatment of metatarsal pain will depend on the etiologic source of this pain. Metatarsal callosities, keratoses, and corns are a serious problem in the elderly because they are often associated with marked atrophy of the metatarsal fat pad. They are difficult to treat by conservative measures such as shoe modifications and orthoses.

The surgical approach that has been found to be highly successful is a proximal osteotomy of the involved metatarsal through a small longitudinal incision and the removal of about a 1 mm section of bone with a dorsally based wedge. The use of a no. 2 chromic catgut suture through two small dorsal openings to prevent rotation has worked satisfactorily. Postoperatively, the use of a firm-soled shoe or perhaps a shoe cast if deemed advisable for 2 or 3 weeks with early weight bearing is adequate postoperative management.

Other sources of metatarsal pain that respond to surgical management are the presence of interdigital neuromas. This diagnosis should be established by the usual findings of local interdigital pain on manual pressure and a carefully documented history. The excision of the neuroma through a dorsal incision and division of the intermetatarsal ligament is a useful procedure. Since interdigital neuroma is easy to overlook as a source of pain when there are other obvious bony deformities, the possibility of this condition as a source of metatarsal pain should be kept in mind in planning other bone reconstructive work in a particular foot.

CASE HISTORIES

Case 1. A 72-year-old patient with rheumatoid arthritis was seen in August of 1982 with the following symptoms: inability to walk, metatarsal pain, corns, and callosities. The patient had experienced no relief with custom-made shoes. The history included a total hip replacement (right) in 1975 and a total knee replacement (right) in 1978.

A preoperative examination indicated a pes planovalgus, a hallux valgus of 60 degrees, with a 60-degree pronation of the great toe. There was also a large bunion, hallux rigidus, and dislocation of the metatarsophalangeal joint of the second through fifth toes (Fig. 13-1). The examination also revealed atrophy of the metatarsal fat pads and incarcerated metatarsal heads.

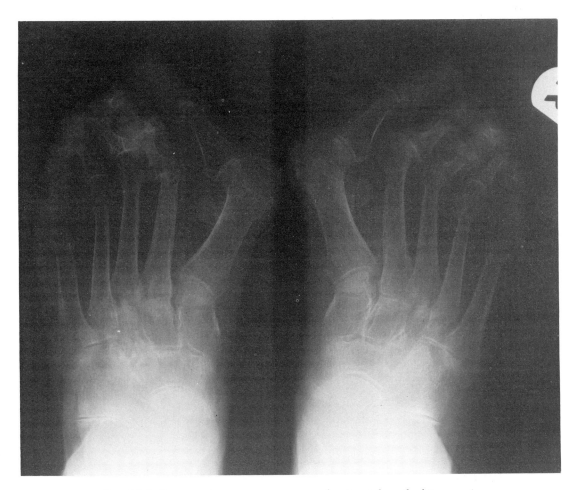

FIG. 13-1. Preoperative roentgenograms of patient described in case 1.

A bilateral operation was performed in stages 1 week apart. The procedure included arthroplasty of the metatarsophalangeal joint of the great toe (double-stemmed hinged Silastic implant), proximal phalangectomy of the second and fifth toes, and proximal hemiphalangectomy of the third and fourth toes. Syndactyly of the second to third toes was carried out. Metatarsal heads two, three, four, and five were resected. Finally Z-plasty lengthening of the extensor hallucis longus tendon was performed. (See Fig.13-2.)

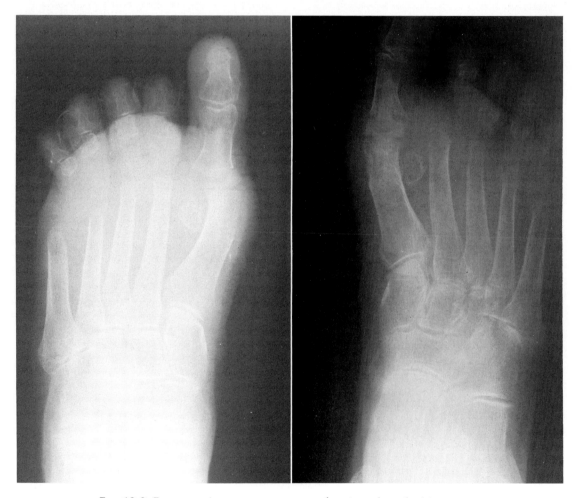

FIG. 13-2. Postoperative roentgenograms of patient described in case 1.

Case 2. A 62-year-old patient had symptoms of pain in the right foot from a bunion, interdigital callosity, and "blister," involving the great toe and the second toe.

The preoperative examination revealed a 10-degree hallux valgus, with hallux pronation between 15 and 20 degrees, a large bunion, deformity of the second toe, and an interdigital corn between the great toe and the second toe (Fig. 13-3).

Surgery was indicated. A Mitchell osteotomy was performed, with a proximal interphalangeal joint resection of the second toe (Fig. 13-4).

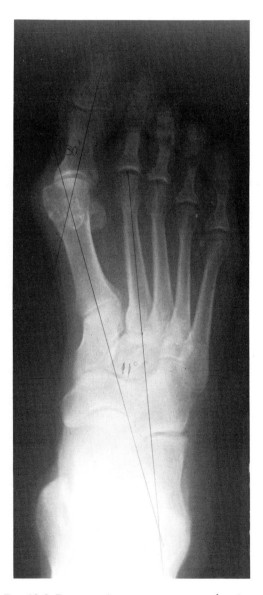

FIG. 13-3. Preoperative roentgenogram of patient described in case 2.

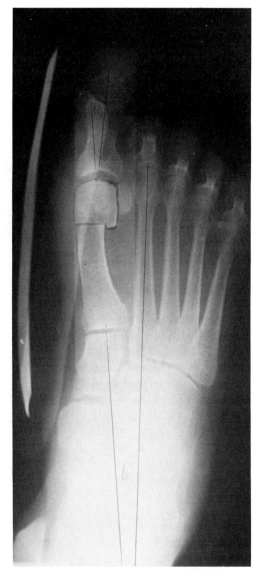

FIG. 13-4. Postoperative roentgenogram of patient described in case 2.

Case 3. A 70-year-old patient had a preoperative painful bunion of the right foot and pain in the third toe and the metatarsal region.

The examination showed moderate pronation, hallux valgus of 15 degrees, a large bunion, a large tender bursa with fluid, and interdigital tenderness between the second and third toes and the third and fourth toes (Fig. 13-5).

Treatment included aspiration of the bursa and, 2 months later, surgery:

1. Osteoplasty of the head of the first metatarsal bone
2. Z-plasty lengthening of the extensor hallucis longus tendon
3. Capsuloplasty of the metatarsophalangeal joint of the great toe
4. Proximal crescent osteotomy of the first metatarsal with 0.062 pin fixation
5. Excision of an interdigital neuroma between the second and third toes and one between the third and fourth toes

The postoperative result is shown in Fig. 13-6.

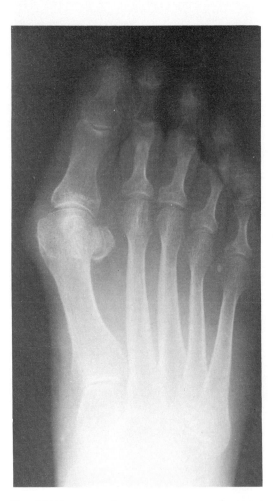

FIG. 13-5. Preoperative roentgenogram of patient described in case 3.

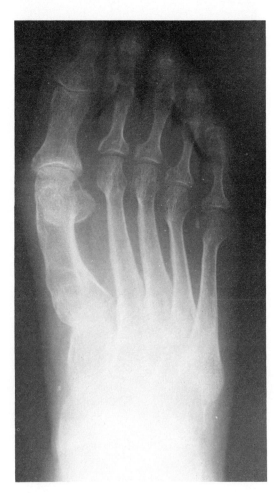

FIG. 13-6. Postoperative roentgenogram of patient described in case 3.

Case 4. A 68-year-old patient had a painful bunion of the left foot and complained of an inability to walk even half a block without pain. There was also a problem with shoe fitting. The patient also had pain in the right foot from the "instep" and ankle.

A preoperative examination of the left foot revealed the following: hallux valgus of 45 degrees; a large bunion; 45 degrees of dorsiflexion and no plantar flexion of the metatarsophalangeal joint of the great toe; the great toe overlapping the second toe; hammertoe of the second toe; tailor's bunionette of the fifth metatarsal; and pes planovalgus and splay foot (Fig. 13-7). The right foot was free of hallux valgus, but the great toe had a large metatarsophalangeal joint, and there was midtarsal dorsal exostosis.

Surgery of the left foot was indicated, and a modified McBride procedure was performed:

1. Adductor tenotomy and adductor tendon transfer to the neck of the first metatarsal
2. Osteoplasty of the head and neck of the first metatarsal bone
3. Excision of the fibular sesamoid
4. Z-plasty lengthening of the extensor hallucis longus tendon
5. Capsuloplasty of the metatarsophalangeal joint of the great toe
6. Proximal crescent osteotomy of the first metatarsal and 0.062 pin fixation
7. Chevron osteotomy of the fifth distal metatarsal, with 0.045 pin fixation

The postoperative result is shown in Fig. 13-8.

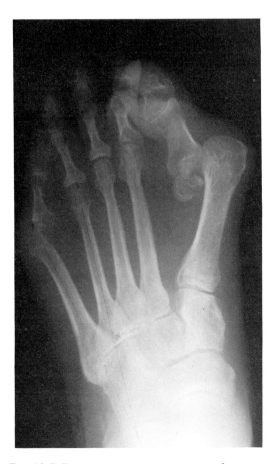

FIG. 13-7. Preoperative roentgenogram of patient described in case 4.

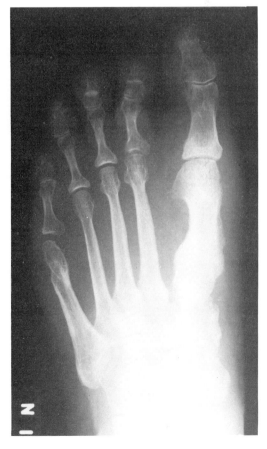

FIG. 13-8. Postoperative roentgenogram of patient described in case 4.

part III

ASSOCIATED DISORDERS OF THE MUSCULOSKELETAL SYSTEM

chapter 14
METABOLIC BONE DISEASE

Joseph M. Lane

Metabolic bone disease was introduced as an entity by Albright and Reifenstein[1] in 1948 to describe a series of skeletal alterations caused by humoral abnormalities. Over the years since their initial entrance into the field of metabolic bone disease, considerable advances have been made in understanding the physiology and pathophysiology of bone remodeling and the various subsets of metabolic bone disease.[2,15-17,22] Osteoporosis, nutritional osteomalacia, subtle hormonal abnormalities affecting the skeleton, and marrow-packing disorders can all lead to a constellation of osteopenia and compression fractures of the spine in the elderly. It is the purpose of this chapter to describe the currently accepted concepts of skeletal metabolism and to apply this understanding to the most common geriatric metabolic bone diseases. The discussion of these disorders will include the pathophysiology, diagnosis, and treatment.

The skeleton consists of calcium hydroxyapatite and collagen as the mineral and organic phases, respectively; 99% of the calcium and 85% of the phosphorus in the body is situated in the skeletal system.[16] Even after the epiphyseal plates have closed, the skeletal dimensions continue to change with time. There is a gradual increase in the outer (periosteal) diameter as well as the inner (endosteal) diameter of bone.

In addition to the anatomic changes, there are morphologic changes within the bone mass itself. Bone can be divided into cancellous and cortical bone. Both cancellous and cortical bone consist of lamellar bone in which mineralization occurs on top of well-aligned collagen lamellal.[15] Bone is normally turned over throughout life. The bone is initially resorbed by osteoclasts and new bone formation occurs in the sites of previous resorption. Osteoblasts first produce osteoid and then become incorporated within the collagen matrix as the mineralization process proceeds. These incorporated osteoblasts are known as osteocytes. There are small canaliculi that connect the osteocytes to each other and to the outer surface or Haversian systems. Although most of the mineral is isolated from the general circulation, a significant surface area is readily available for transfer of calcium and phosphorus ions. Most areas of cortical bone are remodeled every 2 to 4 years. The necessity for the remodeling of the osteons within the cortex is unclear and may be the result of fatigue fractures of the osteon unit or some humoral factor released by the osteocyte. The cortical thickness undergoes thinning with aging. In men the progressive loss is of a more gradual nature than in postmenopausal women, and usually it does not lead to marked weakening of the cortex as it does in women.

The regulation of bone formation and bone resorption appears to be affected by physical mechanical requirements, local humoral factors, and the general hormonal status of the individual. Frost[6] was one of the initial advocates of the idea of a coupling phenomenon in which the turnover of bone consists of a close sequential coupling of osteoclastic resorption followed by osteoblastic formation. Only on the periosteal surface does bone formation proceed without prior osteoclastic activity. Metabolic bone diseases occur when there is an imbalance in the rate of bone resorption and bone formation.[2,6,16,17,22]

Bone has three primary functions: structural support for the individual, a metabolic bank containing calcium and phosphorus for the organism, and the marrow cavity as an environment in which blood elements are made. There is a continual conflict between these three roles. The remodeling and removal of bone can be retarded by structural demands placed upon it. The loaded vertical trabeculae of the vertebral bodies are retained while the stress-shielded horizontal trabeculae are removed preferentially. The horizontally placed trabeculae bear much less structural support than the vertical trabeculae. Situations in which the marrow cavity must be expanded to provide additional blood elements will affect those areas of bones that have a high cellular surface area and are more prone to increased metabolic bone activity when calcium demands are increased. This is most clearly seen in the metaphysis of bones.

Bone metabolism appears to be affected by most hormones either directly or indirectly.[15-17] Three prominent hormones in this process appear to be parathyroid hormone (PTH), vitamin D, and calcitonin. Vitamin D is indeed a hormone. It is produced sequentially first in the skin in the form of vitamin D, converted in the liver to 25 hydroxy vitamin D, and last in the kidney to 1,25 dihydroxy vitamin D (see diagram below). This metabolite stimulates calcium absorption across the gut and potentiates the PTH bone-resorbing action. This metabolite also stimulates phosphorus absorption across the gut. The production of active 1,25 dihydroxy vitamin D metabolite is stimulated by the presence of PTH. In the absence of the PTH, the metabolite 24,25 dihydroxy vitamin D is produced by the kidney. The role for this metabolite has not yet been described, although it may have a function such as stimulating mineralization of the osteoid. The precursor metabolites such as vitamin D and 25 hydroxy vitamin D have little or no effect on calcium absorption across the gut.

The PTH is produced in the parathyroid glands in response to calcium deficiency.[1,16] It is synthesized as a precursor, pro-PTH, and converted to active PTH in the circulation. In this active form it only lasts for a short period of time and it is then converted into an inactive shortened c-terminal fragment that may persist for up to 2 to 3 weeks within the same serum. The PTH has no direct effect on the gut. It acts by stimulating the production of 1,25 dihydroxy vitamin D in the kidney and it encourages increased resorption of calcium and excretion of phosphate by the kidney. Within bone the PTH stimulates osteoclastic bone resorption and osteocytic osteolysis. Actual numbers of osteoclasts are increased and their activity per osteoclast is enhanced. The PTH's action in bone is enhanced by the presence of 1,25 dihydroxy vitamin D.

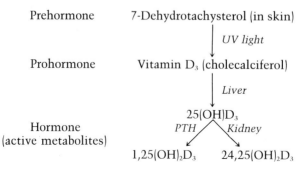

Metabolism of Vitamin D

Calcitonin's role in bone metabolism under normal circumstances is uncertain. It is a potent hypocalcemic agent and its site of action is in bone where it shuts down osteoclastic activity. Its presumed use occurs in the growing child where it is called upon after a high calcium-containing meal. Calcitonin is produced in the thyroid gland in humans.

Other hormones have a role in bone metabolism, probably in an indirect manner. For example, estrogen has been closely associated with bone metabolism.[19,25] The deficiency of estrogen that follows menopause has been coupled to bone loss. Since no binding sites for estrogen have been identified to date in bone cells, it is presumed that estrogen is probably indirectly affecting bone metabolism.

OSTEOPENIA

Osteoporosis is rapidly becoming a problem of major significance in the geriatric population.[16,17] As the relative proportion of individuals beyond the age of 65 increases, the actual number of patients with osteoporosis has risen. Osteoporosis is that condition of the skeleton in which there is a loss of bone mass, including the mineral and the organic components equally. The loss can be caused by any defect in the biochemical makeup of bone, including the collagen and minerals. The defects in collagen, such as in the states of scurvy and

osteogenesis imperfecta, are quite rare, particularly in the geriatric population. Most cases of osteoporosis have no obvious attributable biochemical defect. Conditions of augmented bone resorption over formation, depressed information in the presence of normal resorption, or a combination of both can all lead to osteoporosis.[2]

In contrast to osteoporosis, a failure in mineralization of the osteoid leads to conditions of osteomalacia (Fig. 14-1). Marrow-packing tumors or endocrine disorders can also lead to osteopenia. The rest of this chapter will discuss the pathophysiology of the major subgroups of osteopenia, characterize the clinical manifestations, describe the various diagnostic modalities available to the clinician, and identify current modes of treatment.

Definitions

Osteopenia in adults is defined as decreased radiodensity on a planar x-ray film, often highlighted by accentuation of the vertical trabecular pattern and by wedge fractures of the thoracic spine and "codfish" compression fractures of the lumbar spine (Fig. 14-2).[15-17] This general heading of osteopenia includes four major subgroups: osteoporosis, osteomalacia, endocrinopathy, and marrow-packing disorders. *Osteoporosis* occurs most commonly in 15% of the postmenopausal white women beyond the age of 65. Most osteoporosis is grouped under the heading of senile or postmeno-

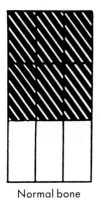

Normal bone

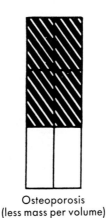

Osteoporosis
(less mass per volume)

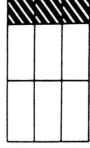

Osteomalacia
(failure to mineralize osteoid)

FIG. 14-1. Schema of normal bone, osteoporosis, and osteomalacia. Dark areas represent mineralized bone and clear areas unmineralized osteoid.

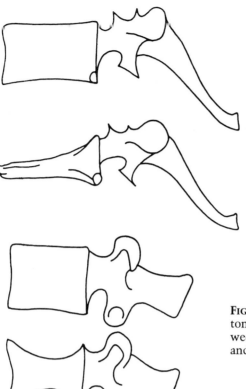

FIG. 14-2. Typical spinal fractures. Top to bottom: normal thoracic vertebral body, thoracic wedge fracture, normal lumbar vertebral body, and lumbar codfish deformity.

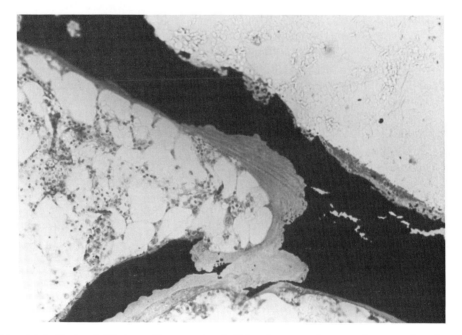

FIG. 14-3. Undecalcified von Kossa stained slide of osteomalacia with mineralized matrix black and osteoid grey.

pausal, but there are other conditions that can cause osteoporosis. These include estrogen-deficiency states, increased alcoholic intake, immobilization, and a whole series of endocrinopathies.[7,9,16]

Avioli, Baran, Whyte, and Teitelbaum[2] have identified 8% of their osteopenic patients as having frank evidence of osteomalacia. *Osteomalacia* is the failure to mineralize collagen and osteoid (Fig. 14-1) and is classically seen in vitamin D–deficiency rickets.[15-17] It is most commonly seen in adults with nutritional deficiencies, malabsorption syndromes, and advanced states of vitamin D degradation, including those resulting from phenytoin (Dilantin) therapy. Alterations in calcium and phosphorus metabolism as well as the inborn error of hypophosphatemia have also been indicated as playing a significant role in this disorder. Microscopically, there is a marked increase in unmineralized bone (Fig. 14-3) and there is a demonstratable decrease in the rate of mineralization. Clinical x-ray films may be normal in mild cases or give evidence of osteopenia. Osteomalacia occurs quite frequently, particularly in the group of patients with hip fractures. There is a large subset of patients with osteoporosis who have mildly increased osteoid.[2] Their values of osteoid are too low to be included in clear cases of osteomalacia, and these individuals have been designated as *hyperosteoidotic* patients. There is a close association between these people and mild chronic calcium-deficiency states. Scileppi et al.[29] have identified a 33% incidence of hyperosteoidosis in patients over 50 years old with femoral neck fractures.

Endocrine disorders can give rise to osteopenia.[15-17] The most common dysfunctions include hyperthyroidism, hyperparathyroidism, and hypersteroidism. In both hyperparathyroidism and hyperthyroidism there is increased osteoblastic and osteoclastic activity with a net effect of bone loss. Hypersteroidism has been identified with decreased absorption of calcium across the gut and the inducement of secondary hyperparathyroidism. Other endocrine disorders associated with osteopenia include congenital 17 hydroxylase deficiencies, estrogen deficiencies, diabetes mellitus, and acromegaly.[9,19,25]

Although not fully understood, marrow-packing disorders can give rise to osteopenia. Multiple myeloma, leukemia, and thalassemia characteristically will expand the marrow cavity at the expense of trabecular bone volume. Specific humoral factors leading to bone resorption have been identified with hematologic elements. An osteoclastic-activating factor derived from lymphocytes and monocytes has been shown to be quite effective in promoting bone resorption and may play a role when increased numbers of these cell elements are present.

Iatrogenic factors have been clearly identified as causing osteopenia. Agents such as chronic heparin use, corticosteroid therapy, hydantoins, methotrexate, and other antimetabolites have all been shown to lead to significant osteopenia.

Connective tissue disorders may uncommonly give rise to osteoporosis. These should be suspected especially in patients in the younger age groups, but such disorders may also not be clearly present until the patient has become elderly. Entities that fall under this category include osteogenesis imperfecta, homocystinuria, and adult hypophosphatasia.

Pathophysiology

After excluding conditions such as malabsorption, liver and renal disease, inadequate sunlight, alcoholism, and steroid therapy, all of which may contribute significantly to abnormal bone metabolism, there remains a significant population who suffer from severe loss of bone mass. It is known that the bone mass decreases with age in all individuals with a net loss of cortical thickness, particularly after the menopause in women. The mechanism of this bone loss is poorly understood, but specific genetic and environmental factors seem to play a significant role.

Women have a greater incidence of osteoporosis than men.[16,17] This occurs mostly in the postmenopausal age group. White women particularly from a northwestern European ethnic background have a much higher incidence than those of Mediterranean descent. Black populations have a higher ratio of cortical-to-cancellous bone than white populations (61% versus 35%); therefore osteoporosis is rare in blacks. Osteoporotic individuals frequently have skimpy builds and are not usually obese. Other hallmarks of an osteoporotic individual include a fair complexion, freckles, blonde or red hair, hypermobility, and scoliosis. Nutrition has been suggested as a key element in the initiation of osteoporosis.[7] Studies have indicated that in the initial stages of osteoporosis there is an increased urinary calcium, and this frequently correlates well with increased bone resorption. Riggs et al.[27] have shown that 15% of osteoporotic individuals have an increased immunoassay of parathyroid hormone (secondary).

A poor calcium intake has been identified in a significantly higher population of patients with osteoporosis than in the general population.[4,7] Requirements for calcium vary with age (Table 14-1).[16] Women who have breast fed their children have been shown to have on the order of 10% less bone mass than non-breast-feeding peers. Goldsmith and Johnston[9] postulated that the cause of this decreased bone mass was inadequate calcium supplementation during the breast-feeding period. A clear figure for the postmenopausal calcium requirements is only indirectly suggested by the studies of Recker, Savile, and Heaney.[25] In studying postmenopausal and perimenopausal women, they found that 1500 mg of calcium per day could prevent bone loss for periods of up to 3 to 6 years.

The geriatric population frequently is quite deficient in calcium intake.[4,7] The most common sources of calcium are dairy products and leafy green vegetables. One dairy portion will contain approximately 250 mg of elemental calcium. Not only do most elderly women have an inadequate calcium intake, but also they have poor adaptation to a low-calcium diet. In addition, the elderly are less efficient in absorbing calcium across the gut (30% to 60% decreased efficiency). Lactase deficiency has been identified in a high percentage of

TABLE 14-1
Daily requirements for calcium

Category	Daily requirements
Child	400-700 mg
Adolescent	1000-1300 mg
Young adult	400-500 mg
Pregnant female	1500 mg
Lactating female	2000 mg
Middle-aged adult	750-800 mg
Postmenopausal female	1500 mg
Elderly adult	1500 mg

white patients with osteoporosis.[4] It has been documented that patients who are lactase deficient frequently have a low calcium intake. This may be an excellent marker to identify a chronic calcium-deficiency state and its contribution toward osteoporosis.

There is a close association between bone loss and the menopausal state. Meema, Bunker, and Meema[19] have shown that following the onset of menopause, there is significant bone loss, irrespective of the age at which menopause occurs. Patients who have entered menopause 20 years before their peers will have appreciably lower bone mass than their peers. Although most women have decreased estrogen following menopause, only 20% have more than a fourfold decrease. Almost all postmenopausal women have estrogen levels below those of comparably aged men. Estrogen has therefore been implicated as having a key role in the initiation of postmenopausal osteoporosis. However, as noted previously estrogen does not seem to have a receptor site on bone cells. Consequently, it may have only an indirect effect on the skeletal system. Antiestrogen metabolic conditions such as hyperprolactinemia can give rise to a state of osteopenia comparable to that found in deficient estrogen states.

Not all postmenopausal women get osteoporosis although all people do lose bone with age.[16,17] In postmenopausal women and only gradually in elderly men the endosteal diameter increases more rapidly than the periosteal diameter, leading to net cortical bone loss. Within this framework, increased cortical and trabecular bone loss seems to lead to a high risk of fractures in approximately 15% of the postmenopausal population. High rates of thoracic wedge fractures and lumbar crush fractures occur in patients in whom the trabecular bone volume (marrow, osseous fraction) is less than 11%.[22] At the Hospital for Special Surgery 50% of patients with crush fractures of the spine had trabecular bone volumes of 15% or less and only rare individuals had crush fractures when the iliac trabecular bone volume was greater than 22%.[16]

Patients over 50 years of age with femoral neck fractures have a high incidence of underlying osteopenia and 60% of women and 70% of men have either hyperosteoidosis (30%), osteoporosis (30%), and/or increased resorption (30%).[29] Those patients with a trabecular bone volume of 15% or less had successful union in only one third of the cases as compared to a 90% success rate when metabolic bone disorders were minimal or absent.

The concept of morphologic homogeneity of the nonosteomalastic osteoporotic adult is no longer justified.[2,22] Multiple workers inluding Muniere have studied iliac bone biopsies of large osteoporotic populations. Muniere et al.[22] have found that 10% of the patients with a collapsed vertebral body and low trabecular bone volume had high bone remodeling rates within the biopsies, 33% had depressed osteoblastic activity, and 57% had pathology indistinguishable histologically and dynamically from nonosteoporotic senile subjects. These studies have indicated that, in fact, there are multiple groups of patients who fit within the overall heading of osteoporosis. Studies are currently underway in multiple centers to clarify these categories so that appropriate therapeutic modalities can be directed at each one of the special groups.

It has been found that 30% of the bone can be removed from the vertebral body before evidence of osteopenia can be identified on classical anteroposterior and lateral plan radiographs. All previous remarks in this chapter do not diagnostically differentiate clearly osteoporosis from osteomalacia, endocrine dysfunction, or neo-

plastic or hypoplastic marrow-packing conditions. Specific diagnostic tools have been developed to help in the differentiation and quantitation of osteopenia and they fall within the loose headings of invasive and noninvasive techniques. These special studies are only warranted when historical and clinical settings suggest osteoporosis.

Clinical presentation

The clinical presentation of osteoporosis is frequently noted to be associated with back pain and fractures.[15] Vertebral compression fractures (often multiple and most commonly T5-8 and T11-L2), proximal femur fractures (femoral neck and intertrochanteric), distal radial fractures, and pelvic fractures are the most common fracture types and locations (Fig. 14-4). Kyphosis and loss of height secondary to multiple vertebral fractures are quite characteristic of the osteoporotic patient. The patient has a history often revealing early menopause, low dietary calcium, malabsorption symptoms, lactation, steroid therapy, northern European heritage, fractures, and back pain. The physical examination keynotes kyphosis, scoliosis, loss of height, and localized bone tenderness particularly in the spine. Laboratory studies including the serum calcium, phosphorus, and alkaline phosphatase are usually normal. Urinary calcium may be high initially at the onset of osteoporosis and usually becomes normal or depressed in chronic osteoporotic circumstances. The radiographic findings of osteoporosis include early changes of osteopenia, particularly in the spine and pelvis, and loss of horizontal trabeculation in the vertebral bodies. The spinal compression fractures known as biconcave codfish deformities are common, particularly in lumbar and wedge fractures in the mid and low thoracic spine. Small Schmorl's nodes, including disc protrusion through the vertebral end plate, are frequently seen. No focal lytic or blastic lesions occur in osteoporosis. In cases in which patients have the above mentioned history, physical examination, laboratory findings, and radiographic manifestations, diagnostic invasive and noninvasive techniques may be help-

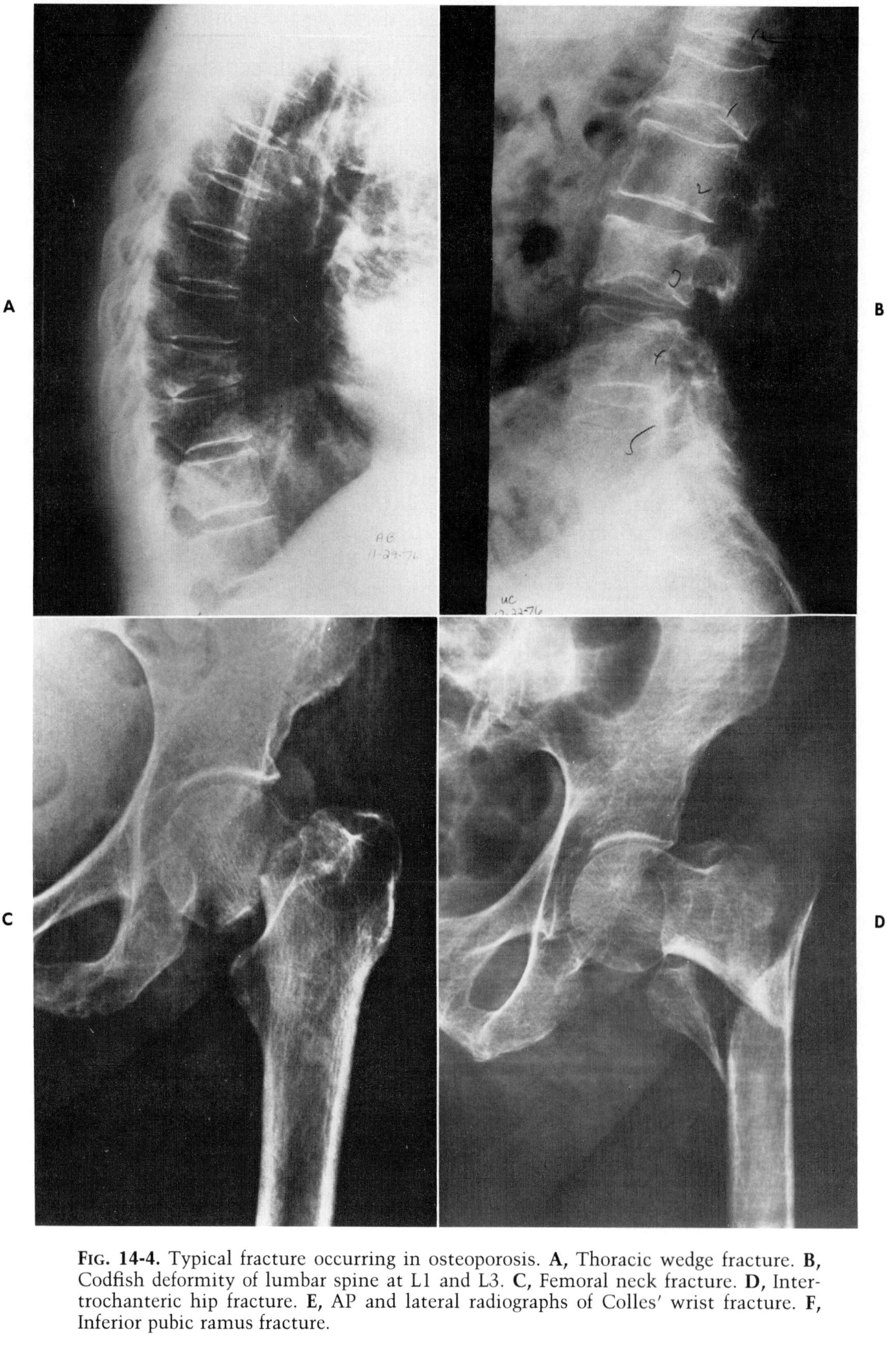

FIG. 14-4. Typical fracture occurring in osteoporosis. **A,** Thoracic wedge fracture. **B,** Codfish deformity of lumbar spine at L1 and L3. **C,** Femoral neck fracture. **D,** Intertrochanteric hip fracture. **E,** AP and lateral radiographs of Colles' wrist fracture. **F,** Inferior pubic ramus fracture.

ful in discerning the etiology of the osteopenia.

Differential diagnosis of nonosteoporotic osteopenias.[15-17] Patients who have chronic back pain from repeated vertebral fractures or asymptomatic patients with osteopenia found by chance all deserve a careful diagnosis as noted above. Osteopenic disorders other than osteoporosis must be excluded because their treatment is quite different from osteoporosis. The differential diagnosis of osteopenia does frequently include specific disorders that will be discussed at this time and these include multiple myeloma, metastatic malignancy, genetic disorders, hyperthyroidism, hyperparathyroidism, osteomalacia, renal osteodystrophy, and gastrointestinal disease.

Multiple myeloma would be suggested with findings of decreased alkaline phosphatase and monochromal gammopathy, lytic lesions on the x-ray films, and generalized bone tenderness. Some of the lesions may be negative on the bone scan. A bone marrow biopsy is the most accurate diagnostic technique for this entity.

Metastic malignancy may be manifested by increased alkaline phosphatase, hypercalcemia, cortical erosions, particularly of the pedicles, on x-ray films, localized rather than generalized osteopenia, and positive bone scans. Tumors most frequently found in bones are breast cancer, hypernephromas, and lung cancer. A history of a tumor in the 2 to 5 years before the first appearance of these symptoms without other evidence of metastases requires tissue confirmation to prove the diagnosis of a tumor. Unrecognized hidden malignant tumors initially appearing as bone metastases may elude ultimate diagnosis; at Memorial Hospital 15% to 20% of primary tumors were never identified even at autopsy.

Genetic disorders masquerading as osteoporosis include various forms of osteogenesis imperfecta. Most of these disorders can be identified by history, physical ex-

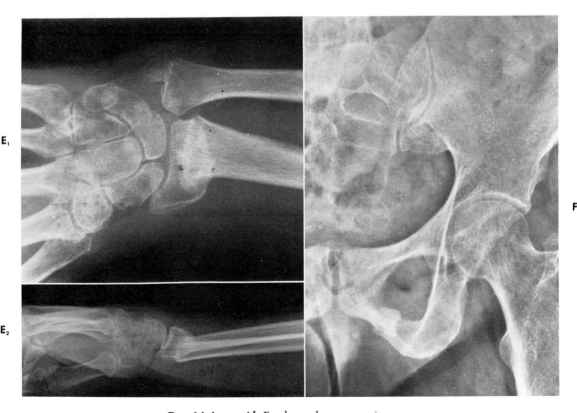

FIG. 14-4, cont'd. For legend see opposite page.

amination, and characteristic radiographs. Mild forms of osteogenesis imperfecta, however, may be quite misleading and should be suspected in the presence of blue sclera and dentinogenesis.

Hyperthyroidism is suggested by weight loss, heat intolerance, elevated serum thyroxin, and elevated urinary calcium and hydroxyproline. Elderly patients with hyperthyroidism often will not have exophthalmos. Many elderly people have a tremor and have difficulty with heat and cold intolerance. The hallmark of this disease is a suspicion raised by significant weight loss and possibly tachycardia.

Hyperparathyroidism (primary) is suggested by elevated serum calcium, decreased serum phosphorus, and elevated parathormone levels. Availability of the immunoparathormone assay has significantly helped in making the diagnosis of this disorder. Radiographic evidence of endosteal and periosteal resorption, particularly in the phalanx, and the "salt-and-pepper" skull are suggestive. Biopsies often reveal osteoitis fibrosis cystica, an increased number of resorbing osteoclasts, and dissecting resorption of the bone trabeculae from within.

Osteomalacia is often recognized by the presence of low or low-normal serum calcium level and a depressed phosphorus level. Elevated alkaline phosphatase is found in the most virulent forms. Radiographs reveal pseudofractures. Biopsies reveal increased osteoid seams and decreased mineralized matrix volume. There may be a number of patients with osteopenia who have hyperosteoidosis at a level somewhere between frank osteomalacia and osteoporosis. Most of these patients have a poor dietary calcium intake and low-normal vitamin D levels. They respond quite rapidly to calcium and vitamin D supplementation.

Renal osteodystrophy is becoming more prevalent in light of extensive dialysis programs. Often osteodystrophy is quite obvious from the history and from blood serum studies showing an elevated blood urea nitrogen (BUN), elevated phosphorus, decreased calcium, decreased creatinine clearance, and ectopic mineralization in widespread disease. PTH will often be elevated, in response to the low calcium, in the form of secondary hyperparathyroidism.

Symptoms of malabsorption or a history of previous gastrointestinal surgery, particularly Billroth II procedures, suggest decreased calcium absorption as a cause of osteopenia. Following gastric bypass procedures 60% of patients will have microscopic osteomalacia within 10 years following the treatment.

Noninvasive techniques

The noninvasive techniques for determining the extent and etiology of osteopenia have utilized various modalities of roentgenology.[15-17] Anteroposterior, lateral, and occasionally planar tomography will identify the extent of fractures in the thoracic and lumbar spine. Bone scans are extremely sensitive in identifying an old versus a relatively new fracture (Fig. 14-5). Usually crush fractures of the vertebral spine will remain positive for 1 to 2 years. There is a progressive diminution of radioactivity as the fracture consolidates, and this can be identified through serial bone scans. These scans can also identify a pattern more consistent with metastatic disease as well as highlight areas that were not recognized initially as sites of fractures. This latter situation is most pertinent in unrecognized nondisplaced fractures of the hip. The hallmarks of osteomalacia are lucent lines, which are symmetrical stress fractures. These are most readily visible on scans and can further be identified by coned down x-ray films and occasionally by planar tomography.

Singh, Riggs, Beabout, and Jowsey[30] have utilized the femoral trabecular pattern as an index for osteoporosis. It has been found to be fairly sensitive in identifying patients with osteoporosis versus the general population. However, there is a broad overlap in degrees of osteoporosis and there is only a moderate correlation between the Singh index and bone density.[16] Radiographic photodensity attempts to estimate bone mass by measuring the optical density of the radiograph. The relative exposure of the bone image on the radiograph presumably reflects the mass of bone absorbed by the radiographic beam. Radiographic morphology, on the other hand, utilizes the measurement of cortical thickness in relationship to its width as a measure of density. This latter technique suffers from measurement imprecision while the former technique does not adequately compensate for such factors as soft tissue thickness. Absorptiometry utilizing monoenergetic radiation passed through the bone has recently become widely used. It is accurate with a high degree of reproducibility and has been successfully used in predicting bone mass. However, the degree of correlation is dependent on the anatomic site. Techniques utilizing two monoenergetic radionucleotides (duo-photon absorptiometry) are currently coming into vogue and may be more sensitive tools. Serial examinations using photon absorptiometry in the same patient may be of considerable assistance in following the osteoporotic patient under treatment. They are also an ex-

cellent tool for grossly separating patients who fall into fracture risk groups versus the general population. Unfortunately, photoabsorptiometry of the wrist does not correlate exactly with the bone mass in the vertebral spine, and this has been somewhat misleading particularly in men. Most recently, the CT scanner (fourth generation) has demonstrated 3% to 5% precision and accuracy in determining bone mass in the vertebral spine.

Invasive techniques

Invasive techniques center on laboratory diagnostic studies specifically directed at identifying endocrine dysfunction, calcium balance, malabsorption, liver and renal function, and hematology. The Metabolic Bone Unit at the Hospital for Special Surgery performs preliminary screening laboratory studies in an effort to identify significant metabolic dysfunctions (See box on p. 246.) It must be recognized that most cases of osteoporosis have normal studies because of the slow chronicity of the evolv-

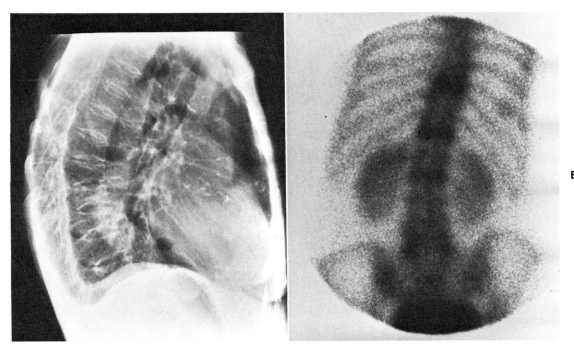

FIG. 14-5. Radiograph and bone scan of thoracic spine. **A,** Lateral thoracic spine radiograph illustrating multiple thoracic crush fractures. **B,** AP bone scan demonstrating that only 1 lumbar and 2 thoracic fractures are recent (< 1 year).

PRIMARY SCREENING TESTS FOR OSTEOPOROSIS
(Metabolic Bone Disease Unit, The Hospital for Special Surgery)

Radiographs
1. Thoracic and lumbar spine: AP, lateral
2. Skull: sella, lateral
3. Hands: AP
4. Pelvis and hips: AP

Total body bone scan (technetium diphosphonate) to distinguish new from old fractures
Bone density (Cameron) of wrist to determine bone mass
Blood and urine studies
1. BUN, creatinine (rule out kidney disorders)
2. Bilirubin (rule out liver disorders)
3. Calcium, phosphorus, alkaline phosphatase, 1,25 dihydroxy vitamin D, and 24-hour urinary calcium, hydroxyproline (rule out mineralization defects)
4. T3, T4, c-terminal PTH, estrogen, cortisol (rule out endocrine disorders)
5. Serum and urinary proteinelectrophoresis, CBC, differential and sedimentation rate (rule out hematopoietic disorders and bone marrow tumors)

TABLE 14-2
Diagnoses suggested by initial laboratory results

Laboratory study	Values	
	Increased	*Decreased*

Serum calcium	Primary hyperparathyroidism
	Multiple myeloma (60%)
	Immobilization (10%)
	Neoplasm
	  Metastases
	  Ectopic parathyroid hormone
	Hyperthyroidism (15%)
		Vitamin D–deficiency states
		  Malabsorption
		  Dietary deficiency
		  Anticonvulsants
		Calcium deficiency
		  Lactose intolerance
		  Dietary
		  Utilization (growth, pregnancy, lactation)
		Renal osteodystrophy

Serum phosphate	Renal osteodystrophy
	Immobilization
	Widespread metastases
		Hypophosphatemic rickets
		Vitamin D–deficiency states
		  Malabsorption
		  Dietary
		  Vitamin D–dependent rickets
		  Anticonvulsants
		Primary hyperparathyroidism
		Neoplasm
		Phosphate deficiency

TABLE 14-2
Diagnoses suggested by initial laboratory results—cont'd

Laboratory study	Values	
	Increased	*Decreased*

Alkaline phosphatase	Paget's disease
	Renal osteodystrophy
	Vitamin D–deficiency states
	  Malabsorption
	  Dietary
	  Vitamin D dependent rickets
	  Anticonvulsants
	Primary hyperparathyroidism
	Hypophosphatemic rickets
	Widespread metastases
		Hypophosphatasia

24-hour urinary calcium	Hypercalcemia
	  Primary hyperparathyroidism
	  Neoplasm/myeloma
	Cushing's disease/steroids
	Immobilization
	Hyperthyroidism
	Hypophosphatasia
	Renal tubular acidosis (loop diuretics)
	Phosphate deficiency
		Renal osteodystrophy
		Hypophosphatemic rickets
		Vitamin D–deficiency states
		  Malabsorption
		  Dietary
		  Vitamin D–dependent rickets
		  Anticonvulsants
		Calcium deficiency
		  Lactose intolerance
		  Dietary
		  Utilization

Creatinine	Renal osteodystrophy Multiple myeloma	
Creatinine clearance		Renal osteodystrophy Poor urine collection
Hemoglobin	Cushing's disease	Neoplasm/myeloma
WBC (differential)	Leukemia (abnormal differential) Cushing's disease ($\downarrow$ lymphocytes)	Thyrotoxicosis (Graves' disease) ($\uparrow$ lymphocytes)
Electrolytes Chloride	Neoplasm without bone metastasis Renal tubular acidosis	Multiple myeloma Metastatic neoplasm
Potassium Carbon dioxide		Renal tubular acidosis Renal osteodystrophy Renal tubular acidosis
Urinalysis pH Glucose	Renal tubular acidosis Cushing's disease Franconi's syndrome Multiple myeloma	
Protein	Renal osteodystrophy	
T4	Thyrotoxicosis	Phenytoin (Dilantin)

Serum protein electrophoresis
  Paraprotein
  Albumin
	Multiple myeloma	Hypocalcemia

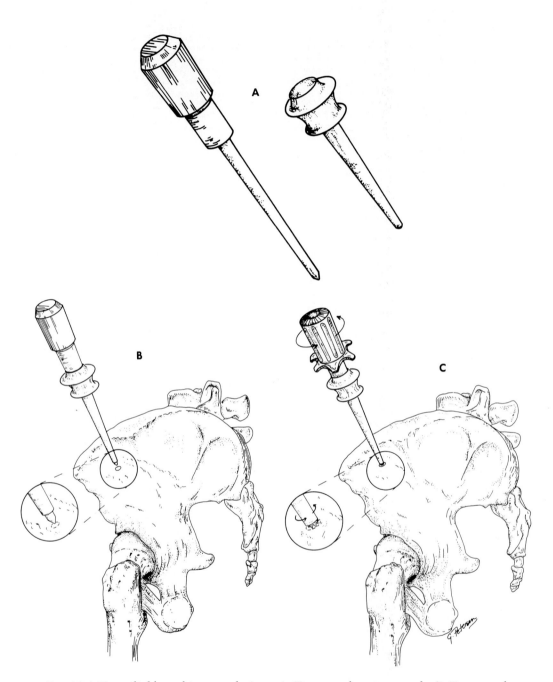

FIG. 14-6. Transilial bone biopsy technique. **A,** Trocar and outer cannula. **B,** Trocar and cannula have been directed through skin to anterior superior iliac crest. **C,** Bone-biting cutter then removes 5 to 6 mm core of ilium (two cortices and trabecular marrow). **D,** Core is removed. **E,** Biopsy site is filled with wax or thrombin-soaked Gel foam. (From Gartsman, G.M., and Lane, J.M.: A simple method of obtaining bone graft by bone biopsy trocar, J. Hand Surg. **6:**627-628, 1980.)

ing disease process. The screening studies at the unit include a serum calcium, phosphorus, alkaline phosphatase, and a 24-hour urinary calcium and hydroxyproline determinations. These are for identifying mineral and collagen turnover disorders. Renal function is evaluated by BUN and creatinine clearance. Endocrine function studies include 1,25 dihydroxy vitamin D (for vitamin D content and cascade), c-terminal PTH (parathyroid gland function), T3 and T4 (thyroid gland function), plasma cortisol (adrenal corticosteroid status), and fasting glucose (diabetes mellitus). The marrow hematopoietic evaluation includes blood count, sedimentation rate, Bence Jones protein, serum electrophoresis, albumen, and total protein. If any of these studies suggest further investigation, second-line studies specifically directed toward the suspect disorders such as malabsorption may be performed (Table 14-2).

The most critical invasive study is the transilial bone biopsy performed 2 cm cau-dal and posterior to the superior anterior iliac spine (Fig. 14-6). A cancellous cortical core biopsy is taken and the material is then evaluated by undecalcified histomorphometric techniques. Bone mass and rate of turnover can be determined by an internationally accepted methodology. Numerous investigators in metabolic centers feel that the transilial bone biopsy is the most reliable method for indicating the status and diagnosis of a generalized skeletal disease. The biopsy has a low complication rate and hematopoietic tissue can be also analyzed in the specimen. The utilization of double labeling with autofluorescent tetracycline antibiotics given at two separate times allows the rate of bone formation and reabsorption to be determined by the method of Frost.[6] Most importantly the biopsy is the only sensitive method for determining the presence of osteomalacia in a patient with osteopenia.[2,15-17,22] A discussion of the methodology is not pertinent for the purposes of this chapter. However, phy-

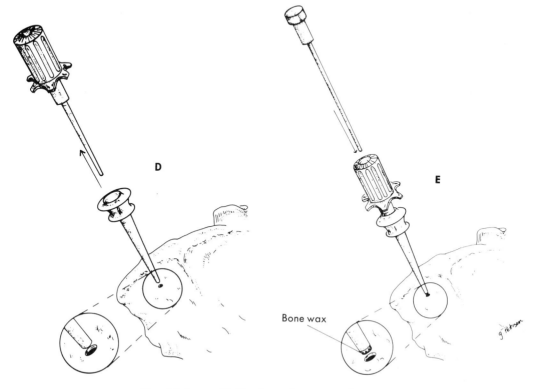

FIG. 14-6, cont'd. For legend see opposite page.

sicians treating geriatric skeletal disease should recognize the methodology as the most sensitive tool for diagnosis. At the Hospital for Special Surgery 25% of patients with a diagnosis of osteoporosis had a plethora of other disorders only recognized through the biopsy. These included premalignancies, mild osteomalacia, multiple myeloma, and marginal endocrinopathy. Laboratory studies in all these patients were quite equivocal and, in fact, misleading. Only the biopsy was able to identify these subgroups so that appropriate therapy could be established.

Treatment

The treatment for the osteoporotic patient involves (1) care of the acute fracture, (2) treatment of the osseous consequences of osteoporosis including kyphosis, foreshortening of the lumbar spine, and traumatic arthritis of the spine, and (3) correcting the underlying metabolic bone disease.[15-17]

Often, the diagnosis of osteopenia may be identified incidentally in the course of a routine chest x-ray examination or through the physician's awareness of a progressive loss of height. Also, fractures and back pain may lead to an awareness of the disorders. There have been great strides in the treatment. Consequently, once the diagnosis of osteopenia has been made, a more positive approach toward the care of the geriatric patient is indicated.

Acute vertebral fractures are best treated by rest, heat, mild muscle relaxants, and then early mobilization. Sometimes, back supports may be necessary to get the patient out of bed. It should be recognized, however, that braces are counterproductive and may lead to further loss of bone from immobilization of the affected skeleton. According to Wolff's law of function, if the vertebral body does not bear weight, it will undergo further loss of bone mass. Frequently, a girdle with minimal supporting stays will be sufficient to get elderly patients up and about. Progression from a walker to a single cane with the support of heat and rest are sufficient. Most fractures will become controllable within 5 weeks

and if pain persists beyond that period of time, the possibility of additional new fractures or underlying metastatic disease must be considered. Once the patient has recovered from the acute fracture episode, diagnostic studies should be initiated to resolve the problems of the differential diagnosis of osteoporosis, osteomalacia, endocrinopathy, or marrow-packing tumors.

Treatment of primary osteoporosis. * Once the etiology of the osteopenia has been identified and true osteoporosis has been established, treatment is directed both at the osseous injury and at the underlying metabolic bone disease. In particular, the adult with the back pain is treated with a program of selective analgesics, appropriate bed rest, and a progressive program of exercises. Flexion and extension exercises of the Williams variety and pool therapy have been most successful in the long run in strengthening muscle mass and stimulating retention of mineral within the stressed bone. Height is usually not regained; however, the progressive stooping within the day can be prevented as muscle mass improves. Acute fractures of the spine will heal with conservative care within 5 weeks. Bracing is rarely indicated unless the patient cannot be mobilized without support.

The medical treatment of osteoporosis is not standard. Part of the problem resides with the clinical diversity of the osteopenic disorders and the morphologic heterogeneity. Physical activity has definitely been shown to benefit osteoporosis by stimulating retention of mass. However, in terms of the nutritional factors, there is a certain degree of choice.[7,15-17,25] Replacement calcium, even in patients in whom osteoporosis can be attributed to calcium deficiency, does not lend itself to increased bone mass although it will decrease bone loss. Provision of 1.5 g of elemental calcium will help to mineralize unmineralized osteoid and turn off any secondary hyperparathyroidism. The result of calcium therapy is to shut down any augmented bone resorption and facilitate progressive mineralization. Recker, Savile, and Heaney[25] study-

*References 7, 13, 15-17, 19, 22, 25, 27.

ing perimenopausal nuns have shown that women shortly after menopause can effectively stop bone loss for up to 6 years. It is not sure whether prolonged calcium augmentation carried out into late postmenopausal periods such as the 80s will remain as effective. The studies at the Hospital for Special Surgery have suggested that bone loss will again occur, but at a decreased rate, in the very elderly. Estrogen, 0.625 mg of conjugated estrogen per day, when given to the perimenopausal woman will in a similar manner stop bone loss but will not lead to bone formation.[19,25] However, estrogen administered to women 6 years beyond menopause had only a marginal effect in reducing bone loss. Recent studies have suggested that estrogen supplementation even in small doses increases the risk of uterine cancer up to ninefold. Therefore, unless the patient taking estrogen is observed carefully for uterine abnormalities, estrogen supplementation may be hazardous. Calcium has never been identified with any propensity for malignancy. Calcium carbonate, however, may lead to constipation and may also be contraindicated in patients with renal stone history. Urinary calcium maintained at 100 to 250 mg for 24 hours indicates that adequate calcium supplementation has been achieved, yet this is below the level necessary for stone formation. The constipation occasionally associated with calcium carbonate can often be improved by roughage within the diet and the use of tomato juice. Calcium lactate and calcium gluconate contain only 15% of elemental calcium per pill versus the 40% in calcium carbonate. Therefore, instead of taking 6 pills of calcium carbonate, 650 mg per day, the patient taking calcium lactate or calcium gluconate would need to take 15 to 18 tablets per day. The use of these alternate calcium forms has led to difficulty with patient compliance. Vitamin D, in the form of 400 to 800 units per day, should be provided. Higher doses may potentiate secondary hyperthyroidism. In frank osteomalacia with documented deficiency of 1,25 dihydroxy vitamin D, higher vitamin supplementation is indicated, such as 50,000 units of

vitamin D per week for malabsorption or 1,25 dihydroxy vitamin D itself in patients with renal disease. Vitamin D and estrogen will not lead to bone accretion but should delay the usual physiologic bone resorption in the postmenopausal population. For many patients with a lactase deficiency or low dietary calcium intake, calcium carbonate supplementation is indicated even in the premenopausal female. Patients who are undergoing pregnancy or breast feeding require high calcium supplementation in the order of 1500 and 2000 mg per 24 hours, respectively. It is critical that the physicians treating these women at risk should be aware of the nutritional requirements and do a careful dietary history of these patients.

Active bone accretion has been achieved with sodium fluoride in doses of 1 mg/kg/day, corrected for creatinine clearance.[13,16,17,27] The dose is decreased by a percentage of the decreased creatinine clearance. At the Hospital for Special Surgery, sodium fluoride increased trabecular bone volume by 15% to 20% per year at this dosage level when supplemented with calcium, 1500 mg of elemental calcium per day, and low dose vitamin D, 400 units per day (Fig. 14-7). Unopposed sodium fluoride while increasing bone mass may lead to a considerable increase in the amount of unmineralized bone component. Presence of the calcium and vitamin D has been found in our unit as well as in those of Riggs and Jowsey to prevent these problems.[13,16,27] In a carefully screened population at the Hospital for Special Surgery, spinal fractures decreased from more than 800/1000 patient years before treatment to 50 fractures/1000 patient years after 15 months of therapy. No fractures occurred after 18 months of treatment. The long-term effects of sodium fluoride and the need for continued administration are still undetermined at this time. It has been our feeling that once the trabecular bone volume has reached 25%, sodium fluoride can be discontinued and the patient maintained on only calcium and vitamin D.

Sodium fluoride has a number of local and general complications.[13,16,17] Sodium

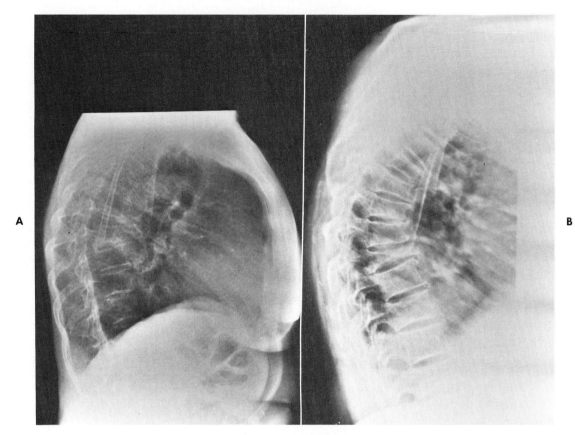

FIG. 14-7. Effect of sodium fluoride treatment on bone mass. **A,** Pretreatment thoracic spine. **B,** Posttreatment thoracic spine.

fluoride can cause some gastric indigestion and nausea though these mild gastric complaints may be resolved by choosing an appropriate vehicle for the sodium fluoride. Sodium fluoride given in the form of a liquid such as 15 mg per teaspoon and dissolved in juice, particularly tomato juice, and taken at the time of meals has often been well tolerated. The sodium fluoride can also be placed in capsules for utilization in the duodenum. Other complications include a possibility of ankle edema and plantar fasciitis. These resolve with symptomatic care and may not, in fact, be related to the sodium fluoride per se but to a general well being in the patient and increased activity. Brittle bones can occur in the presence of sodium fluoride therapy when calcium and vitamin D supplementation is not maintained. Sodium fluoride must be terminated when and if the patient stops taking supplemental calcium and vitamin D.

Other agents now under experimental protocols are being tested for efficacy in osteoporosis. These include new forms of diphosphonates, calcitonin, PTH, vitamin D metabolites, and anabolic steroids such as Stanizol.[16] These agents have been applied in an attempt to exploit experimental animal evidence showing decreased bone resorption as a result of diphosphonate and calcitonin and increased bone turnover from PTH, and formation from Stanizol. These agents are still not available for the general population but may become so in the next 3 to 5 years.

At this time, the careful diagnosis of the patient with osteopenia will allow a clarification of the etiologic factors. The treatment of acute fractures should be quite successful, but the prevention of new fractures rests on revising the underlying metabolic bone status. Calcium and/or estrogen plus maintenance vitamin D have been quite effective in preventing or decreasing the physiologic bone loss of postmenopausal women. Sodium fluoride appears to be an efficacious agent in increasing bone mass and probably in preventing fractures. Further drugs may be coming on the scene, but even so at this time hope should be voiced for patients with the problem of osteopenia. Improved nutrition and physical exercises should be encouraged in the osteopenic population and the patient's quality of life can certainly be improved with a little attention to the simple modalities.

PAGET'S DISEASE

Robert L. Merkow
Joseph M. Lane

Sir James Paget originally presented five cases of a bone disorder he called "osteitis deformans" in 1876. Although this disorder is not truly inflammatory and deformity is not always present, his original descriptions are remarkably accurate and quite eloquently characterize the disease:

It begins in middle age or later, is very slow in progress, may continue for many years without influence on the general health, and may give no other trouble than those which are due to changes of shape, size, and direction of the diseased bones. Even when the skull is hugely thickened, and all its bones exceedingly altered in structure, the mind remains unaffected.

The disease affects most frequently the long bones of the lower extremeties and the skull, and is usually symmetrical. The bones enlarge and soften, and those bearing weight yield and become unnaturally curved and misshapen. The spine, whether by yielding to the weight of the overgrown skull, or by change in its own structures, may sink and seem to shorten with greatly increased dorsal and lumbar curves; the pelvis may become wide; the necks of the femora may become nearly horizontal, but the limbs, however misshapen, remain strong and fit to support the trunk.

In its earlier periods, and sometimes through all its course, the disease is attended with pains in the affected bones, pains widely various in severity and variously described as rheumatic,

gouty, or neuralgic, not especially nocturnal or periodical. It is not attended with fever. No characteristic conditions of urine or feces have been found in it. It is not associated with syphilis or any other known constitutional disease, unless it be cancer.

In three out of five well-marked cases that I have seen or read of, cancer appeared late in life; a remarkable proportion, possibly not more than might have occurred in accidental coincidences, yet suggesting careful inquiry.[24]

Paget's disease of bone is defined as a process of increased bone remodeling; the primary event is increased resorption (osteoclastic activity) followed by subsequent reactive bone formation (osteoblastic activity). The disease may be monostotic or polyostotic. It is usually assymetric and may or may not cause symptoms.

Epidemiology

Paget's disease of bone is more common than once thought. It has been detected in certain populations with an incidence of 3% to 4% in middle-aged patients and 10% to 15% in the elderly population. There are definite racial and geographic variations. The disease is seen more frequently in Great Britain, the United States, Australia, New Zealand, Germany, and France. It is rare in Scandinavia, Switzerland, Japan, China, the Middle East, and Africa. In most reports men are affected more commonly than women.[11] Although no definite hereditary pattern has been established, a familial clustering has been reported and a positive family history is present in approximately 15% of cases. Paget's disease has occasionally been reported in younger patients. In those instances it takes an extensive and severe form.

Etiology

The inciting cause of Paget's disease is unknown. Paget believed that a form of chronic inflammation was responsible for the enlargement and deformity of the bones. Over the past century numerous hypotheses have been proposed including inflammatory, neoplastic, vascular, genetic, traumatic, endocrinologic, immunologic, and infectious etiologies. Recent evidence appears to support a virus as an important etiologic factor. Histologically, giant multinucleated osteoclasts and intranuclear inclusion bodies (viruslike particles) have been identified in Paget's bone. Familial and geographic clustering as well as a long latent period could be explained by a slow virus etiology. However, no definite virus has been isolated, and therefore, the exact cause of Paget's disease remains to be elucidated.

Pathology and pathophysiology

Paget's disease of bone is a focal disorder characterized by increased bone resorption and secondary new bone formation that is architecturally abnormal. This increased rate of turnover results in newly formed vascular bone that is poor in structural integrity, often deformed, and prone to pathologic fractures. Radiographically, lytic or blastic or combination lesions may be present. Early in the process, a "flamed-shaped," advancing osteolytic front may be seen, particularly in long bones (Fig. 14-8). Grossly, the involved bone appears spongy with generalized enlargement, thickened cortices, and coarsened trabeculae, frequently with bowing because of poor structural integrity (Fig. 14-9). Histologically, one sees a pattern of irregular segments of mature (lamellar) bone with increased cellularity, multinucleated osteoclasts, and irregularly arranged cement lines (Fig. 14-10). Cement lines imply reversal of osteoclastic resorption and subsequent new bone formation. The resultant "mosaic" pattern is diagnostic of Paget's disease. Microscopically, this pattern is identified with an irregular patchwork appearance of bone plaques highlighted by prominent cement lines (Fig. 14-11).

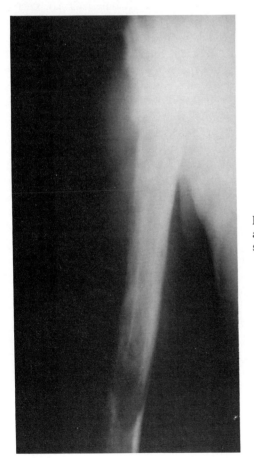

FIG. 14-8. Radiograph of humerus demonstrating advancing "flame-shaped" osteolytic wedge seen in early Paget's disease.

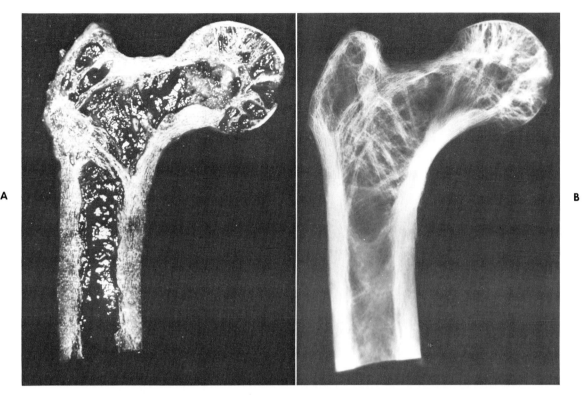

FIG. 14-9. A, Coronal section of gross specimen from proximal femur. Note varus deformity, thickened cortices, and coarse scant trabeculae. B, Radiograph of same specimen demonstrating thickening of cortical bone and distorted architectural pattern. (Courtesy of P. Bullough.)

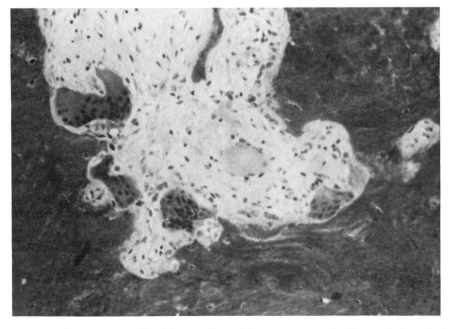

FIG. 14-10. Photomicrograph of bone affected by active Paget's disease. There is increased cellularity, numerous osteoblasts, and multinucleated osteoclastic giant cells. (Courtesy of P. Bullough.)

Pathophysiologically, Paget's disease has been divided into two major phases: the "active phase" and the "inactive phase." Early in the active phase osteoclasts are hyperactive, resorbing bone at a high rate causing destruction, osteoporosis, and fibrovascular hyperplasia. This intense resorption will stimulate osteoblastic activity and in the "mixed phase" bone resorption and formation are balanced, generating histologically abnormal bone. Late in the active phase, osteoblastic activity exceeds that of the osteoclasts and sclerotic ivory-hard bone is formed. In the inactive phase bone remodeling and turnover decrease towards normal. Enlarged, sclerotic, structurally abnormal, and often deformed bones remain.

Clinical presentation

In the majority of cases of Paget's disease, the focal bony changes are asymptomatic since they usually occur deep in the soft tissues of the spine, pelvis, or femora, where deformity may go unnoticed. The diagnosis is often discovered accidentally during a radiologic or laboratory examination for unrelated complaints. When symptoms arise, they depend upon the site and the extent of skeletal involvement. The most frequent sites of Paget's involvement include the spine, femora, cranium, pelvis, and sternum (Table 14-3).

The most common complaints are pain, skeletal deformity, and change in skin temperature. Pathologic fractures, neurocompression, arthritis, and symptoms resulting from vascular shunting also occur frequently. Additionally, systemic, metabolic, or rheumatic manifestations have been noted in the literature. Hypercalcemia and hypercalciuria may occur especially after fractures and immobilization[5] and may contribute to the formation of renal stones. Hyperuricemia and symptomatic gout as well as calcific periarthritis have been associated with Paget's disease in some reports. Cardiovascular complications including high-output congestive heart failure are only manifested in patients with greater than 30% of skeletal involvement. Apathy, lethargy, and easy fatigability may

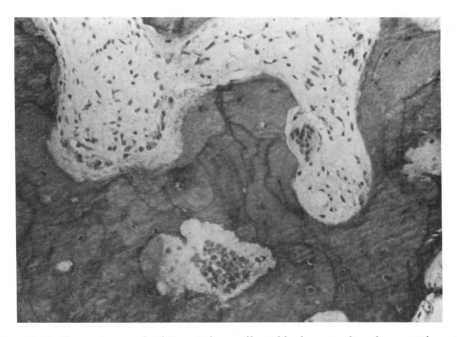

Fig. 14-11. Photomicrograph of Pagetic bone affected by longstanding disease. There is increased cellular activity and prominent "mosaic pattern" of irregularly arranged cement lines. (Courtesy of P. Bullough.)

also be seen in patients with extensive Paget's disease. The "Pagetic steal syndrome," where blood is shunted from the brain to the external carotid system, is also occasionally seen. Malignant degeneration occurs in less than 1% of all Paget's cases.[14] However, in elderly patients with bone sarcomas, 20% to 30% are associated with Paget's disease. The tumor types vary from the highly malignant osteosarcoma or fibrosarcoma to more benign lesions such as giant cell tumors. Paget's sarcoma may occur at any site. Clinically a marked increase in pain arises and, radiographically bone destruction, extracortical extension, and/or a soft tissue mass may be apparent (Fig. 14-12). The serum alkaline phosphatase need not be excessively elevated in secondary Paget's sarcoma.

TABLE 14-3

Sites of Paget's disease involvement in the skeleton

Sites of involvement	Percent of cases
Sacrum	56
Spine (lumbar, most frequently)	50
Cranium	28
Femur	23
Sternum	23
Pelvis	21
Clavicle	13
Tibia	8
Ribs	7
Humerus	4

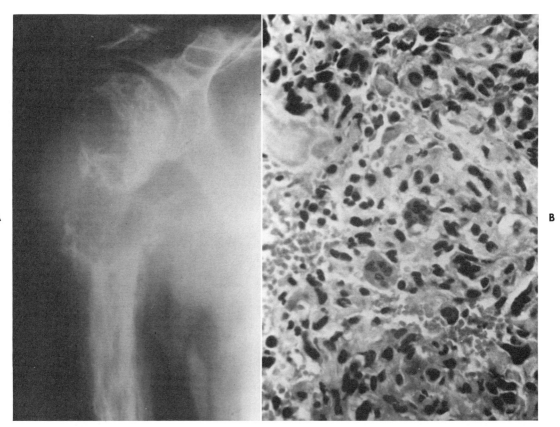

FIG. 14-12. A, Radiograph of Paget's sarcoma involving proximal humerus. Note bone destruction, extracortical extension, and soft tissue mass. **B,** High-power micrograph of biopsy specimen from same pathologic fracture. It shows a pleomorphic spindle cell tumor with many giant cells, the typical histologic appearance of Paget's sarcoma. (Courtesy of P. Bullough.)

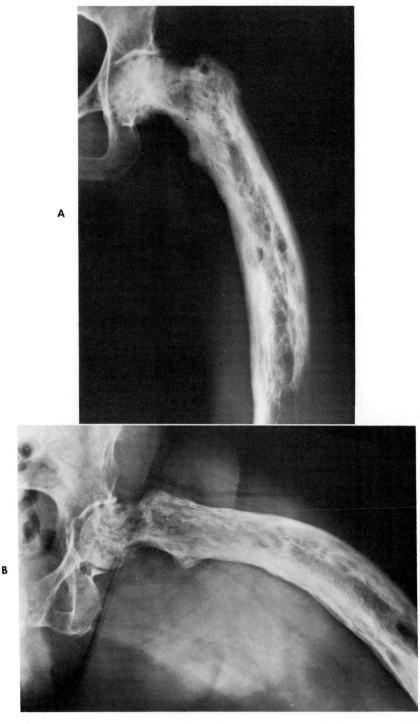

FIG. 14-13. **A,** X-ray film of Paget's femur demonstrating marked anterior and lateral bowing deformity. **C,** X-ray film after corrective biplane osteotomy transfixed with intramedullary nail. **D** and **E,** X-ray film 1 year postosteotomy after removal of rod demonstrating corrected alignment and solid bony union.

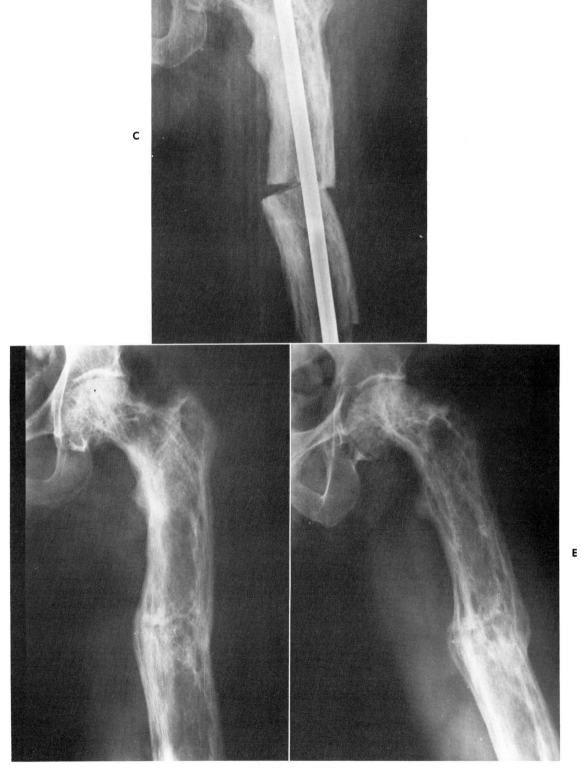

FIG. 14-13, cont'd. For legend see opposite page.

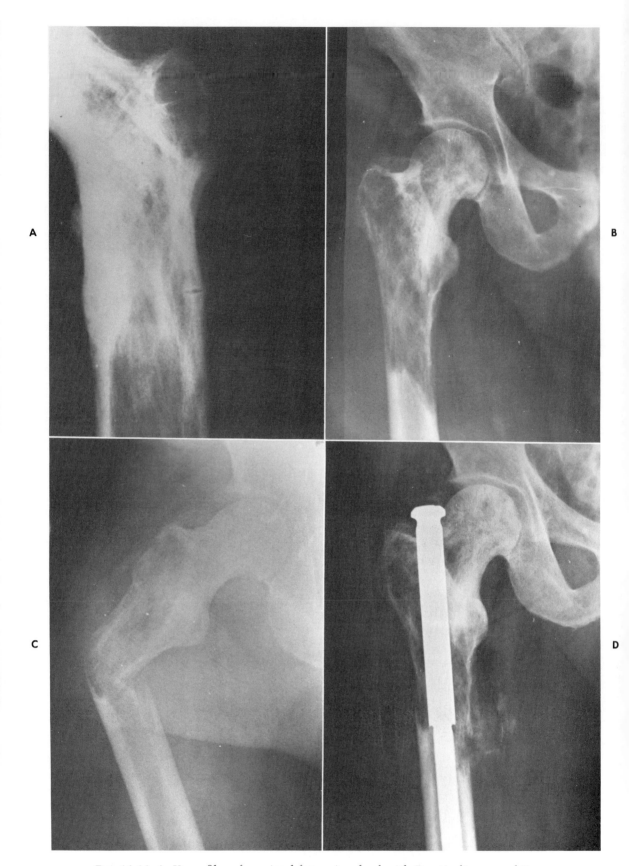

FIG. 14-14. A, X-ray film of proximal femur involved with Paget's disease and "pseu-dofracture" on the "tensile cortex" in subtrochanteric region. **B,** X-ray film demon-strating lytic Paget's disease in proximal femur. **C,** Pathologic fracture and displacement occurred after incident of minimal trauma. **D,** Reduction and intramedullary fixation of fracture.

The bone pain in Paget's disease is usually a deep aching pain, most often mild to moderate in severity and worsened by weight bearing when it occurs in the lower extremeties. Bony impingement on the dura or nerve roots because of enlarged, deformed vertebral bodies, particularly in the lumbar and thoracolumbar areas, is a frequent cause of back pain. This occasionally causes severe local pain with typical radicular radiation into the legs. Pain may also be the result of associated or complicating arthritis, most commonly in the hips and knees. The pathogenesis of the arthritic changes associated with Paget's disease is not established. However, evidence suggests that disturbance of subchondral bone formation related to hyperemia and secondary derangement of joint mechanics may be responsible for the arthropathy seen in Paget's disease.[8] Radiographically, the hip joint typically demonstrates loss of medial joint space before superior narrowing in contradistinction to primary osteoarthritis. Arthritic pain is worse with motion and weight bearing. Painful symptoms may be the result of a combination of factors, including (1) metabolic activity of the disease, (2) neurologic impingement, (3) impending fracture, and/or (4) secondary arthritis. Careful evaluation of the patient's complaints and systematic trials of treatment(s) are used for dealing with these specific cause(s) in a particular case.

Skeletal deformities are typically characterized by an increased size and abnormal shape of the affected bones. The deformities in the cranium and long bones are most readily appreciated on routine examination. In the lower extremity the femur tends to bow laterally and anteriorly (Fig. 14-13) and the tibia anteriorly and internally because of muscular imbalances and weight-bearing forces. The increase in skin temperature most often seen about the involved tibia is the result of increased vascularity and blood flow to the soft tissues.

Pathologic fractures may be the initial manifestation or a complication in a patient with known Paget's disease and they occur with an incidence of between 10% and 30%. Fractures most frequently occur in the long weight-bearing bones of the lower extremities. The femoral neck, subtrochanteric, and tibial regions are the most common sites (Fig. 14-14). Fractures may also occur in the humerus, vertebral column, or the pelvis. They are usually transverse or short oblique, often occur after a minor trauma, and at times appear at the site of pseudofractures (transverse lucent lines on the convex border of long bones) (Fig. 14-14). Pseudofractures may or may not be symptomatic; when they are locally painful and tender, impending pathologic fracture is likely. Although a pathologic fracture in Paget's disease may be treated by either closed or open means, the incidence of delayed union, nonunion, or refracture is significant. Treatment with calcitonin during the healing phases is recommended to bring the metabolic environment back toward normal.[21]

Neurologic complications resulting from cranial disease include mechanical compression on the neural foramena of the exiting cranial nerves, particularly I, II, V, VII, and VIII; infiltration into the inner ear causing neurosensory deafness; softening and basilar invagination, which may cause vascular compression; pagetic steal syndrome; brainstem or cerebellar compression; or blockage of cerebrospinal flow with resultant hydrocephalus.

Laboratory findings

In polyostotic Paget's disease the marked elevation in bone turnover is reflected in the elevation of the serum alkaline phosphatase and 24-hour urinary hydroxyproline. The alkaline phosphatase activity is an indicator of bone formation and it reflects the number of active osteoblasts; the urinary hydroxyproline level is an indicator of collagen turnover correlating with the number of osteoclasts triggered. In monostotic disease these values, and the serum calcium and urinary excretion of calcium may be normal since bone formation is usually balanced with the increased rate of resorption. However, in patients with fractures for whom bed rest was prescribed, elevation of the serum or urinary calcium may occur.

Radiographic findings

Radiographic pictures of Paget's disease can be pathognomonic. Typically, there are focal areas of bone resorption and formation that appear as radiolucencies and densities. The overall bone size and mass are enlarged and the cortices are thickened; the trabecular pattern is coarsened and irregular (Fig. 14-9). A "flame-shaped" osteolytic front extending from the ends of long bones may be seen early in the disease (Fig. 14-8). Bowing deformities, elongation, and incomplete transverse pseudofractures, as well as pathologic fractures, are frequently seen in the long bones (Figs. 14-13, 14-14). Joints with adjoining pagetic bone may show changes up to and often involving the subchondral surfaces with secondary arthritic changes (Fig. 14-15). The arthritic pattern in the hip disease usually shows medial or concentric joint-space narrowing with minimal osteophyte formation and commonly a protrusio acetabuli deformity.[12] Specific radiographic findings and clinical symptoms vary, depending upon the location and extent of the disease process (Table 14-4).

Bone-seeking radioisotopc scans are more sensitive and accurate than conventional x-ray films in diagnosing early Paget's disease and in evaluating the extent of the disease as well as in monitoring its response to treatment. The high degree of bone turnover takes up more radioisotopic material, making the lesion appear "hot" on the scan.[14] With treatment or during the sclerotic "burnt-out" phase, the scan may appear minimally abnormal. Hot lesions may also be seen in osteomyelitis, healing fractures, fibrous dysplasia, or bone tumors. Conventional x-ray films and/or a biopsy may be needed to differentiate between these lesions.

Treatment

Most patients with Paget's disease are asymptomatic and in these individuals, if the chemistries are near normal and weight-bearing bones are uninvolved, no treatment is indicated. Baseline assessment of the extent of the skeletal involvement using whole body bone scanning and appropriate conventional x-ray films is prudent. Biopsy of the involved bone is needed

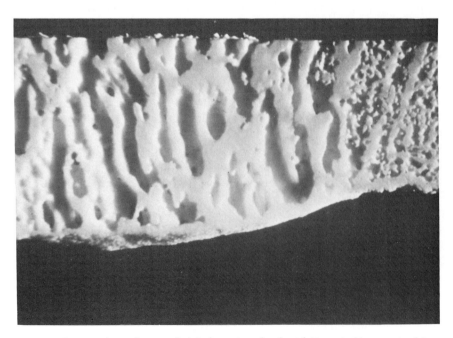

FIG. 14-15. Cut specimen from arthritic knee involved with Paget's disease. Architecture of subchondral bone is distorted, showing enlarged irregular trabeculae and uneven surface. (Courtesy of P. Bullough.)

only if the clinical and radiographic diagnosis is in doubt. Nonhistiocytic lymphoma and metastatic prostatic cancer can mimic Paget's disease although neither has elevated alkaline phosphatase levels or bone expansion.

Patients with symptomatic Paget's disease must be thoroughly evaluated as to the extent of the bony disease, the nature of their symptoms, the metabolic activity of the disease, and any associated problems and/or referred pain syndromes from distant neurologic impingement. Additionally, rheumatic manifestations commonly associated with Paget's disease,[5] such as rheumatoid arthritis, ankylosing spondylitis, gout, and calcific periarthritis, must be recognized and appropriately treated.

Indications for treatment. The primary indication for treatment is pain. This may be the result of the metabolic activity of Paget's disease, neural irritation, arthritis, or a combination of these causes. It is important to differentiate as much as possible between these etiologies since arthritis may require additional treatment modalities. Significant elevation of biochemical indices (e.g., alkaline phosphatase elevated to twice the normal levels) also warrants treatment because this may help control the metabolic activity and thus the degree of architectural distortion and integrity of the bones and joints. This is particularly important when Paget's disease involves the weight-bearing bones of the lower extremities, the spinal column, and/or areas

TABLE 14-4
Radiographic and clinical manifestations of Paget's disease of bone

Location	Radiographic findings	Clinical symptoms
Skull	Osteoporosis circumscripta Cranial enlargement Basilar invagination	None Occasionally painful Occipital neuralgia; lower cranial nerve impingement; medullary compression; syringomyelia with ventricle obstruction and increased intracranial pressure; vertebral basilar artery insufficiency
Facial, jaw bones	Temporal bone involvement Auditory ossicle involvement Unilateral radiographic changes	Hearing loss Hearing loss Proptosis; trigeminal neuralgia; displacement of teeth
Spine (enlarged)	Enlarged "window frame" vertebra(e)	Nerve root compression; spinal stenosis; spondylitis
Pelvis, hip joint	Acetabular and femoral head disease with articular degeneration; protrusio acetabuli; sacroiliac joint ankylosis	Pain; end-stage arthritis; fracture
Knee	Distal femoral involvement with bone and joint deformity	Pain; arthritis: fracture
Tibia, femur, humerus	Bowing, with or without fracture; change in joint geometry	Pain; arthritis; fracture
Any site of involvement	Marked destruction of bone; extracortical extension; possible soft tissue mass	Marked increase in pain; neoplasia must be ruled out

TABLE 14-5
Indications for pharmacotherapy

Major	Minor
Pain	Asymptomatic involvement in weight-bearing bone
Deformity	Increased alkaline phosphate less less than twice the value of normal
Increased alkaline phosphatase that is twice the value of normal; increased urinary hydroxyproline that is twice the value of normal	Treatment not indicated for asymptomatic disease in non-weight-bearing bones in patients with normal biochemistries
Neurologic compression	
High output of congestive heart failure	
Pathologic fracture	
Osteotomy/arthroplasty	

close to major weight-bearing joints. Radiographic disease in these locations is a secondary indication for treatment in order to attempt to prevent bowing deformities, fractures, or joint destruction (Table 14-5).

Neurologic deficits, fracture, elective skeletal surgery, progressive disease, congestive heart failure, and polyostotic disease are additional indications for suppressive pharmacotherapy. Further orthopaedic treatment may be indicated for (1) severe disabling arthritis (particularly of the hip, knee, or shoulder); (2) severe bowing deformities of the femur or tibia; (3) pathologic fractures; or (4) sarcomatous degeneration. Neurosurgical treatment is rarely indicated for brainstem or spinal cord compression. Treatment is not indicated for patients with asymptomatic disease in non-weight-bearing bones or monostotic involvement with normal alkaline phosphatase.

The two major therapeutic agents available for the treatment of Paget's disease are the calcitonins[18] (porcine, salmon, or human) and the diphosphonates (disodium etidronate). The aim of such therapy is to control the metabolic activity of the disease, to normalize the biochemical parameters, and to ameliorate the clinical symptoms. However, symptomatic relief may be achieved without control of biochemistries. Both agents work by inhibiting osteoclastic activity. Calcitonin is a small polypeptide hormone that acts through a spe-cific receptor mechanism in the osteoclasts to alter cell function by a cyclic adenosine monophosphate (AMP)–mediated system. Diphosphonates are the newer agents. They act as analogs of pyrophosphate and interfere with the growth and dissolution of hydroxyapatite crystals.[31] They also appear to impair osteoclast function directly. In high doses diphosphonates may impair normal mineralization of osteoid and cause an increased incidence of pathologic fractures. Serial or combination treatments using calcitonin and diphosphonates have been shown to enhance their therapeutic effectiveness and to ameliorate side effects.[3] Mitromycin, a third agent, is an antibiotic with cytotoxic properties. It is a strong inhibitor of osteoclasts and osteoblasts and has been shown to be effective in rapidly relieving the bone pain caused by Paget's disease, often in 4 to 5 days. However, it has significant side effects with toxicity to the liver, kidneys, gastrointestinal tract, and platelets, and for these reasons I recommend its use only for Paget's paraplegia. In such cases, it is administered intravenously, 15 mg/kg/day for a 10-day period.

For the major indications, I recommend serial treatment with calcitonin, 50 units subcutaneously three times a week for 6 months, followed by diphosphonate, 5mg/kg/day for 6 months, with the agents overlapping for 1 month. Occasionally, the diphosphonate is continued longer until the alkaline phosphatase plateaus (it may never return to normal) and the urinary hydroxy-proline is normal.

In the Hospital for Special Surgery's Metabolic Bone Disease Clinic two thirds of the patients treated according to this regimen achieve remission without relapse for 5 years. If relapse should occur, I recommend repeating the cycle of treatment. Alternatively, low-dose diphosphonate, 5mg/kg/day, may be given alone for 6 months, or high doses, 20mg/kg/day, may be given in monthly pulses every 4 months.

For elective orthopaedic procedures, such as osteotomy or arthroplasty, I recommend beginning the treatment protocol 3 months before surgery.

For minor indications I recommend treatment with diphosphonate alone, 5mg/kg/day for 6 months. However, diphosphonates are not recommended initially in the presence of fracture or osteotomy since they impair bone healing.

Laboratory tests of alkaline phosphatase and urinary hydroxyproline levels are followed initially every 3 months for the first year, then every 6 months (or sooner if the patient becomes symptomatic) for 5 years; thereafter annual testing is sufficient.

Orthopaedic surgical procedures

Surgical intervention in Paget's disease is indicated for (1) selected fractures; (2) severe, disabling arthritis; and (3) extreme bowing deformities causing malalignment of weight-bearing joints.

Fractures. *Stress* or *pseudofractures* occur most frequently in the tibia and proximal femur. They often appear in metabolically inactive bone but may be tender and painful especially with weight bearing. Treatment by bracing or protection from weight bearing for a period of several weeks to months can often relieve symptoms and allow healing. Persistent pain for more than 3 to 6 months may be an indication for prophylactic surgical treatment.

Completed fractures are usually transverse or short oblique. Most femoral fractures are best treated by operative methods,[23,26] preferably with intramedullary devices when possible. Treatment with calcitonin, 50 units subcutaneously three times per week, is recommended to aid in fracture union. Femoral neck fractures are a problem and frequently do not heal, especially when displaced or biomechanically unstable.[10] In such cases, replacement arthroplasty is preferable.

Intertrochanteric and subtrochanteric fractures will usually unite after appropriate fixation with either a sliding nail and screw-plate or an intramedullary device. Technical problems may be encountered because of the enlarged, sclerotic, or softened bone, which is often deformed. Routine treatment with calcitonin is recommended.

Tibial fractures can frequently be managed closed without difficulty because of the transverse stable configuration of these fractures in Paget's disease. Surgical stabilization is indicated for unstable fractures. Intramedullary fixation is desirable but, again, there may be technical difficulties present as a result of medullary and cortical sclerosis and deformity.

In general, fractures in Pagetic bone heal with abundant callus; however, re-fracture is occasionally seen, and delayed or nonunion is more frequently encountered when the bone is in the sclerotic phase.

Arthritis. Severe arthritis of the hip or knee may require total joint reconstruction. Replacement arthroplasties have been performed with a high degree of success, and stable fixation of prosthetic components for periods of 2 to 10 years has been achieved (Fig. 14-16).

Careful preoperative evaluation of the patient's complaints is mandatory. Differentiating the cause(s) of pain about the hip or knee in patients with Paget's disease can be very difficult. Possible factors contributing to the pain in addition to mechanical malalignment and arthritis include the metabolic activity of Paget's disease, neural compression both local and/or remote, and numerous rheumatic manifestations frequently associated with Paget's disease. Specific trials of medication, either anti-inflammatory or anti-Paget's, and/or an intra-articular injection with an anesthetic agent can be helpful in determining the cause(s) of pain.

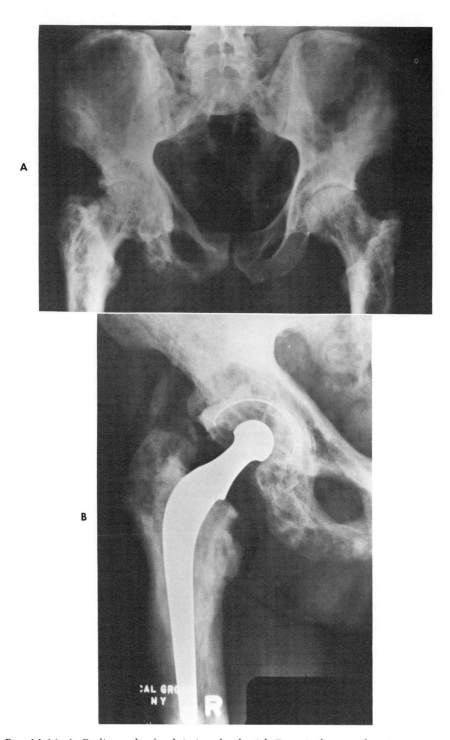

FIG. 14-16. A, Radiograph of pelvis involved with Paget's disease showing concentric type Paget's arthritis of right hip. B, Same patient 4 years following total hip replacement showing stable fixation of components.

Technical problems encountered in total hip replacements include increased bleeding; sclerotic bone, making reaming difficult; and bony deformities requiring careful preoperative planning and surgical techniques. A varus neck-shaft angle and bowing of the proximal femur are frequently associated with Paget's disease and they predispose the patients to an undesirable varus placement of the femoral component. The transtrochanteric approach is recommended in such cases in order to achieve a neutral or valgus placement of the stem and appropriate muscle tension and adductor lever arm. Protrusio acetabulum is frequently associated with Paget's coxarthrosis. Acetabular bone grafting and/or reinforcement, although rarely required, should be performed whenever necessary to place the socket laterally and inferiorly as close as possible to its normal anatomic location. An increased incidence of postoperative heterotopic ossification has been reported.

No well-controlled studies have documented beneficial effects of perioperative treatment with anti-Paget's medication in patients undergoing joint replacement surgery. However, on theoretical grounds I recommend serial perioperative treatment with calcitonin followed by diphosphonate for patients with either active Paget's disease or in those where a trochanteric osteotomy is planned.

Osteotomy. Osteotomy to correct deformity and improve weight-bearing joint mechanics may be indicated for symptomatic malalignment of the hip or knee. Relatively well-maintained lateral and patellofemoral compartments and ligamentous stability in the knee and congruence in the hip are prerequisites to osteotomy. A course of calcitonin should be given first to relieve bone pain resulting from the metabolic activity of the Paget's disease. If arthritic symptoms persist, osteotomy may be indicated. Calcitonin should be continued postoperatively until bone union is achieved. Tibial osteotomy for medial compartment Paget's arthrosis can be expected to relieve pain and improve ambulation in a high percentage of patients.[21] The results of intertrochan-teric osteotomy for Paget's coxarthrosis are not as predictable, and their prognosis is comparable to the outcome of osteotomy done for primary osteoarthritis.[28]

References

1. Albright, F. and Reifenstein, E.C., Jr.: The parathyroid glands and metabolic bone disease: selected studies, Baltimore, 1948, The Williams and Wilkins Co.
2. Avioli, L.V., Baran, D.T., Whyte, M.P., and Teitelbaum, S.L.: The biochemical and skeletal heterogeneity of "post-menopausal osteoporosis." In Barzel, U.S., editor: Osteoporosis II, New York, 1978, Grune and Stratton.
3. Bijvoet, O.L.M., et al.: Treatment of Paget's disease with combined calcitonin and diphosphonate (EHDP), Metab. Bone Dis. Rel. Res. **1**:251-261, 1978.
4. Birge, S.J., Jr., Keutmann, H.T., Custrecasas, P., and Whedon, G.D.: Osteoporosis, intestinal lactase deficiency and low dietary calcium intake, N. Engl. J. Med. **276**:445-448, 1967.
5. Frank, W.A., Bress, N.M., Singer, F.R., and Krane, S.M.: Rheumatic manifestations of Paget's disease of bone, Am. J. Med. **56**:592-603, 1974.
6. Frost, H.M.: Tetracycline-based histological analysis of bone remodeling, Calcif. Tissue Res. **3**:211-237, 1969.
7. Gallagher, J.C., and Riggs, B.L.: Current concepts in nutrition, N. Engl. J. Med. **298**:193-195, 1978.
8. Goldman, A.B., et al.: Osteitis deformans of the hip joint, Am. J. Roentgenol. Radium Ther. Nucl. Med. **128**:601-606, 1977.
9. Goldsmith, N.F., and Johnston, J.O.: Bone mineral: effects of oral contraceptives, pregnancy and lactation, J. Bone Joint Surg. **57A**:657-668, 1975.
10. Grundy, M.: Fracture of the femur in Paget's disease of bone, J. Bone Joint Surg. **52B**:252-263, 1970.
11. Handy, R.C.: Paget's disease of bone, 1981, Praeger Publishers.
12. Harris, W.H.: Paget's disease involving the hip joint, J. Bone Joint Surg. **53B**:650-659, 1971.
13. Jowsey, J., Riggs, B.L., Kelly, P.J., and Hoffman, D.L.: Effect of combined therapy with sodium fluoride, vitamin D and calcium in osteoporosis, Am. J. Med. **53**:43-49, 1972.
14. Krane, S.M.: Paget's disease of bone, Clin. Orthop. **127**:24-36, 1977.
15. Lane, J.M.: Metabolic bone disease and fracture healing. In Heppenstall, R.B.: Fracture treatment and healing, Philadelphia, 1980, W.B. Saunders Co.
16. Lane, J.M., and Vigorita, V.J.: Osteoporosis—definition, pathophysiology, diagnosis and treatment. Current concepts review, J. Bone Joint Surg. **65A**:274-278, 1983.
17. Lane, J.M., Vigorita, V.J., and Falls, M.: Diagnosis and treatment of osteoporosis—an update, Geriatrics, 1984. (In press.)
18. McIntyre, I., et al.: Chemistry, physiology, and therapeutic application of calcitonin, Arthritis Rheum. **23**:1139-1147, 1980.
19. Meema, S., Bunker, M.L., and Meema, H.E.: Preventive effect of estrogen on postmenopausal bone loss, Arch. Intern. Med. **135**:1436-1440, 1975.

20. Merkow, R.L., Pellicci, P.M., Hely, D.P., and Salvati, E.A.: Total hip replacement for Paget's disease of the hip, J. Bone Joint Surg., **66A:**752-758, 1984.

21. Meyers, M.H., and Singer, F.R.: Osteotomy for tibia vara in Paget's disease under cover of calcitonin, J. Bone Joint Surg. **60A:**810-814, 1978.

22. Muenier, P.J., et al.: Bone histomorphometry in osteoporotic states. In Barzel, U.S., editor: Osteoporosis II, New York, 1978, Grune and Stratton.

23. Nicholas, J.A., and Killoran, P.: Fracture of the femur in patients with Paget's disease, J. Bone Joint Surg. **47A:**450-461, 1965.

24. Paget, J.: On a form of chronic inflammation of bones (osteitis deformans), Med. Chir. Trans. **60:**37, 1877.

25. Recker, R.R., Savile, P.D., and Heaney, R.P.: Effect of estrogens and calcium carbonate on bone loss in postmenopausal women, Ann. Intern. Med. **87:**645-655, 1977.

26. Resnick, D., and Niwayama, G.: Paget's disease. In Diagnosis of bone and joint disorders, vol. 2, Philadelphia, 1981, W.B. Saunders Co.

27. Riggs, B.L., et al.: Effect of the fluoride/calcium regimen on vertebral fracture occurrence in postmenopausal osteoporosis, N. Engl. J. Med. **306**(8):446-460, 1982.

28. Roper, B.A.: Paget's disease of the hip with osteoarthritis: results of intertrochanteric osteotomy, J. Bone Joint Surg. **53B:**660-662, 1971.

29. Scileppi, K.P., et al.: Bone histomorphometry in femoral neck fractures, Surg. Forum **32:**543-545, 1981.

30. Singh, M., Riggs, B.L., Beabout, J.W., and Jowsey, J.: Femoral trabecular-pattern index for evaluation of spinal osteoporosis, Ann. Intern. Med. **77:**63-67, 1972.

31. Siris, E.S., Jacobs, T.P., and Canfield, R.E.: Paget's disease of bone, Bull. N.Y. Acad. Med. **56:**285-304, 1980.

32. Stauffer, R.N., and Sim, F.H.: Total hip arthroplasty in Paget's disease of the hip, J. Bone Joint Surg. **58A:**476, 1976.

chapter 15
FRACTURE MANAGEMENT OF THE ELDERLY PATIENT

John P. Lyden

With the dramatic increase in the size of the geriatric population in the past few decades and the concomitant increase in their life expectancy, the problem of fractures in the elderly is a growing concern. Not only has the number of patients increased but so have their (and their families') expectations, often in spite of patient fragility. The number of hip fractures, for example, in this country today, their bed requirements, and the need for extended care facilities or home care will continue to strain our resources. In contradistinction to elective reconstructive surgery, the fracture patient is totally unprepared for the accident. The socioeconomic impact of a broken hip can so disrupt an elderly person's measured world that many never return to their former functional status. As a corollary to that disruption, patient mortality in the succeeding year rises dramatically. Although the in-hospital mortalities have been reduced, the trauma to the individual is almost impossible to overcome. Many elderly live alone, often far from any family, and with marginal financial resources. Even a Colles fracture can devastate such a tenuous existence and lead to great hardship or institutionalization.

COMPLICATING FACTORS

Patients over 70 are already faced with progressive multiorgan failures. Their balance is often poor because of cerebral degenerative disease, vestibular dysfunction, or cardiovascular disease. If they arise quickly, turn suddenly, or slide on a wet surface, their protective reflexes are slow. Their eyesight is deteriorating either from cataracts or from progressive macular degeneration. All too often the loss of function in one eye leads to poor depth perception to which they have difficulty adjusting. Cardiac function itself is often marginal. Whether the patient collapses and then breaks the hip or trips first is often unclear.

For these reasons, I feel that it is important to observe the elderly fracture patient in the hospital for at least 24 to 48 hours preoperatively to rule out any occult organic problem. A transient ischemic attack, cerebrovascular accident, myocardial infarction, or electrolyte imbalance can cause the fracture and be neglected or even aggravated further in the rush to repair it. All too often "rapid fixation" to permit mobilization and decrease morbidity may result in the missing of an evolving myocardial infarction or cerebrovascular accident. A balanced approach to the patient includes an evaluation of why the injury occurred, what events preceded it, and whether the patient is in the midst of an additional evolving medical problem. Elderly patients will never be ideal anesthetic risks; there are always abnormalities present. It requires experience and judgment to know when to proceed with surgery. The elderly patient with severe pain from an unstable hip fracture who cannot use the bedpan or even move around comfortably in bed will deteriorate over the succeeding days. Decubiti or pulmonary or bladder complications may then make surgery even more risky. The trauma of bed rest must be thoughtfully weighed against the trauma of surgery.

Shoulder Fractures

A fracture of the shoulder is a common injury seen by a triage officer in the emergency room setting. Luckily the injury is often an isolated one and occurs from a low-energy fall on the outstretched hand of an elderly person. The anatomy of these fractures may vary widely as a result of the degree of osteoporosis, the energy of the fall, and the direction of impact. The approach to fractures in the shoulder region should be based on the patient's realistic goals, bearing in mind that the shoulder actually only functions to place the hand in space. An overly aggressive approach to a shoulder fracture can leave a stiff, painful, restricted arm; the physician should treat these patients with modest immobilization, early motion, and a minimum of surgical intervention. Considerable angular deformity can be accepted in return for early fracture healing and a rapid return to activity.

The neurovascular status of the arm should be checked at the outset and throughout treatment. The axillary sheath and its contents are vulnerable to compression or stretching, especially if a dislocation or fracture dislocation has gone untreated. A laceration of the axillary artery or vein from injury or occurring during reduction is an emergency situation, and this possibility should always be kept in mind. Loss of the peripheral pulse that does not return immediately after reduction necessitates an immediate vascular exploration.

After the initial clinical examination of the shoulder, the x-ray films should be obtained. I have found the trauma series recommended by Neer[10] to be very helpful. This includes an anteroposterior view of the glenohumeral joint and a lateral view of the scapula. The axillary view is also informative if the situation is still unclear. Fractures of the proximal humerus may be classified by their location or the parts involved: (1) greater tuberosity, (2) lesser tuberosity, (3) surgical neck. In addition, they may be classified by the Neer system.[10,11] This classification depends on the displacement or angulation of the fragments of the proximal humerus. The pieces examined are the head fragment, the greater and lesser tuberosities, and the humeral shaft.

Of the fractures of the proximal humerus 80% are impacted or minimally displaced, and are therefore classified as one-part fractures (Table 15-1, Fig. 15-1). They are treated by immobilization for 2 weeks, and then by gradual, progressive range-of-motion ex-

Table 15-1
Shoulder fractures

Type of fracture	Frequency	Author's treatment
One part: The fragments are together with less than 1 cm displacement or 45 degrees of angulation	80%	Progressive exercises as tolerated
Two part: Two fragments with more than 1 cm displacement or 45 degrees of angulation	10%	Usually closed treatment
Three part	3%	Open reduction and internal fixation
Four part	4%	Open reduction and internal fixation of prosthesis
Head split or crushed	3%	Prosthesis

ercises of the Codman type. This immobilization, especially during the first week, should hold the humerus firmly against the chest both for fracture protection and patient comfort. This treatment can be difficult because of associated injuries, restricted pulmonary capacity, pendulous breasts, and the realities of a person coping, often alone, with the activities of daily living. If the injury is in the dominant arm, the problems are even worse, and a brief period of hospitalization or home assistance may be necessary. In the beginning, I prefer to use a deluxe sling-and-swathe (Zimmer) for im-

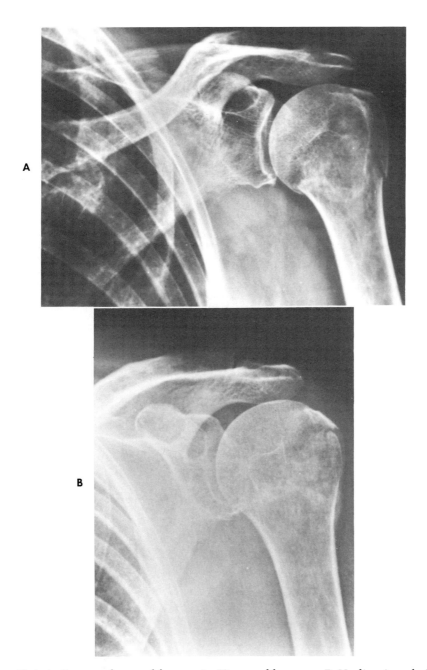

FIG. 15-1. A, One-part humeral fracture in 82-year-old woman. B, Healing 4 weeks later, immobilized with a sling.

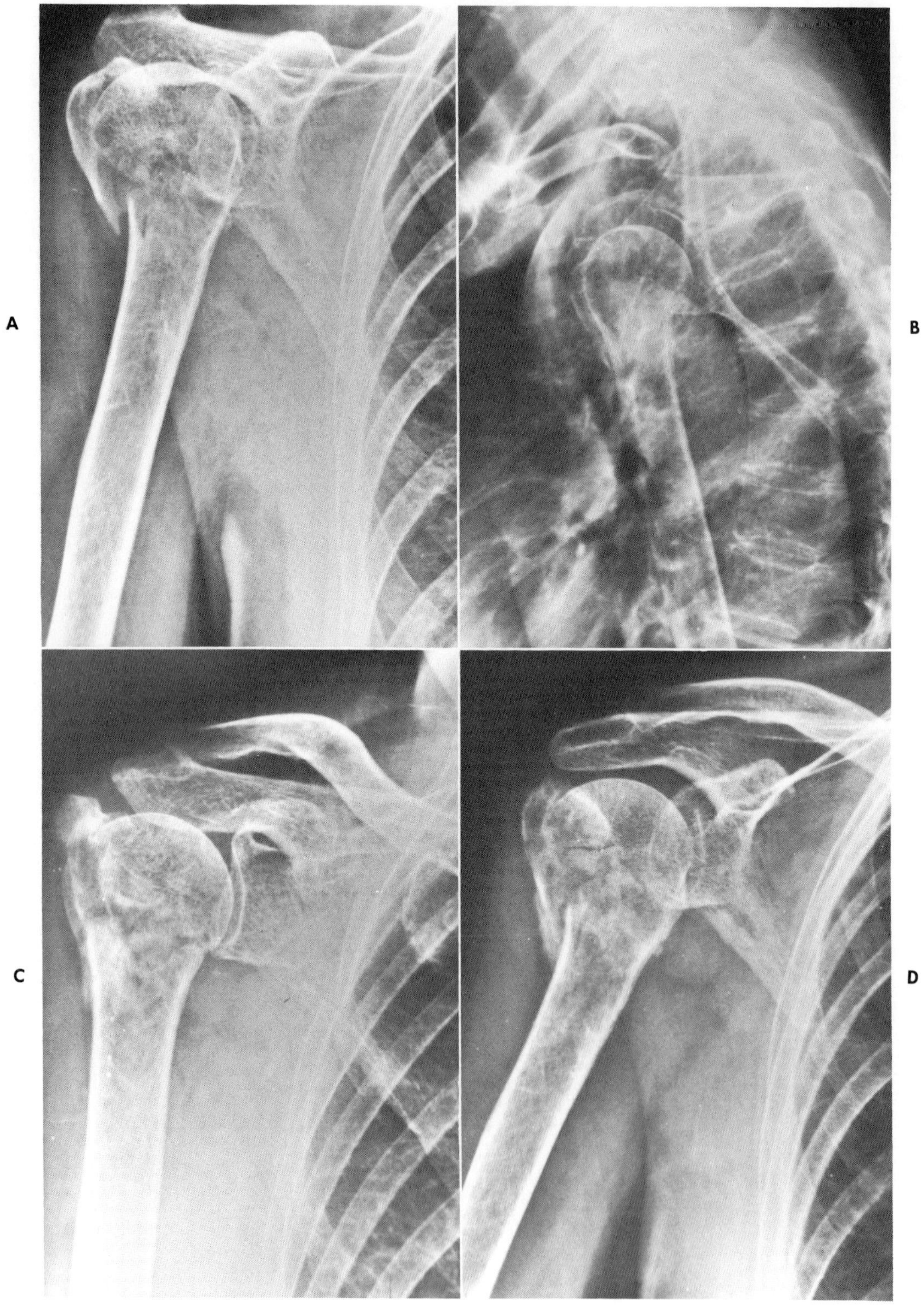

FIG. 15-2. A and B, Three-part fracture in 75-year-old woman. C and D, Fracture healed 6 weeks later with a deluxe sling and swathe.

mobilization because it has Velcro fasteners and is therefore easy to use. After 1 to 2 weeks, I switch to a simple sling or scarf for occasional support and encourage increased use of the arm. Throughout this treatment, the elbow and hand are watched and exercised to prevent the development of edema, stiffness, and reflex dystrophy.

If, however, the displacement of the head fragment from the humeral shaft is excessive or if the tuberosities are widely displaced, then consideration must be given to reduction either by closed or open means. One must remember that the alignment of these fractures, but not their displacement, will often improve with time as gravity is allowed to overcome the surrounding muscle spasm. Once the muscles have fatigued, the soft tissue envelope will often improve the alignment. Thus, a week of observation and evaluation of the patient is often helpful before an operation is recommended.

Most surgeons agree on the basic surgical techniques for fixation of various fractures. Some are more aggressive than others when deciding which patients to operate upon, but the wires, Rush rods, and AO screws and/or plates are utilized in a fairly standard fashion. The major argument arises over the three-part or four-part fractures of Neer. In these fractures, where the anatomic head is without its soft tissue attachments, the chance of avascular necrosis and stiffness of the shoulder is increased. These fractures may also be further complicated by the degree of osteoporosis and/or preexisting rotator cuff disease. The alternatives are to accept the fracture as it is, to reduce the fragments and fix them internally, or to discard the humeral head and insert a prosthetic replacement. The younger the patient, the better the alignment wanted, and the less liable the surgeon is to resort to a prosthesis. If one choses the first option, the patient is immobilized for 2 to 3 weeks and then begun on progressive range-of-motion exercises (Fig. 15-2). There will be some loss of forward flexion and internal rotation so activities like eating, hair combing, and toilet care may be compromised.

Unfortunately, the amount of restriction is unpredictable. It is often impossible to state at the outset how significant the disability will be.

The opposite extreme is the use of a prosthesis (cemented or noncemented) of the Neer variety. This provides a concentric head and enables rapid mobilization of the shoulder. The tuberosities and the rotator cuff muscles that are attached to them are attached to the prosthesis at the time of surgery. The proponents of this treatment emphasize early aggressive rehabilitation to prevent stiffness or subluxation of the prosthesis, and they believe that the improved function justifies the operation. The results are, however, unpredictable and therefore many surgeons perfer not to use the prosthesis.

I prefer to use internal fixation, when necessary, with Rush rods, wires, and/or screws. If possible, I keep the humoral head and still achieve enough stability to allow early motion within the first few weeks after surgery. If I cannot achieve this degree of stability then, selectively, I will use a prosthesis. One must always keep in mind the fact that many elderly patients have had restricted shoulder function before their fractures; they already had difficulty flexing their shoulder above 100 degrees or abducting it beyond 90 degrees. Given this baseline functional level, it becomes apparent that extensive surgical reconstruction, particularly in the truly elderly patient, is unwise.

PELVIC FRACTURES

Few injuries require greater multispecialty cooperation than the pelvic fracture. Here the damage to multiple organ systems dictates smooth cooperation between abdominal, vascular, neurologic, urologic, and orthopaedic specialists. From the outset evaluation, stabilization, and reconstruction must proceed smoothly. The injuries may vary from the mildest nondisplaced pubic fracture in an elderly woman to the total disruption suffered by a pedestrian who is struck by a motor vehicle.

While the elderly patient would not be expected to have suffered significant associated soft tissue injuries, the pedestrian could well have a perforated viscus, bladder rupture, urethral tear, or significant iliac vessel injury. If the bone fragments have been significantly displaced, then the surrounding venous plexus may be grossly disrupted, and significant retroperitoneal bleeding will ensue. Such massive bleeding is difficult to control by either closed or open means, and hence it carries a high mortality rate.

There are several different classifications of pelvic fractures. I prefer the classification of Key and Cauldwell:[8]
1. Fractures of individual bones without a break in the continuity of the pelvic ring
2. Single break in the pelvic ring
3. Double breaks in the pelvic ring
4. Fractures of the acetabulum

In general, pelvic fractures may be thought of in their high-energy and low-energy forms. The former tend to occur in younger people, often with other concomitant injuries; the patient may even by unconscious. The evaluation begins with an anteroposterior pelvic x-ray film. On this film the physician should check the sacroiliac joints, acetabula, and general innominate configuration. Areas of tenderness, abrasions, or crepitus are all helpful in the initial examination. A rectovaginal examination should be performed, and the urine must be checked for any signs of hematuria. If there is any doubt, a general surgeon should be called upon to evaluate the abdomen since it may deteriorate rapidly in the succeeding hours either from visceral injury or retroperitoneal bleeding. Stabilization of the pelvis by sandbags, traction, or an external fixator should be considered, particularly if hemorrhage becomes a major problem. In these instances, many methods have been tried, unfortunately, each with mixed success. These methods include:
1. Arterial/venous embolization
2. Abdominal exploration and ligation of the hypogastric vessels
3. Pressure suits

Absolute anatomic reduction is not of critical importance except to reconstitute the acetabulum for later weight bearing or to prevent excessive leg shortening in cases of double vertical (Malgaigne) fractures. These

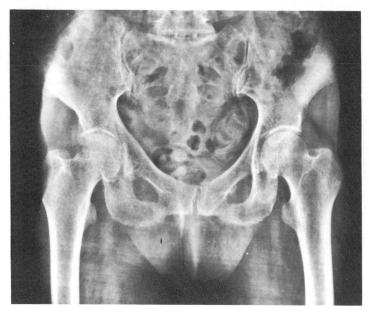

FIG. 15-3. Fracture of ischium in 82-year-old-woman healed uneventfully.

are both readily dealt with after the initial several days of stabilization.

The other group of pelvic fractures are those resulting from a low-energy injury. These occur usually in the elderly osteoporotic patient who stumbles and falls. These injuries can easily be overlooked or confused with hip fractures. Rotation tests of the hip, heel percussion, and finally x-ray films may not differentiate such injuries clearly, and therefore a bone scan 2 or 3 days later is needed to make the diagnosis. All too often the patient is sent home after an initial negative x-ray film, only to be found later on to have had either a pelvic, or worse still, an unrecognized hip fracture. The combination of osteopenia, intestines distended with feces and gas, old healed fractures, and the triage officers' fear of acquiring a disposition problem causes errors. These patients are often only marginally independent. With a seemingly minimal pelvic fracture, they become unable to care for themselves.

The treatment for such patients once hospitalized consists of mild analgesics, (minimal narcotics), prophylaxis against pulmonary emboli, prevention of ileus, and ambulation as soon as the pain can be tolerated. Rarely is traction or surgical treatment required; these fractures do not tend to be widely displaced or unstable (Fig. 15-3). The pain is slow to resolve, and since these people are fragile, it often takes them several weeks to regain independence. The fracture lines disappear slowly when evaluated by x-ray films, but the patient should be gently mobilized anyhow to prevent the many complications of bed rest and prolonged hospitalization. Ambulatory aids play a major role in helping restore confidence, security, and hence, mobility. The walker is the mainstay of my therapy program for these people. Some patients may cautiously progress to Canadian crutches or a cane, but the security of a walker is not to be dismissed lightly. Often families will want to have the patient progress rapidly to a cane as a sign of independence and progress, but this should be discouraged.

HIP FRACTURES

Hip fractures are primarily a problem of the elderly. At the New York Hospital these patients average 70 years of age. The injury is often caused by a simple fall with minor trauma; few result from a major injury. The bone that fractures is in a sense pathologic since it usually shows microscopic changes of osteoporosis and/or osteomalacia. Hip injury accounts for such morbidity and mortality that the geriatric population fears it above all others. Until the 1940s mortality was nearly 50%, but with more modern methods the in-hospital survival rate is over 90%.

These fractures can be divided into two prime groups—intracapsular (subcapital) or extracapsular (peritrochanteric). The two types occur with approximately equal frequency but are quite different in terms of treatment and prognosis. In an intracapsular hip fracture, the fragments are contained by the capsule, and therefore the bleeding is minimal and hypovolemic shock is uncommon. The problems arise later on with nonunion or avascular necrosis causing pain and disability.

The surgeon can either internally fix the fracture and allow healing to occur or replace the femoral head with a prosthesis (Austin-Moore, bicentric, total hip replacement). In most instances, I prefer internal fixation with Knowles pins as recommended by Arnold, Lyden, and Minkoff.[1] These pins hold the fragments in position and allow the patient to be up and out of bed while healing occurs. This technique is quick and relatively atraumatic and can be performed percutaneously under local anesthesia if necessary. Bleeding and wound complications are virtually nil. A good reduction of the fracture is essential. This is performed with traction and internal rotation, and verified by either x-ray films or an image intensifier. The calcar femorale should support the femoral head without excessive valgus. Three pins are enough for an impacted fracture, while four are recommended for a fracture that had been displaced. The impacted fracture, if left untreated, may displace later (at 2 or 3 weeks) and therefore it should be surgically fixed.

The Knowles pins should be placed into the subchondral bone of the femoral head for the best purchase, that is, to within 1 cm of the hip joint. They should be parallel to allow settling to occur as the fracture heals. If not, the pins will lock by converging or diverging and prevent impaction, leading to a nonunion. The actual configuration of the pins is not critical, but they should be parallel to the line of the femoral neck or be in slight valgus, and preferably one pin should lie along the calcar femorale. Elderly patients rarely can adhere to a program of non-weight-bearing. For these reasons, stable fixation should be achieved at surgery, or a primary hip replacement should be considered. It is unreasonable to assume that there will be minimal stresses in these fracture fragments postoperatively during the early recuperative phase. The forces across the hip that are caused by merely raising the leg in bed or lifting oneself onto a bedpan are high (1 to 2½ times body weight). If slippage does occur soon after surgery, the wisest course is to proceed with a femoral head replacement at that time. Since elderly patients make far less demands on their hips than young people, avascular necrosis with minimal segmental collapse is often, in fact, an acceptable result. Nonunion, however, requires revision in a patient with any more than minimal activity, assuming that the patient is not senile and was capable of walking before the fracture.

Not all intracapsular fractures, however, should be reduced and pinned. If a joint has already been affected by arthritis (osteoarthritis or rheumatoid), if the osteopenia is severe (such as from steroids, alcohol, malnutrition, or metastatic disease), if the patient's life expectancy is short, or if comminution of the femoral neck prevents a stable reduction of the head on the calcar, then the femoral head should be replaced at the primary operation. I prefer the cemented bicentric-type hemiarthroplasty (Osteonics) (Fig. 15-4). This allows immediate full weight bearing, prevents prosthetic migration in the femoral canal

thanks to the methylmethacrylate fixation, and in our elderly patients it has not yet required revision to a total hip replacement for later acetabular wear. At surgery the hip is approached through the standard Southern incision without removing the greater trochanter. Care is exercised to preserve the piriformis, conjoined tendon, and posterior capsule for repair at the end of the operation by reinsertion into the greater trochanter. This repair prevents a postoperative dislocation. A cement restrictor, cement gun, and pressurization technique allow excellent stem fixation even in the large, thin-walled femoral canals often encountered in the elderly. The new Osteonics prosthesis offers heads in 1 mm increments, a snap-on locking cap, and an offset center of rotation that prevents the head from shifting into excessive varus.

Since flexion and adduction is the position of least hip stability and since nurses often roll patients onto their sides by pulling on the opposite knee, I routinely apply a knee immobilizer postoperatively to reduce the chance of a dislocation. The other precautions in these patients are similar to those used during recovery from a total hip replacement. Patients are allowed to dangle their legs over the side of the bed on the second day, and they ambulate with a walker on the third day with weight bearing as tolerated.

Peritrochanteric hip fractures are different. Here problems appear immediately, but delayed failures are less frequent. These fractures occur extracapsularly and hence there is much more bleeding (500 to 1500 ml). Hypovolemic shock is not uncommon in these patients, especially if they were dehydrated or anemic and there is a delay before surgery. Restoration of an adequate intravascular volume with attention to hemodilution and electrolyte abnormalities should take priority in treating such patients. The patient needs to be stabilized and then, in most cases, internal fixation should be performed. If the initial evaluation reveals an evolving myocardial infarction, cardiac arrhythmia, progressive cerebral ischemia, or occult sepsis, these should

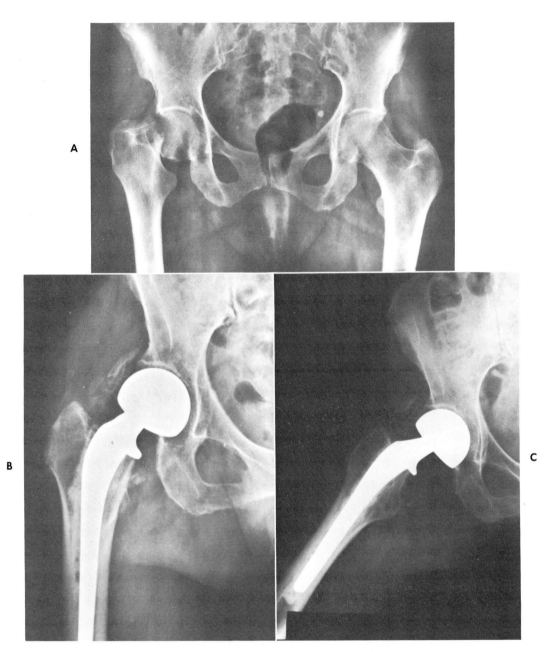

Fig. 15-4. A, Displaced intracapsular hip fracture in 72-year-old woman. **B** and **C,** Osteonics hip replacement.

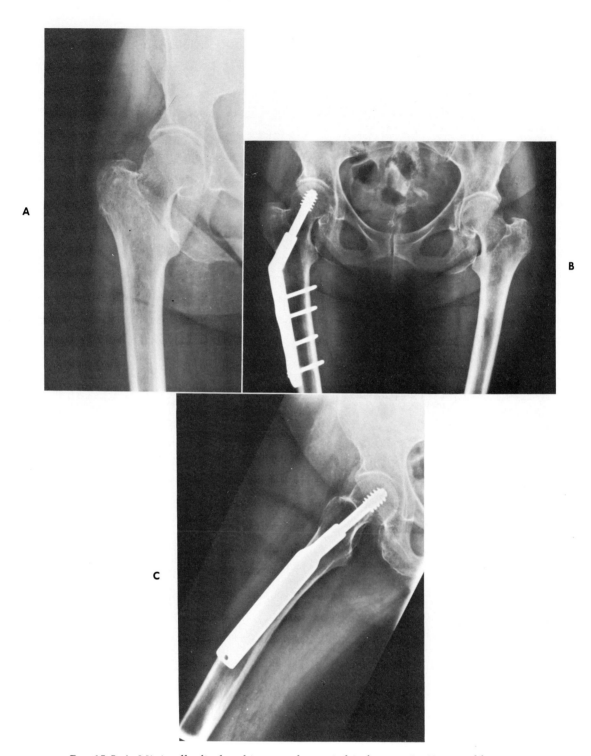

FIG. 15-5. **A,** Minimally displaced intertrochanteric hip fracture in 60-year-old woman. **B** and **C,** Fracture healed after compression screw fixation.

be treated before surgery. In general, it is best to fix the fracture if possible within 24 or 48 hours of admission assuming that the patient is stable.

I prefer the hip compression screw system (HCS) for intertrochanteric fractures (Fig. 15-5). The HCS provides good restoration of anatomy, firm fixation, flexibility, and ease of insertion. However, the Ender nail, which is an alternative device, has several distinct advantages. Such nails require a smaller incision, infections or wound problems are less likely, and healing is more rapid because the hip fracture is never directly operated upon. The periosteum and muscle insertions are not stripped away from around the fracture, and hence the callus forms far more rapidly. In young people where anatomic restoration may be desirable, where shortening or external rotation are unacceptable, or in the elderly where preexisting knee or femoral deformities prevent intramedullary nailing, then the HCS is preferable. In certain special conditions, such as Parkinson's disease with a severe tremor, the HCS fixation is also preferable.

The patient with an intertrochanteric hip fracture can be anesthetized with either spinal or general anesthesia and then placed supine on the fracture table. The affected hip is in extension, slight abduction, and neutral rotation. The image intensifiers are positioned, and the fracture reduction is evaluated. The appearance of the hip fracture is often quite different at this point because the original film in the emergency room usually shows the femur lying in 90 degrees of external rotation. The greater trochanter and lateral buttress can now be visualized more fully; this is important for achieving a stable fixation and for reducing the tendency for the fracture to displace medially. I allow the fragments to settle into a position of maximal stability by themselves. I rarely do a formal medial displacement osteotomy. The Dimon-Hughston osteotomy[2] was popularized in the era of fixed length devices (e.g., Jewett, McLaughlin). At that time, since the fracture fragments could not impact further after the operation, surgeons were plagued with

nails cutting out, pin breakage, and devices loosening from the femoral shaft. The HCS system has virtually eliminated most of these problems. As long as a single hole is cut in the femoral head for the lag screw and the screw is long enough to go in the subchondral bone and still extend down nearly the entire barrel of the side plate, then failure is rare.

Fixation should be performed in at least 135 degrees of valgus to promote sliding, impaction, stability, and hence safe, rapid healing. There are several technical points to be remembered:

1. Use a threaded guide wire to prevent inadvertent extraction with the reamer.
2. Aim for a bull's eye screw placement into the center of the femoral head.
3. Lock the reamer sleeve carefully to avoid drilling into the acetabulum.
4. Ream carefully with the barrel portion to prevent fracturing the greater trochanter.
5. Do not use too short a lag screw; the tail should be just about at the lateral cortex when fully inserted.
6. If the femoral head is osteoporotic, do not overtighten the compression screw and thereby pull out the lag screw.
7. Use the short barrel side plate if you expect considerable impaction.

In fragile patients where the incision should be minimal, the Ender nails offer distinct advantages (Fig. 15-6). Biomechanically, the forces are shifted into greater valgus, the lever arm at the fracture site is diminished, and impaction can occur more readily. Since the fracture is not opened and the fragments are not stripped of their blood supply, the hip heals rapidly. Callus is visible on x-ray films in 3 to 4 weeks with this "closed" method of treatment. This callus indicates early stability, which allows the patient to be mobilized more aggressively at that time. There are, however, several contraindications to the use of the Ender nails:

Absolute contraindications:
1. A deformed femoral canal that will not accept the intramedullary Ender nail

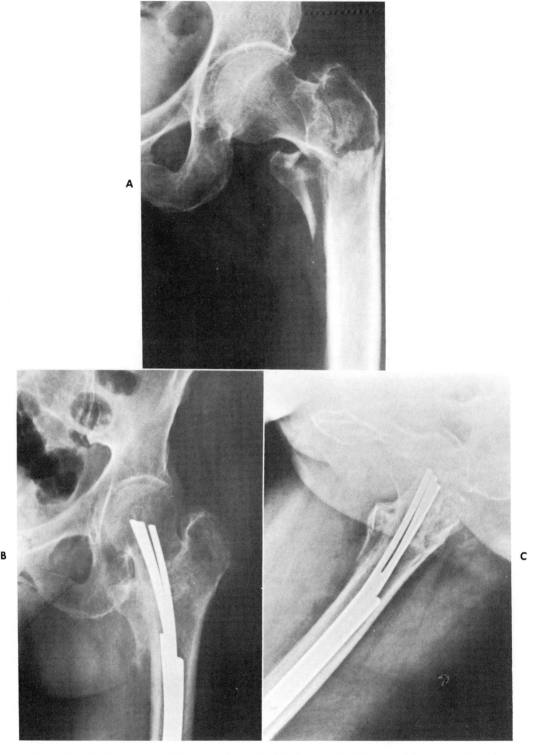

FIG. 15-6. **A,** Comminuted intertrochanteric hip fracture in 68-year-old woman. **B** and **C,** Fracture healed with Enders rod fixation.

2. Fractures at the base of the femoral neck because they tend to collapse into varus and heal slowly

3. Image intensification not available since it is impractical to insert the nails with only x-ray control

Relative contraindications:

1. A young patient in whom you need an anatomic reduction
2. A slender femoral canal
3. Poor quality of the femoral head (metastases)
4. Severe osteoarthritis of the knee

The patient who is to undergo Ender nailing is positioned as previously described for the HCS on the fracture table with the legs extended, and the affected leg is abducted about 10 degrees and is in neutral rotation. The image intensifiers are positioned at the hip for anteroposterior and lateral views, and the reduction is checked. The incision is medial and parallel to the patella, and the superomedial geniculate artery at the metaphyseal flare is the landmark for the nail insertion hole. This hold should be ovoid and approximately 2.5 by 1.5 cm. If a patient has a large femoral canal on the x-ray film, then the hole should be slightly larger transversely because five to six pins might be needed to fill the femoral canal. Using several drill holes and the rongeur, rather than the awl, prevents any splitting of the fragile cortex. The following technical tips should be kept in mind:

1. The fracture should be reduced in valgus to help nail insertion.
2. Slight external rotation of the leg helps reduce the fracture and makes insertion easier.
3. A crutch may be placed beneath the thigh to overcome posterior sag of the femoral shaft.
4. A gentle fan of the nails in the head is sufficient. Do not overbend them since this makes insertion too difficult.
5. If the nail penetrates the femoral head into the joint, pull the nail back to the fracture site and then reintroduce it into a new tract in the femoral head; otherwise the nails will penetrate again as settling occurs.

6. The femoral canal needs to be firmly packed with nails in order to prevent them from sliding out in spite of a small crack that often develops along the femoral shaft at the insertion site.

7. Postoperative traction is often required after Ender nailing for a period of from 1 to 4 weeks. This is a recognized part of the procedure and not a technical failure.

Ender nails are an internal splint similar in many ways to a Knowles pin. They align fragments, but the bone and the subsequent callus provide the true stability. This stability issue is its main difference from the HCS system. There are advantages and disadvantages to each system, as listed above, and the surgeon must decide what system best suits a particular patient. Both devices require familiarity on the part of the operating surgeon to make an intelligent selection for each patient.

Subtrochanteric hip fractures are seemingly very similar to the intertrochanteric type but, in fact, they behave in a far more unpredictable fashion. The incidence of failure here is far higher as a result of nonunion, malunion, and device failure. The chief reasons for the trouble are the higher bending moments at the fracture site and the slow healing properties of the cortical bone located in the subtrochanteric region. When stripped of surrounding muscles and blood supply, this bone can take as long as 4 months to heal. Meanwhile, the fixation device is being repeatedly loaded and stressed, and sooner or later it will fracture. For these reasons, an intramedullary device such as the Ender nail has tremendous appeal. The fracture does not have to be opened when the Ender nail is used, and the device actually shifts the forces to the bones (i.e., a bad-sharing device) and therefore carries little stress itself. These fractures often require postoperative traction to achieve reasonable stability. This may take from 4 to 6 weeks, depending on the anatomy of the fracture. The patient should be adequately observed to minimize the complications of bed rest. Because these factors are better understood today, the morbidity and mortality from this fracture, even in the elderly, are now low.

SUPRACONDYLAR FRACTURES OF THE FEMUR

Fractures of the supracondylar region of the femur are a relatively uncommon but difficult problem combining soft tissue and skeletal elements. While the injury in young people usually represents high-energy trauma as in a motor vehicle accident or a fall from a considerable height, the elderly can develop such fractures from a simple fall to the floor. Younger patients tend to have more splintering and displacement of the fragments, often with a T-shaped configuration (intracondylar), and with fragments of the bone projecting into the quadriceps mechanism. Of the various classification systems, the most widely accepted is that of Neer et al.[12] They described a series of transverse, oblique, T, and Y fractures with their expected patterns of deformity. If the fracture is only minimally displaced, it may be treated by balanced suspension with a tibial pin and traction for 4 to 6 weeks, followed by a cast brace.

Closed treatment of this fracture is, however, complicated by muscle forces acting at the fracture site; the quadriceps and hamstrings tend to shorten, the gastrocnemius muscle flexes the distal fragment, and the adductor magnus pulls it into varus and internal rotation. During the initial traction phase, therefore, extraordinary care must be taken to adjust and align the traction so that malunion does not result. X-ray films taken during this period are notoriously misleading and should be carefully supervised and interpreted to avoid mistakes. As a result of problems with fragment displacement and internal rotation or angulation at the fracture site, many surgeons prefer open reduction and internal fixation.

In the elderly the situation is often complicated by osteoporosis, stiffness of the knee, and occasionally the presence of preexisting devices such as a total hip or total knee replacement with projecting metal components and methylmethacrylate bone cement. One must remember that nonunion, with or without open reduction and internal fixation, may occur in the elderly. These fractures occur through metaphyseal spongy bone and should heal readily, but the crushing that occurs at the fracture site and the difficulty of achieving truly rigid fixation in soft bone can lead to failure. The cast brace, which is such a good adjunct to closed or open treatment in the young, is often not practical in the elderly patient. The tissue of their thighs is often so flabby that even with careful fitting it is questionable whether the cast brace helps immobilize the fracture or whether it actually magnifies the problem by wobbling.

Neurovascular complications should always be kept in mind since the femoral artery runs along the femur in Hunter's canal near the fracture site, and the sciatic, tibial, and common peroneal nerves lie posteriorly. The pulses, sensation, and motor function distally should be evaluated initially and followed carefully thereafter. In the elderly, however, these neurovascular problems rarely arise. It is the widely displaced high-energy, shattering fractures of youth that pose the major danger to these nearby structures.

My preferred method of treatment in the elderly is, therefore, balanced suspension with tibial pin traction or cast (fiberglass cylinder) immobilization with or without closed reduction for an initial 4 to 6 weeks. Thereafter, a long leg brace is used for an additional 6 weeks of protected motion. This allows rapid mobilization of the patient, early discharge, and a minimum of incapacitation during the healing phase. If the cast is too large or heavy, many of these frail patients would be unable to cope outside the hospital. Knee stiffness with this regimen is kept to a minimum by avoiding postoperative adhesions. The splint or cast brace will allow gentle motion of the knee to begin once the fracture is sticky. The orthosis has the added advantage of being lighter than a conventional cast and allows greater functional independence.

If, however, the fracture has a displaced

intracondylar component or if it angulates or interferes with smooth quadriceps and patellar function, then open reduction and internal fixation should be performed. Occasionally an open wound, fat emboli, or thrombophlebitis will delay surgery. The surgical procedure is extensive, and a pelvic bone graft should be used if there is excess comminution at the fracture site.

For these reasons, careful preoperative evaluation and stabilization are essential before proceeding with the fixation. I prefer to use the Richard screw and a 90-degree supracondylar side plate for fixation. This two-part device is more forgiving than the AO 95-degree angled blade plate. It seems to me to give a firmer grip in the condyles. Poor fixation in the osteoporotic distal fragment is a problem and can lead to nonunion and failure. Supplemental cancellous screws in the condyles or interfragmentary screws along the shaft and metaphysis help. Postoperatively, these patients should be managed in balanced suspension and then gradually mobilized, depending on the quality of fixation. Large, firm fragments securely fixed in a cooperative patient can be protected by a brace, as mentioned before, and the patient can be restricted to a walker for 2 to 3 months. If, however, the fixation is not that stable and if there are multiple fragmented areas through the cortical bone, then the surgeon should keep the patient in balanced suspension with tibial pin traction for 4 to 6 weeks to allow early healing. During this time the knee should be regularly exercised to maintain as much motion as possible while the fracture is healing.

Crutches are fine for the young; a walker is far safer for the elderly. Although young people use crutches quite readily, the elderly lack the coordination and confidence necessary and do far better with an inherently stable form of support. The patient should not progress beyond the walker for the first several months especially if the doctor is attempting to maintain partial weight bearing.

As these patients are followed, certain problems should be kept in mind—knee stiffness, degenerative arthritis, thrombophlebitis, chronic edema, and delayed union or nonunion of the fracture. Attention to detail and frequent follow-up visits are necessary to watch their progress and to recognize problems when they arise. These fractures, particularly if they have been operated upon, heal slowly because of the periosteal stripping required at surgery. The physician must bear in mind that it may take 3 to 4 months before firm consolidation has occurred.

PATHOLOGIC FRACTURES

Pathologic fractures as discussed in this section, are those resulting from primary or secondary (metastatic) malignant tumors in bone. In the elderly population fractures caused by malignant tumors are frequent. Until the last few decades the outlook for these people was bleak, but with improvements in hormone therapy, chemotherapy, radiotherapy, and orthopaedic technology, the situation has improved a great deal. The pathologic fracture, especially of the lower extremities (hip or femur), is now amenable to surgical stabilization, and this results in greatly reduced pain and suffering for the patient. The physician faced with an elderly patient suffering from a pathologic fracture has several questions to consider before recommending a treatment.

The patient's general medical status and the extent of the disease (including pulmonary, cerebral, and cardiac function) will roughly define the life expectancy. A precise number is not required, but it should be determined if the patient will most likely survive for a matter of weeks or months. Depending on the pain and nursing problems resulting from the particular fracture and bearing in mind the fact that the cure of the underlying tumor is not possible, a philosophical decision has to be made as to whether or not to submit the patient to an operation. There are two absolute contraindications to surgery, namely cerebral involvement such that the patient is unaware of his condition or general medical fragility that makes anesthesia impossible. My preference is to operate if the patient would be severely incapacitated (bedridden) for more than 1 month and if the patient can reasonably undergo the procedure. To be confined to the bed in plaster, splints, or traction for longer than that period of time seems unkind especially since many of these fractures will never heal. The goals of surgery would therefore be to decrease pain, to increase function, and to mobilize and discharge the patient as soon as possible to his home or to an alternative care facility. Between 1960 and 1970 the published mean survival of these patients after their first long bone fracture was 7.2 months, but by the end of the next decade this number has risen to 18.8 months. In this group, those suffering from lung cancer had survivals of 3.6 months, while those with metastatic breast disease had a mean survival of 22.6 months.[3,4] This is a highly significant increase that is clearly related to the type of primary tumor and its response to treatment.

There are several modes of treatment that should be considered for a patient with a pathologic fracture and each has its applications:

Hormone therapy
Radiotherapy
Chemotherapy
Stabilization (internal, such as nails or a prosthesis; external, such as a cast or braces)
Block excision
Amputation

In fact, to maximize the result for a given patient, there is often a place for using several together (e.g., internal stabilization and chemotherapy). Radiotherapy, chemotherapy, and surgery all interact. It requires careful control to prevent one from adversely affecting another, but with foresight they can be orchestrated effectively. If surgery is being considered, in addition to life expectancy one should also evaluate the following factors:

Extent of disease (bone scan)
Renal function (creatinine, creatinine clearance)
Serum calcium
Coagulogram (e.g., prothrombin time, platelets)

Methylmethacrylate

The advent of methylmethacrylate in the past decade has revolutionized the care of pathologic fractures. The problem of poor bone stock from large lytic areas can be overcome by removal of the tumor tissue and instant fixation with bone cement. The problem of waiting for the bone to heal or for bone grafts to incorporate in the face of radiation, chemotherapy, and a debilitated patient has been eliminated. The cement fills the cavity and stabilizes the fracture during the operative procedure. When used in conjunction with rods or prostheses, it allows immediate mobilization of the patient since the irregular spaces are eliminated, and a solid unit is created that can withstand the stresses of immediate weight bearing.

Hip

The most frequent pathologic fracture is a hip fracture. These occur at the intracapsular, intertrochanteric, and, most importantly, the subtrochanteric levels. While pins, nail-plate devices, or hip compression screws are excellent in the benign fracture, they are dangerous in the pathologic one. In such cases the bone stock is poor, the fractures heal slowly if at all, and weight bearing would be delayed. For these reasons, I prefer prosthetic replacement, if possible, supplemented by methylmethacrylate for firm fixation.[6,7,9] Before surgery it is important to check, using x-ray films, above and below the fracture; i.e., the acetabulum and distal femur. For the intracapsular and intertrochanteric fractures, I prefer a cemented bicentric (Osteonics) type of prosthesis. If the acetabulum is involved, a total hip replacement may be required, but the hemiarthroplasty does remarkably well if the acetabulum is relatively intact. While the acetabulum may go on to degenerative changes in a patient with a benign fracture, that is rarely a problem with these patients with their reduced demands, weakened condition, and short life expectancy. The morbidity from the hemiarthroplasty is less, and the stability of the prosthesis is excellent.

The benign intertrochanteric fracture can be fixed by a spectrum of internal screws, bolts, or nails, but in pathologic cases such devices often fail because of delayed union, poor fixation in osteoporotic or permeated bone, or impaction of the fragments. Some surgeons treat these fractures by using methylmethacrylate around a nail, but if the patient survives for more than 1 year (as with breast tumors or myeloma), the tumor cavities will expand and the device may undergo delayed failure. For these reasons, I prefer an endoprosthesis and bone cement with or without an acetabular replacement. If the patient survives for a prolonged period and the femoral bone stock deteriorates, the prosthesis may settle into the femoral canal, but this is usually acceptable in light of the patient's general condition.

The subtrochanteric hip fracture is even more difficult, and all the reasons for failure in the benign fracture are only magnified in the cancer patient. There is usually a significant loss of cortical bone stock, and it is very difficult to achieve good bone apposition for support. The bending moment at this level in the femur is high. The integrity of the femur proximal and distal to the fracture may be poor. For these reasons, I use either the Ender nail from below or a prosthetic hip replacement. Many would consider removal of an intact femoral head to insert a prosthesis heresy, but it provides a quick, simple solution to a difficult problem, particularly if the femoral head already has been weakened by metastases. In one bold stroke, the problem of nails cutting out, perforating, or breaking is eliminated. In this case, a long-stem cemented femoral component and then the bicentric head or an acetabular replacement, depending on the extent of pelvic disease, would be used. If, on the other hand, the patient seems frail and the femoral bone stock appears adequate in the head and distally, then Ender nails are a quick, relatively atraumatic solution. They may be judiciously supplemented by methylmethacrylate in a pathologic fracture, thereby allowing early weight bearing. On several occasions, I have inserted Ender nails into both femora at one operation with a dramatic, symptomatic improvement.

Humerus

Another common site of pathologic fractures is the humerus. Here as elsewhere there is a choice of operative versus nonoperative treatment. Since weight bearing is not affected, the patient can be relatively independent in spite of an unhealed fracture. If the fracture involves the humeral head or articular surface, then a prosthetic replacement is usually necessary. In the shaft, however, one may splint the fracture, and if the tumor is radiosensitive, irradiate it, expecting that if the tumor cavity is not excessively large, the fracture will heal. If the tumor has destroyed considerable cortical bone and is not responsive to radiotherapy or chemotherapy (as with lung tumors), then surgery is preferable. In the humerus, as in all bone with metastatic disease, plates are to be avoided in favor of intramedullary devices. Screw fixation is usually suboptimal, the plate prevents impaction, and if the fracture does not heal quickly, the plate will eventually fail. For these reasons, an intramedullary nail supplemented by cement is the treatment of choice. The operation is relatively atraumatic, and the return of arm function is rapid.

Spine

The patient with metastatic spinal disease will develop pain that is progressive. This may be controllable with local irradiation, but it can progress rapidly to severe pain, kyphosis, and spinal cord involvement. Paraparesis or paraplegia is a frequent occurrence along the long downhill road of disseminated malignancy, especially since long bone fractures are now responding better to orthopaedic stabilization. The modalities available for the spine include braces, casts, radiation with or without steroids, decompressive laminectomy, or surgical stabilization. Statistics are difficult to unravel in these circumstances because of the multiple factors lumped together under outcome. As patient survival is prolonged, spinal stabilization with or without decompression is more and more often required.[5]

With the advent of CT scanning a much better picture of the fracture is possible, and a decision can be made about the various contributing factors such as direct tumor involvement, posterior or anterior bone impingement, and the quality of the nearby bone. With this information, the surgeon can decide whether to use a posterior laminectomy, an anterior approach, or both. If the vertebral body has collapsed and the kyphosis or retropulsed material is obstructing the canal, then an anterior approach is required to decompress the spinal canal and reconstruct the vertebral column using bone cement and/or Harrington rods. The composite of bone, cement, and metal makes an instant repair that is capable of weight bearing without the need for "time to incorporate." When bone grafts were the only material available, the anterior approach had a more limited expectation since the incorporation was slow and unpredictable. Now the prognosis for a successful repair is better. The anterior stabilization can be supplemented posteriorly at a second operation if the patient's life expectancy warrants the extra stability. Previously these patients were offered body jackets or casts as the only means of controlling their painful instability. Underlying this newer, aggressive approach, however, is the understanding that metastatic disease is usually far more extensive in the spine then is apparent on the plain x-ray films. It takes extensive bone destruction and replacement in these osteoporotic patients before the metastases become visible. For this reason, the surgeon must check carefully above and below the most obvious lesions before attempting an operative stabilization procedure.

Prophylactic fixation of impending fractures

Finally, there is the question of management of an impending long bone fracture. When there is over 50% destruction of the bone cortex at a level and the patient's pain is localized to the lesion visible on x-ray films and when the pain limits the patient's ability to function, then surgery is indicated. If a lesion has not progressed to this point, radiotherapy is the treatment of choice for a sensitive tumor. Surgically filling all the holes on the x-ray film is unacceptable. When it is known that the lesion will probably fracture with even minimal activities, it seems humane to proceed with surgery. Several surprises may greet the uninitiated at this point, such as the anterior bow of an intact femur. Often, it has the good grace to fracture intraoperatively and thus facilitate intramedullary rodding, but if it does not, the surgeon must beware of putting a long, straight nail in a curved tube. Perforation of the anterior femoral cortex does occur, especially in short women. Rarely the tip of the rod may even remain projecting through the cortex as long as it does not interfere with the function of the quadriceps mechanism. Even though the bone destruction may not appear to be extensive, it is wise to add bone cement for stability and to use a short nail in case the bone shortens later on.

In conclusion, it is apparent that the advances in the treatment of cancer during the past two decades have radically altered both the survival statistics and the means of controlling suffering. Thus the patient who has a subtrochanteric fracture secondary to metastatic breast disease has a chance for survival measured in years not months. Along with medical advances, the orthopaedic armamentarium has improved with the use of methylmethacrylate and joint replacements. As a result of these improvements, pathologic fractures can now be treated more aggressively (operatively), allowing the patients far more comfort and well being.

References

1. Arnold, W.A., Lyden, J.P., and Minkoff, J.: Treatment of intracapsular fractures of the femoral neck with special reference to percutaneous Knowles pinning, J. Bone Joint Surg. **56A:**254-262, 1974.

2. Dimon, J.H., and Hughston, J.C.: Unstable intertrochanteric fractures of the hip, J. Bone Joint Surg. **49A:**440-450, 1967.

3. Douglass, H.O., Shukla, S.K., and Mindell, E.: Treatment of pathological fractures of long bones excluding those due to breast cancer, J. Bone Joint Surg. **58A:**1055-1061, 1967.

4. Harrington, K.D.: The role of surgery in the management of pathologic fractures, Orthop. Clin. North Am. **8:**841-858, 1977.

5. Harrington, K.D. In American Academy of Orthopaedic Surgeons: Instructional course lectures, vol. 4, St. Louis, 1980, The C.V. Mosby Co.

6. Harrington, K.D., et al.: The use of methylmethacrylate as an adjunct in the internal fixation of malignant neoplastic fractures; experience with three hundred and seventy-six cases, J. Bone Joint Surg. **58A:**1047-1055, 1967.

7. Higinbotham, N.L., and Nance, R.C.: The management of pathologic fractures, J. Trauma **5:**792-798, 1965.

8. Key, J.A., and Caldwell, H.E.: Management of fractures, dislocations and sprains, St. Louis, 1951, The C.V. Mosby Co.

9. Lane, J.M., Sculco, T.P., and Zolan, S.: Treatment of pathological fractures of the hip by endoprosthetic replacement, J. Bone Joint Surg. **62A:**954-959, 1980.

10. Neer, C.S. Displaced proximal humeral fractures. I. Classification and evaluation. J. Bone Joint Surg. **52A:**1077-1089, 1970.

11. Neer, C.S.: Displaced proximal humeral fractures. II. Treatment of three part and four part displacement, J. Bone Joint Surg. **52A:**1090-1103, 1970.

12. Neer, C.S., Grantham S.A., and Shelton, M.L.: Supracondylar fracture of the adult femur. A study of one hundred and ten cases. J. Bone Joint Surg. **49A:**591-613, 1967.

chapter 16
MUSCULOSKELETAL INVOLVEMENT IN DIABETES

Richard L. Jacobs

With modern methods of care patients with diabetes survive longer and are more likely to develop some previously uncommon complications. The geriatric patient is particularly at risk because of associated medical and orthopaedic problems concomitant to aging. The peripheral limb manifestations of diabetes are also more troublesome in the geriatric patient who may already have altered vascular and neurologic function.

Such modern developments as pancreas transplants, insulin pumps, synthetic insulin, and immunotherapy may lessen the degree of these complications but they will still exist. Almost any organ system can be involved, but the kidney and eye problems are among the most devastating. More specifically, a diabetic patient with appreciable loss of vision *and* a major amputation will probably be confined to a wheelchair. Further, approximately one third of all diabetics who have a major amputation on one side will have a major amputation on the other side within approximately 3 years.

The most important single factor in the orthopaedic care of the diabetic geriatric patient is education. Sufficient time should be allocated for each new patient to have a frank, leisurely discussion of the physiology of diabetes and diabetic foot problems. The changes in circulation and in innervation, as well as the bony structure of the foot, are discussed in basic nontechnical terms that the patient can readily understand. The patient is taught to check the feet at least once a day and to pay special attention to any areas of redness or to blister, callus, or corn formation. Unexplained warmth or swelling of any part of the foot is important. In fact, any change at all in the foot is important. Such problems should be seen by the physician when first recognized rather than waiting for a few days to "see what happens." Incipient ulcerations can be arrested, early infections can be treated on an outpatient basis with oral antibiotics, alterations in shoes or in activity can be prescribed as needed, or a protective orthosis or cast can be applied to prevent progression of any neuropathic change in the skeleton. The difference of one day in treatment can mean a difference of months in treating a problem. The patient must know this.

A wide range of footwear for diabetic patients is not necessary. The shoe most often used is the extra-depth shoe, which is a laced oxford with a high toe box. There is room for a ¼-inch soft Neoprene rubber insole that helps to protect the plantar surface of the foot from formation of mal perforans ulcers and also gives adequate toe room even when there is marked clawing of the toes. If there is severe enough deformity of the foot, bespoke shoes may be necessary, but this is uncommon.

Despite the best care and good patient cooperation, two major problems complicate the life of the diabetic. These complications are both circulatory and neurologic; the interrelationship can be devastating.

VASCULAR ASPECTS

Diabetic geriatric patients with orthopaedic problems in their lower extremities and any apparent circulatory deficiencies should be evaluated by the vascular surgery service. If pedal pulses are felt, there is usually adequate peripheral flow. In some instances, however, peripheral pulses are palpable only because extensive collateral circulation is present, and a more detailed examination will reveal the problem.

Because microvascular disease is common in the extremities of diabetics, there often is unwarranted pessimism about the value of a peripheral vascular evaluation. The concern has been about major vascular impairments, even though the major peripheral vessels are competent. Karmody and Jacobs[4] have found that if adequate pressure *and* pulsatile flow are present or can be obtained in the extremity, then microvascular disease is not a major determinant in preventing successful healing.

Evaluation

Two simple office procedures help in evaluation of peripheral vascular disease in the geriatric patient. One is *pulse volume recording*, a form of plethysmography. A cuff is inflated to a pressure just above the level of venous pressure and indirectly measures the increase in volume of the distal limb as a function of time. This is recorded on a moving sheet of graph paper. If there is an elastic distal vascular bed, the increase in volume with continued arterial flow leads to an abrupt peak on the tracing. Attempts have been made to integrate the area beneath this peak to measure the actual volume of inflow of blood into the limb during inflation of the cuff, but this has not been accomplished on a reproducible and commercially available basis. Extremities with a poor volume of arterial blood flow and an inelastic distal vascular tree have an entirely different pattern and lack the sharp, abrupt peaks of the more adequately profused limb. Immediately after these recording are taken, *Doppler pressures* (Fig. 16-1) are taken at various levels in the limb and recorded on the same sheet. Wagner[6] has made the useful generalization that when the Doppler pressure at the level of the ankle is at least one half of the Doppler pressure at the axilla, this is a favorable indication of the potential for healing. Still, some individuals have enough sclerosis of the vessels being measured so that the cuff

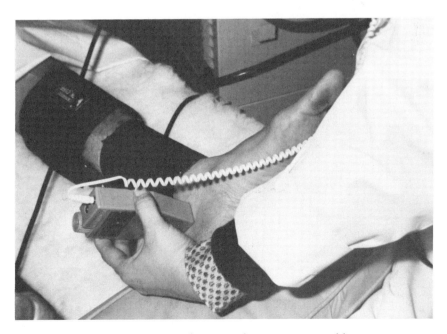

FIG. 16-1. Recording Doppler pressure at ankle.

will not occlude them easily. Doppler pressures much in excess of the axillary pressures may be found (Fig. 16-2). In these cases, the pulsatile peaks are not seen on pulse volume recordings, and the falsely high Doppler pressures are discounted. With greater experience in doing vascular surgery in diabetics, surgeons are more optimistic in recommending surgical treatment. In some instances such treatment can halt the relentless progression of gangrenous changes in a compromised extremity (Fig. 16-3), while in other cases it will enable healing without resorting to major amputations. These two screening tests indicate the degree of the problem.

Arteriograms are usually done only when pulse volume recordings and measurement of Doppler pressures indicate im-

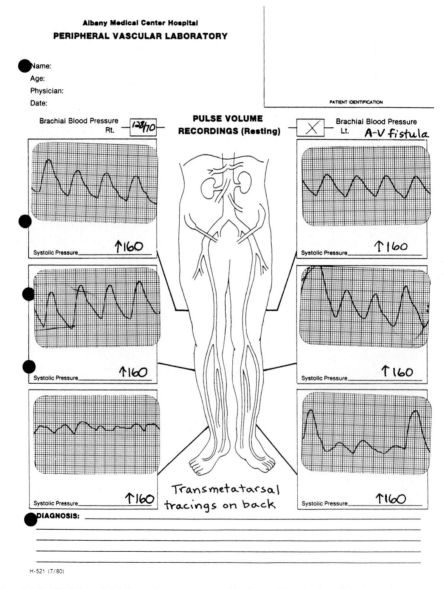

H-521 (7/80)

FIG. 16-2. With brachial Doppler pressure of 128 mm Hg, both ankle Doppler pressures are greater than 160 mm Hg. Pulse volume recordings at ankle are poorly pulsatile, especially on right ankle.

pairment of flow that might be helped by vascular surgery. These radiographic studies delineate the problem and act as a "road map" to determine what, if anything, can be done surgically to augment blood flow. In the past reversed vein bypass grafts were common. More recently in situ venous bypass has become the mode at our hospital. With the indications used for this technique, the number of patients with lesions

amenable to bypass surgery has almost doubled. Synthetic grafts, such as Gortex, or processed bovine grafts are occasionally used. These two materials are used only in situations where adequate vein grafts are not available.

Some common primary vascular problems are seen in geriatric patients. In the "blue toe syndrome" atherosclerotic arterial plaques loosen microemboli showers to

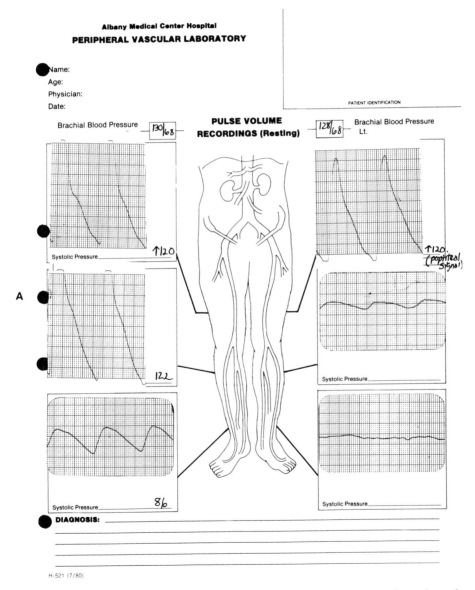

FIG. 16-3. A, No Doppler pressure obtained at ankle preoperatively and flat pulse volume recording on left.   *Continued.*

the affected extremity. The affected embolized toe is blue and cool but not frankly gangrenous. If there are no further emboli, the situation may resolve itself favorably. The vascular surgeon should try to determine if such a condition should be dealt with surgically or with anticoagulants only. Another common situation involves larger emboli that may occlude circulation to a toe or to a much larger area of the foot or leg. Some instances of frank gangrene, such as those involving a single toe, may (infrequently) be left to demarcate and spontaneously separate. The problem involved is one of time. Demarcation and separation may take many months to occur and the patient must be closely watched to be certain that local infection, which can spread more proximally, does not develop. Because of the time involved and because

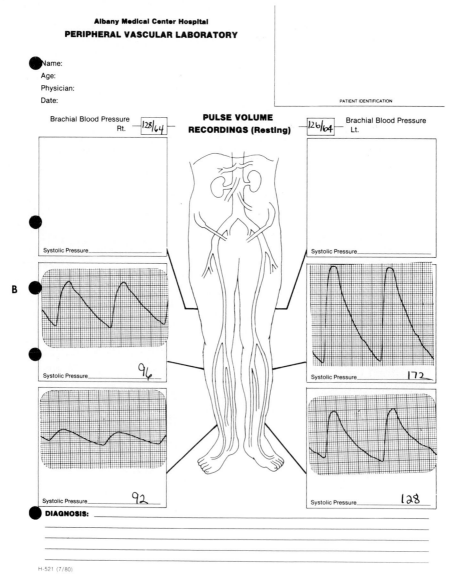

FIG. 16-3, cont'd. B, Same patient after left femoral endarterectomy. Doppler pressure at ankle is 128 mm Hg, and there are new pulsatile waveforms on left.

of the possibility of infection, it is usually better to plan primary amputation of the affected tissue as soon as demarcation is obvious.

DIABETIC NEUROPATHY

This is the second major problem causing orthopaedic complications in diabetics. The etiology of this form of neuropathy has never been clearly defined. It may be on a metabolic basis or it may result from impaired circulation of the peripheral nerves. From whatever cause, the end result is a scattered polyneuropathy. Mild degrees of sensory neuropathy are extremely common in diabetics. This is often described as a "stocking type" of hypesthesia in the lower extremities. Certain peripheral nerves may be much more involved than others; a more anatomic distribution of neuropathy may be apparent on close examination. Loss of proprioception in the toes and pallesthesia (sensation to a tuning fork) are further early manifestations. With partial or complete loss of the protective pain sensation, many common patterns of injury can occur.

Patterns of injury

With an imbalance of weight bearing on the plantar surface of the foot, corns or calluses may occur. Clawing of the toes, probably secondary to loss of intrinsic muscle innervation, is common. As this happens, the weight-bearing function of the toes is lost and more weight is shifted onto the metatarsal heads. With *normal* protective pain sensation, there is sufficient pain so that the problem is attended to either by wearing proper orthotic devices or by debridement of the corns and calluses that form. The diabetic geriatric patient with impaired pain sensation has less premonitory warning pain, and full weight bearing is continued.

The accumulation of keratin may become sufficient to erode through the dermis and cause a plantar ulcer. At first the *epidermis* may be intact, and the patient may not realize anything has happened. Eventually the subepithelial accumulation of se-

rum will simulate the appearance of a blister. When this blister is opened, the underlying ulcer will be found. This ulcer may become infected and purulent drainage is seen from the infected forefoot. This mal perforans ulcer can lead to all sorts of threatening secondary problems. The most common location of mal perforans ulceration is beneath the metatarsal heads. The spread of infection into the forefoot can cause soft tissue necrosis. Inflammation can also cause thrombosis of blood vessels, leading to secondary gangrene of the toes and forefoot. Infection may spread into the leg along the flexor or extensor tendons.

Management

The early mal perforans ulcer without apparent infection can often be treated by protecting the forefoot against further weight bearing until the lesion has an opportunity to heal. The patient can start povidone-iodine dressing changes for the ulcer and use crutches to allow non-weight-bearing on the affected side. Such patients should always be evaluated to make sure that impaired circulation is not a limiting factor in healing. The use of total contact plaster casts has been advocated for treatment of more severe ulcers in the insensitive foot, but I have always been hesitant about this technique and prefer to use an extremely well-padded short leg plaster cast instead. Care must be taken to make sure that the distal edge of the cast does not cut into the dorsum of the foot nor cause pressure areas along the side of the fifth or first toe.

Some clean ulcers that fail to heal because of exposed avascular tendons or the metatarsal head in their depths may be treated by local debridement followed by a split-thickness skin graft at some later time after good granulations have formed.

If such conservative treatment has failed to heal the ulcers, a longitudinal incision is made over the dorsum of the affected metatarsal head and neck, and through this incision the metatarsal head is excised along with any necrotic tissue. The wound is irrigated copiously with a triple antibiotic solution, and a sponge is pulled back and forth through the wound and out through the plantar ulcer to help debride soft tissue in that area. Only the dorsal incision is closed, leaving the plantar ulcerated area open for drainage and to close secondarily by itself (usually within a matter of a few weeks). Systemic antibiotics are continued during healing. Constant vigilance is required thereafter in these patients. They must be fitted with protective insoles that help unload the metatarsal heads and they must inspect their feet daily. When one metatarsal head is excised, more weight must be taken on adjacent metatarsal heads and they are at greater risk than they were before. New mal perforans ulcers may form on one side or the other of an excised metatarsal head.

Some geriatric patients develop large, confluent ulcers on the plantar surface of the forefoot and these spread beneath more than one metatarsal head. Other patients have two or more ulcerations underneath separate metatarsal heads. Some patients who previously had an amputation of a great toe because of gangrene or infection, later develop an ulceration beneath one or more of the residual metatarsal heads. If one of the four remaining metatarsal heads is resected, a much greater load is thrown on the remaining three metatarsal heads and further ulceration beneath these three metatarsal heads is likely. Furthermore, if there are two individual deep ulcerations that require metatarsal head excision, only three metatarsal heads are left and there is a high likelihood of more problems. When two or more metatarsal heads must be excised anyway, problems are avoided by

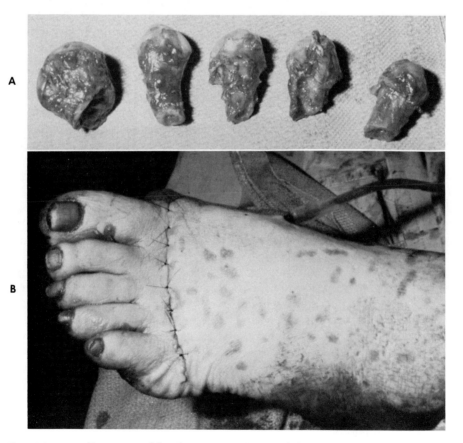

FIG. 16-4. **A,** All metatarsal heads are excised in modified Hoffman procedure. **B,** Hoffman procedure postoperatively, with Jackson-Pratt drain in place.

doing the Clayton modification of the Hoffman procedure,[2] which excises all of the metatarsal heads through a dorsal approach (Fig. 16-4). Vascular consultation is requested. Circulation must be adequate to heal the foot after surgery.

NEUROPATHIC ARTHROPLASTY

Charcot joints or neuropathic arthropathy can also occur secondary to diabetic neuropathy in the elderly. If the problem is not recognized or if the physiology is not understood, this can be a most difficult problem for the physician to treat. The underlying etiology is loss of protective pain sensation. From time to time, any individual with normal mobility will sustain some minor injuries to the bones or joints or supporting structures that will cause at least momentary, transient pain. After such an insult, pain will cause the individual to protect the injured member for a period of time until healing has had a chance to occur and pain diminishes. Protective pain sensation has done its job. If there is peripheral neuropathy, such pain may be diminished or not perceived at all. If the patient is fortunate and does not sustain another injury in a short time, the injury may heal and this often occurs. However, the patient may sustain still another injury before healing is complete and then another injury and there will be a "cascade" effect. Eventually, the sum of these injuries results in damage characteristic of a Charcot joint or of a "spontaneous fracture" of a long bone.

The advanced state of these changes in joints is histologically not different in any way from a severe traumatic arthritis. Once this is understood, treatment becomes less difficult. The whole idea is to recognize such changes early. The characteristic changes are of local swelling and increased local temperature, with or without bony deformity. There may or may not be any associated pain. X-ray films may be negative, and the clinical index of suspicion must be high. Patients should learn self-inspection early before skeletal changes and deformity have occurred. The extremity should be protected to allow the soft tissue and bone to heal, the swelling to be reduced, and the local temperature elevation to subside. Protection may sometimes be accomplished by the use of crutches and, for a short period of time or in more obvious cases, the application of a well-padded short leg cast until the lesion has become quiescent.

These Charcot joints can actually occur anywhere in the body, including the spine and hips. In the diabetic they are most common in the foot and may involve any and all of the joints of the foot. There are characteristic patterns that may involve metatarsophalangeal joints, Lisfranc's joints, Chopart's joints, subtalar joints, and/or ankle joints.[5] Whichever area is involved, the aim of treatment is to immobilize the extremity and to allow healing to occur, just as would be done for a bone or joint injury in a person with normal pain sensation. This is really the key to the whole problem. It is thus wise to take special precautions against further injury. When injuries involve Lisfranc's, Chopart's, or the subtalar joint, the forefoot may deviate laterally, shifting weight bearing to poorly "padded" areas that may subsequently ulcerate. Fixed skeletal deformities of this nature can be almost impossible to deal with, so care must be taken to prevent such changes. A sensible form of protection for such extremities often needs to be no more complicated than a posterior molded polyprophylene splint of the Texas Rehabilitation Institute type (ankle-foot orthosis) along with an appropriate extra-depth shoe.

When there is ulceration and deformity and the only alternative is ablation of the extremity, corrective osteotomies or fusions may be attempted to realign the foot if circulation is adequate. Postoperative immobilization is necessary for prolonged periods of time, *much* in excess of the times necessary in the foot with normal sensation.

An example of this approach and the persistence necessary was seen in a geriatric patient with profound peripheral neuropathy (Fig. 16-5). The patient developed a large mal perforans ulcer beneath the first metatarsal head and an associated plantar abscess. In another hospital, the first metatarsal head and neck were excised. With antibiotic treatment and a local dressing, healing was by secondary intent. No special protection was given after this, and full weight bearing was resumed. Soon, changes of neuropathic arthropathy appeared in the ankle and subtalar joints (the foot was swollen, deformed, and grossly everted). A large ulceration appeared on the medial side of the foot at the level of the malleolus. This communicated with the ankle joint, and

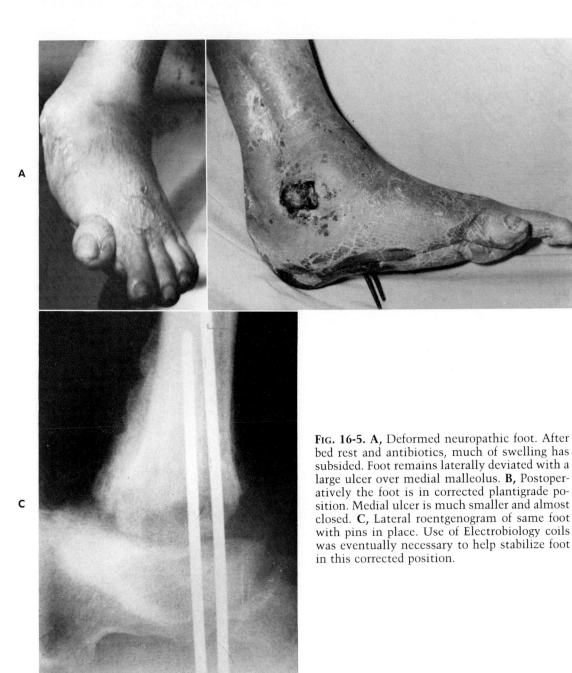

FIG. 16-5. A, Deformed neuropathic foot. After bed rest and antibiotics, much of swelling has subsided. Foot remains laterally deviated with a large ulcer over medial malleolus. B, Postoperatively the foot is in corrected plantigrade position. Medial ulcer is much smaller and almost closed. C, Lateral roentgenogram of same foot with pins in place. Use of Electrobiology coils was eventually necessary to help stabilize foot in this corrected position.

was infected and draining. The patient was referred to our hospital; bed rest and local debridement were started, along with appropriate intravenous antibiotics. The infection was rapidly controlled. Much of the swelling was obviously injury-and-repair reaction. When the ulcer began to granulate, an ankle fusion was attempted through an anterior approach to put the foot in a corrected, plantigrade position Loose cartilagenous and bony debris was removed from the ankle joint and enough of the talus was excised to put the foot in a neutral position. Two heavy threaded pins were driven up through the hindfoot into the distal tibia to hold the foot in this corrected position during healing. A posterior splint was applied with the medial ulcer exposed for dressing changes. With this further immobilization, the ulcer completely granulated and was successfully skin grafted to give a closed wound within several weeks after the original operation. A non-weight-bearing short leg cast was then applied. The pins were finally removed several months after surgery. There was still a great deal of motion in the ankle, and immobilization was continued for several more months. To gain more stability, Electro-biology external coils were applied. There was still a jog of motion at the ankle joint 3 months later, but the mobility had greatly decreased. The patient was fitted with a well-molded ankle-foot orthosis and an extra-depth shoe rather than continuing plaster immobilization and electrical stimulation. After wearing this orthosis for several years with no further sign of ulceration or increased instability of the foot or ankle, the patient feels that the prolonged treatment time was entirely preferable to having an amputation and an artificial limb. He also has both limbs. It is important to remember that what happened on one side can happen on the other.

The lessons illustrated in this case are typical for any neuropathic joint. When fusion operations are attempted, the failure rate is high. Still, the surgery can be counted as a success if the extremity is in a corrected position, it can be stabilized in this position by acceptable orthotic devices, and function is maintained.

Infection

Appearances can be deceptive in diagnosis of infection in patients with neuropathic problems of the extremities. For example, an elderly patient developed a mal perforans ulcer on the forefoot, a temperature elevated to 101° rectally and general feelings of malaise. The entire foot was red, swollen, and warm. There was marked swelling around the lateral malleolus. When the patient was admitted to the hospital, cellulitis of the forefoot was diagnosed, and it was also thought that there was abscess formation along the course of the peroneus longus tendon into the lower leg. There were advanced neuropathic changes of the bones of the ankle and hindfoot. Bed rest was prescribed and then the ulcer was locally debrided and massive doses of parenteral antibiotics were given. The temperature elevation and much of the forefoot erythema rapidly subsided. The swelling of the lateral side of the foot at the level of the malleolus did not go down nearly so quickly. For this reason, a small incision was made under sterile conditions into the fluctuant area. Thick, viscous synovial fluid was obtained. Passage of a probe through the incision showed that the area communicated with the ankle joint. It became quite obvious that there was intense synovitis of the ankle secondary to a Charcot ankle. What originally appeared to be a plantar abscess with extension along the peroneal tendons was mainly traumatic synovitis. With 2 weeks of bed rest and parenteral antibiotics, the foot was substantially improved. Findings that might seemingly indicate amputation were found to be incorrect. This patient was often not cooperative in his own care at home but, in general, if this type of extremity is protected afterward with an ankle-foot orthosis with extra-depth shoes, the foot and leg can be maintained successfully. This implies periodic examination and continuing medical care as well as daily self-inspection of the foot by the patient.

Both these cases emphasize that injury and repair reactions in a neuropathic foot cause swelling, erythema, and a local increase in temperature that can be indistinguishable from massive infection. The destructive roentgenographic changes are often misdiagnosed as being primary osteomyelitis. Experience in treatment will lead to earlier, more precise diagnoses. In the meantime, it is best to err in favor of the diagnosis of Charcot joint changes. Conservative treatment can then continue as long as *favorable progression* is seen and systemic findings indicate control of infection.

Ulceration

Ulceration on the plantar or medial aspect of the great toe can occur in patients with insensitive feet. This is probably a function of rotatory force beneath the great toe as the leg rotates internally and the forefoot goes into relative supination during the push-off of the gait. When ulceration first occurs in this area, it can often be treated successfully by measures to unload the great toe. These can include such measures as arch supports with metatarsal pads and steel shank shoes of sufficient width. Occasionally, a split-thickness skin graft may be needed on the ulcer.

If a persistent ulceration does not respond to simple conservative measures, a modification of the Keller bunionectomy may be needed. No tourniquet is used. A longitudinal, dorsal incision is made just medial to the extensor tendon of the great toe.[1] The incision goes directly down to the bone. With a sharp dissection the base of the proximal phalanx is exposed and delivered from the wound. The proximal half of the proximal phalanx is then excised. The wound is thoroughly irrigated with triple antibiotic solution and the skin is closed with nylon sutures. A soft dressing holds the great toe in a corrected position. Correcting flaps from the abductor tendon are not developed and no further soft-tissue dissection is done. This avoids problems with soft tissue slough. With the great toe thus shortened, the area of the ulcer appreciably decreases right on the operating table as ten-

sion is released. If the ulcer is large, a split-thickness skin graft is applied. This operation decreases the weight-bearing function of the great toe and helps heal the ulcer.

Medial ulcerations can also occur more proximally, directly over the first metatarsal head. This can be treated by simply resecting the first metatarsal head and part of the shaft, letting this cavity granulate, and later applying split-thickness skin grafts (Fig. 16-6). This is cosmetic and leaves the great toe. An equally acceptable alternative is to resect the first ray, using some of the skin from the great toe as a flap to help cover the defect. The patient should help decide which procedure is to be attempted.

Ulceration in the diabetic foot over the heel cord and the os calcis posteriorly is common.[3] Some ulcers obviously occur as a result of excessive pressure in bedridden patients, but more commonly they occur spontaneously in patients with severe peripheral vascular disease. Normal blood supply to this area is not abundant, and when peripheral circulation is impaired, blood supply here can be very poor. Local debridement of such ulcerated areas is done to clean the tissue. After the initial use of a povidone-iodine dressing to control infection, wet-to-dry saline dressings are used until granulations appear. Split-thickness skin grafts are then applied for closure. None of these efforts will accomplish much in the face of inadequate circulation, and vascular bypass surgery is often needed to obtain healing. If the ulcerated area can be closed and the extremity can be salvaged, it is time well spent. There are major problems in protecting the heels, once closed. Some extremities have been successfully fitted with polyethylene-foam-lined boots with a rigid ankle and others with double-upright braces with a cutout heel. There is no one answer for fitting problems, so the services of a skilled orthotist are invaluable.

Elderly diabetics with peripheral vascular disease may have loss of blood supply and gangrene of the skin in rather large areas of the lower extremities even though the underlying bone and muscles may be intact and there may be no problems with infection. Use of skin flaps to obtain coverage for such areas is contraindicated because of possible further skin loss if the flap dies. Instead, the eschar is locally debrided. If there is clean, bleeding soft tissue underlying the eschar, a split-thickness skin graft is applied immediately. If not, wet-to-dry saline dressings can be applied four times a day until a granulating bed appears that is adequate to support a split-thickness skin graft. A Brown dermatome, set for a 0.0010-inch thickness, is used. The graft is tailored to fit the defect and multiple perforations are made to allow exudate to escape. A large graft may be stapled or sewn into place, but the routine, smaller graft can simply be laid in place and covered with one thickness of Xeroform gauze followed by fluff dressings and then held in place by a roller gauze dressing. This dressing is carefully removed in 3 days and any exudate beneath the graft is expressed by rolling over the graft with sterile cotton swabs. The dressing is then reapplied and left in place for about another 3 or 4 days to ensure maximum take of the graft (Fig. 16-7).

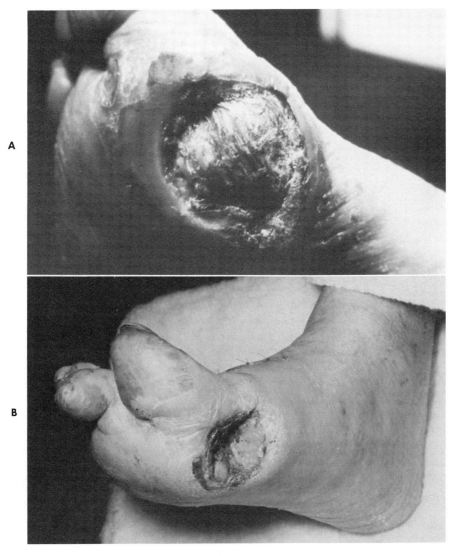

FIG. 16-6. **A,** Large ulcer over first metatarsal head. Underlying bone is dry and devitalized. **B,** After debridement of first metatarsal head and placement of local split-thickness skin graft. A few marginal crusts have yet to separate; foot is healed.

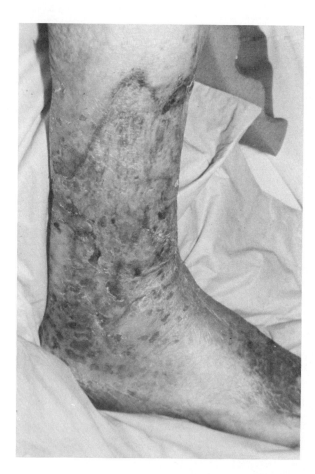

FIG. 16-7. Almost circumferential skin loss. Split-thickness skin grafts saved leg.

Amputation

Major efforts are made to salvage the entire extremity when vascular-neuropathic problems arise in the geriatric diabetic, but sometimes an amputation becomes the most desirable route. Many considerations arise. These may include such factors as the life expectancy, the status of the *other* limb, and the probability of satisfactory function of the affected member if it *is* saved. When amputation becomes necessary, the aim is to preserve the maximum amount of tissue and to ensure best function of the foot. No tourniquet is used since it is helpful to see that there is adequate bleeding from the tissue flaps formed during amputation. Also, the circulation could be further compromised by inflating a tourniquet for any appreciable period of time. A circumferential incision is made just proximal to the dead or inflammed tissue. No inflamed skin is left in the flaps because of the high likelihood that this skin might later thrombose, necrose, and leave a dead flap. The incision is made down to the bone, and soft tissue is reflected from the bone proximally just far enough to allow soft tissue closure as the section through the bone is completed.

In some cases immediate split-thickness skin grafts are applied to allow closure without the necessity for more proximal amputation. An example might be of a gangrenous middle toe where tissue death extends onto the skin of the dorsum of the foot (Fig. 16-8). Metatarsophalangeal disarticulation along with excision of the eschar on the dorsum of the foot and split-thickness skin grafting to the dorsum of the foot may be all that is needed. If there is extensive gangrene of all five toes but circulation seems reasonably good and no problem with healing is anticipated, a circumferential incision is done at the base of the toes to reflect enough soft tissue from the metatarsal necks to allow a relaxed soft tissue closure after the transmetatarsal bone section. In other instances, where there is viable skin at the very base of the toes, I amputate each toe individually through the proximal phalanx and make closure individually (Fig. 16-9). This lessens the magnitude of healing that has to occur and also leaves the weight-bearing metatarsal heads. When all toes are amputated, the patient is usually fitted with a molded insole with a filler for the toes to prevent pumping of the foot inside of the shoe and the possible development of blisters or ulcerations on the heel or residual forefoot.

When more proximal amputation is necessary, a Lisfranc amputation is often done (Fig. 16-10). Because there is some loss of balance in the foot and a tendency toward equinus, a percutaneous section of the heel cord is done at the same time. The heel cord will reconstitute, with some lengthening. Forefoot ulceration may occur if this precaution is not taken and the foot goes into equinus.

If gangrene is proximal enough so that this level cannot be obtained, a Chopart level amputation (Fig. 16-11) can be done, also with heel cord lengthening. With this amputation I employ a specially fabricated polypropylene prosthesis designed and fabricated by Richard LaTorre of Schnectady, New York. This two-part prosthesis encases the limb, and the leg can then be fitted with a regular laced oxford shoe. When this prosthesis is used, many of the objections to a Chopart amputation are overcome. Pumping motion of the stump in the prosthesis is eliminated. Shear forces are minimized and a regular shoe can be worn. The flexible forefoot simulates a normal push-off gait. The full length of the extremity is maintained. The patient can go to and from the bathroom at night without putting on the prosthesis. The prosthesis is the key to a successful amputation at this level.

If there is extremely poor circulation at the level of the ankle, Pirigoff's amputaion (Fig. 16-12), which is disarticulation through the ankle joint with part of the tuber of the os calcis preserved, can be done. The tuber is placed against the denuded plafond of the tibia after cartilage and subchondral bone have been removed. The tuber is held in place with a heavy threaded pin until soft tissue stabilization has occurred, usually on the order of a 1½ to 2 months. Bone healind need not occur across the tuber into the tibia before ambulation is started and a prosthesis is fitted. This amputation avoids the flap necrosis that can sometimes occur as the tuber is dissected off the heel pad in a Syme level amputation, and it does give a little more length to the stump. Function is the same as with the Syme amputation and a below-knee amputation is often avoided. If at the ankle there is Doppler pressure that is at least one half of the brachial Doppler pressure, a routine Syme amputation can be done with less fear of flap necrosis. The Pirigoff amputation is worth trying, even in the presence of very low Doppler pressure at the ankle.

If the heel pad is gangrenous, a modified Syme amputation can be done and length preserved. All available soft tissue is saved as the ankle disarticulation is done. This soft tissue may come from the dorsum or the sides of the foot. After the malleoli are removed, these flaps are brought down around the stump to obtain the best closure possible. After the soft tissue shrinks, the padding for the stump is inferior to that of the classical Syme amputation. A great deal of attention is necessary to obtain a satisfactory prosthetic fitting. The functional result offers no major advantage over a below-knee amputation.

A multitude of possibilities have been discussed for the range of foot problems that may be encountered in treating geriatric diabetic patients. This approach assumes the will to try for the maximum salvage compatible with function and it assumes the will to persist in the effort. To paraphrase an adage, "Success is nothing but a great aptitude for patience."

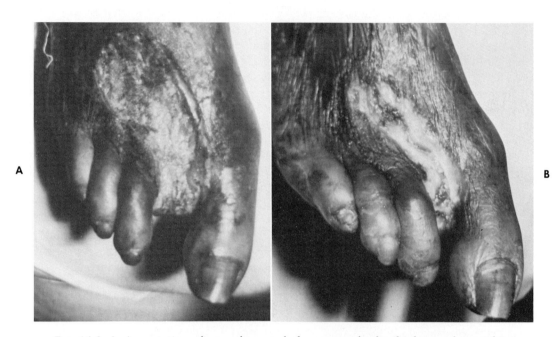

Fig. 16-8. A, Amputation of second toe and placement of split-thickness skin graft on nearly avascular bed after eschar was debrided. B, Grafts failed but did act as a biologic dressing. Wound contracted and healed. This patient now has gangrene of her *other* foot, requiring a below-knee amputation. Time was well spent on treatment of this foot.

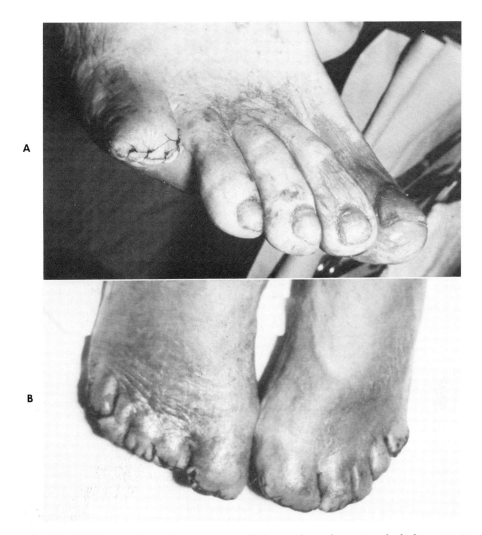

FIG. 16-9. A, Amputation of gangreneous fifth toe through proximal phalanx. **B,** Amputation of all toes on both feet through proximal phalanges. All toes healed without incident.

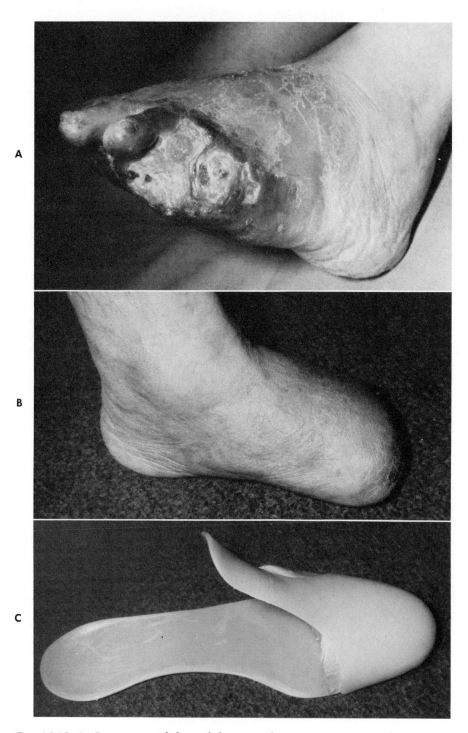

FIG. 16-10. **A,** Gangrene with loss of three toes by autoamputation. There are chronic drainage and failure to heal 6 months after onset. **B,** Same foot, revised to Lisfranc amputation. **C,** Prosthesis for this Lisfranc amputation.

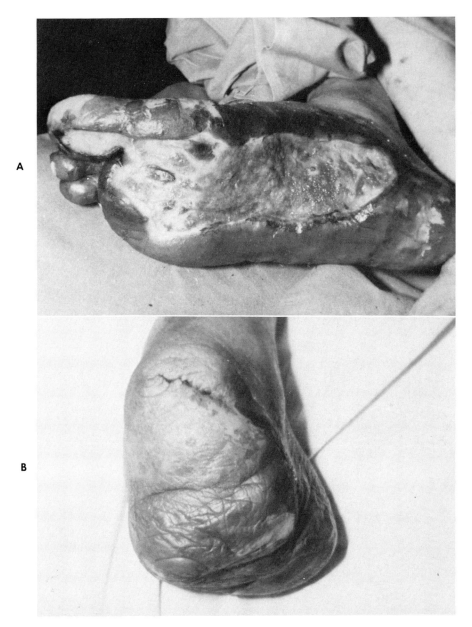

FIG. 16-11. A, Patient developed large plantar abscess and lost almost all soft tissue on plantar surface of foot. Tarsal joints exposed and infected. **B,** Chopart amputation was done, using medial skin flap for closure. Heel cord was percutaneously lengthened.

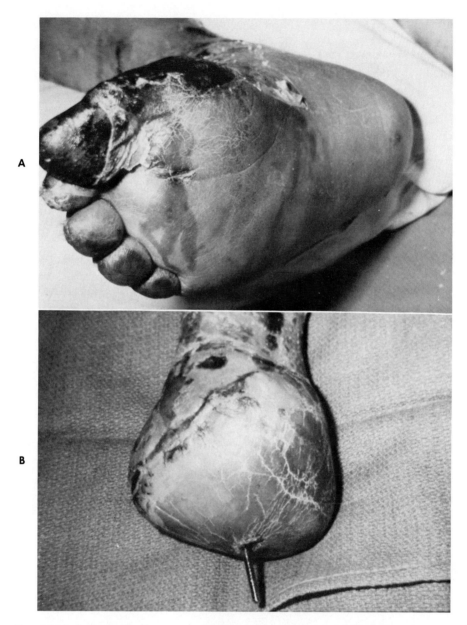

FIG. 16-12. A, Entire forefoot was cold, blue, and gangrenous. No Doppler pressure could be obtained at ankle and pulse-volume recordings were flat. **B,** Pirigoff's amputation was done and a threaded pin used to keep os calcis centered during healing. Pin removed at about 6 weeks. **C,** With pin removed, fibrous tissue gives sufficient stability. Bone healing between os calcis and tibia has *not* occurred. Several months may pass until there is sufficient stability. Posterior plaster splint is kept in place until then. **D,** Pirigoff's amputation prosthesis (fabricated by Richard La Torre). **E,** Pirigoff's amputation prosthesis in place.

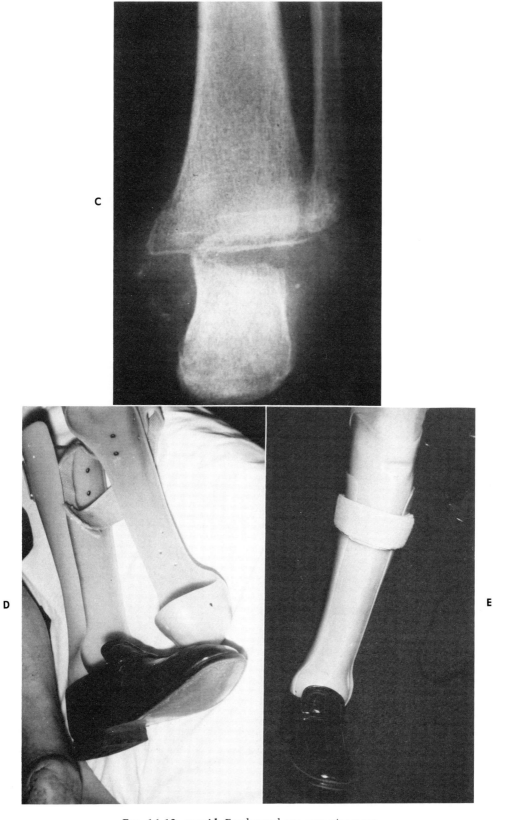

FIG. 16-12, cont'd. For legend see opposite page.

References

1. Downs, D., and Jacobs, R.L.: Treatment of resistant ulcers on the plantar surface of the great toe in diabetics, J. Bone Joint Surg. **64A**:930-933, 1982.
2. Jacobs, R.L.: Hoffman procedure in the diabetic foot, Foot Ankle **3**:142-149, 1982.
3. Jacobs, R.L., and Karmody, A.: Salvage of the diabetic foot with exposed os calcis, Foot Ankle **1**:173-178, 1980.
4. Karmody, A., and Jacobs, R.L.: Salvage of the diabetic foot through vascular reconstruction, Orthop. Clin. North Am. **7**:957-979, 1976.
5. Milgram, J.E.: In Ghormley, R.K., editor: The arthropathies in orthopaedic surgery, New York, 1938, Thomas Nelson and Sons.
6. Wagner, F.W.: The use of transcutaneous Doppler ultrasound in prediction of healing potential and selection of surgical level in dysvascular lower limbs, West. J. Med. **130**:59, 1979.

chapter 17
AMPUTATION SURGERY IN THE AGED

Walther H.O. Bohne

Increasing age brings problems in increasing numbers and severity to the individual in good health. Serious illnesses increase the magnitude of these problems for the aged. Any change in the level of function that interferes with the independence of the aging person can prove devastating and ultimately fatal to the individual. The most obvious is the change in the functional abilities of the individual when an amputation has to be carried out. Unfortunately, the overwhelming majority of amputations in the lower extremities have to be done for the consequences of acute and chronic vascular disease in the geriatric population.[8]

Recently the number of geriatric amputees has been increased as a result of patients with uncontrollable infections of total joint arthroplasties. Not only do these patients belong in the older age group, but also they require amputations at the least favorable levels: at the mid and proximal thigh and disarticulations at the hip.

Therefore, the physician is confronted with two tasks: first and foremost, to eradicate the disease process and, second, to restore function. The amputation sometimes is a life-saving procedure that requires quick decisions as to the timing of the operation, the type of preoperative preparation possible and necessary, and the level and type of amputation. More often, the amputation is an elective procedure that is the final step in a series of procedures aimed at saving the limb. Whether the amputation is done as an emergency procedure or as an elective operation, it should always be viewed as a step in the overall treatment of the patient, which leads to the achievement of second aim of the physician: the restoration of function and, with it, independence for the amputee. Ideally, this process of rehabilitation should start before the actual operation.[18] The rehabilitation of the patient in the most comprehensive sense is best taken on by a team. This team should include the surgeon, a social worker who is willing and able to take on the long-term care of the amputee, a physical therapist who is knowledgeable about the gait training of amputees as well as conditioning training of the aged, and the prosthetist. The leader of the team, however, should remain conversant with the problems of each individual team member, including the amputee, and must deal with them.[22]

PREOPERATIVE CONSIDERATIONS

Clinically, the decision to amputate is rarely difficult. Signs of increasing systemic toxicity and decreasing renal function (in the acute arterial occlusion hemoglobinuria) can require an amputation as a life-saving procedure. In the less acute situation, increased resting pain, dry and especially wet gangrene, and progressive decubitous ulcers lead to the decision to amputate.[21]

It is far more difficult to involve the patient and the family in the decision making

309

and to gain their confidence and cooperation. All too often, the patient is unable to comprehend the seriousness of the situation, either because of senility or emotional reasons. Even when the patient clearly recognizes that the limb is hopelessly diseased, it is a serious step to give up the integrity of the body to which the patient has been accustomed for his entire life. The patient may feel that he is too old to survive the loss of independence and the necessary rehabilitation. Careful and repeated explanations of the social services available and the mechanism of rehabilitation will allay many of the fears of the patient. The family of the senile patient may view the amputation as an unnecessary torment for their relative who is so obviously ailing, and any improvement in his condition may be seen as a prolongation of a life that has become a burden to the suffering relative as well as to the entire family. Despite these objections, amputation, even in the bedridden patient, often has to be considered as a means to decrease the suffering of the patient and as a help in the nursing care.

Level of amputation

Another difficult choice in the decision-making process is determining the level of amputation. Generally, the lower the amputation (i.e., the more joints that can be saved), the more likely it is for the patient to become a prosthesis user through the rehabilitation process. End-bearing stumps are particularly desirable in the geriatric amputee.[2,10,24]

The level of amputation in the patient with a malignant tumor is clearly dictated by the need to eradicate the diseased part. This holds true also in the patient in whom overwhelming infection is the cause for amputation. In the patient with vascular insufficiency, however, the level of amputation is not as clearly defined. Indeed, the extent of the gangrene may only indicate the level to which tissue death has occurred. It does not give an indication for the viability of tissues under the stress of the activities of daily living. Thus, attempts have been made to predict the level at which the amputation wound will heal by

primary intention and where the amputation stump will withstand the rigors of prosthetic wear. Transmetatarsal amputations, Syme amputations, and knee disarticulations should be given serious consideration and should be chosen over the next higher level. Viable and well-vascularized skin remains the most important tissue for the coverage of the amputation stump. Attempts to predict the lowest possible level for the successful amputation are directed toward the evaluation of the skin circulation.

Method of level prediction. Even when the peripheral pulse in the extremity can no longer be palpated, it may be possible to detect it by the use of a Doppler ultrasound flow detector. The pulse pressure can be determined with the use of a slowly deflating pneumatic tourniquet. A systolic pressure of approximately 70 mm Hg seems to be quite adequate for primary healing in the lower extremity.

Radioactive isotopes and in particular xenon 133 have been introduced into the skin to measure the rate of clearing. A flow rate of 2.6 ml/min/100 g of tissue was the minimal acceptable value for primary healing of the amputation wound.[20]

Preparation of the patient for surgery

In the preoperative period the patient should undergo an evaluation by an internist to evaluate the patient's general physical condition, and the appropriate tests for this purpose should be obtained. It is advisable to obtain a second opinion before amputation, not so much because of the difficulty of diagnosis but to substantiate the necessity of the amputation to the patient and family. Internal medical evaluation and a second opinion may become an unnecessary luxury where the patient's rapidly deteriorating general condition requires immediate action to save his life.

The mental preparation of the patient and, where necessary, the family ideally includes an explanation of the procedure and its dangers and complications as well as an explanation of the procedures in the immediate postoperative period. The traction in the case of an open amputation, the rea sons for and advantages of the immediate postoperative rigid dressing, upper extremity strengthening, and unipedal and ultimately bipedal ambulation must be mentioned. Ideally the patient should visit the prosthetist and certainly should have an extensive interview with the social worker.[25] If possible, the patient should speak to a successfully rehabilitated amputee.

AMPUTATIONS
Open amputations

Open amputation in the aging patient is indicated when infection beyond the level of amputation is suspected. Another reason for open amputation is advanced toxicity in an older patient with an ischemic limb. The rationale for this kind of amputation is to ablate the diseased part of the limb, leaving the amputation wound to heal by secondary intention or after secondary closure.

Circular open amputation or guillotine amputation. A circular skin incision is made approximately 1 to 2 cm distal from the intended amputation of the bone. The skin is retracted and the underlying soft tissue is transected down to the bone. Vessels are either clamped and tied as they are encountered or, if amputation is done under tourniquet control, tied after the bone has been transected and the amputation is completed. At this point the nerves are also sought out, dissected free, and cut above the level of amputation.

The dressing consists of nonadherent gauze placed closest to the wound surface with fluffed gauze over it. A stockinette is rolled over the stump and held in place with skin adherent. The open distal end of the stockinette that covers the wound dressing is closed with a cord, which in turn is used for skin traction of 1 to 1.5 kg.

Wound secretions collect under the dependent part of the stump in the postoperative period. To avoid maceration of the skin and skin breakdown, as well as loosening of the stockinette, abdominal pads or chux should be placed under the stump and changed frequently to absorb these secretions. Redressing of the wound should be done for the first time after 2 or 3 days.

Epithelialization of the amputation wound can be hastened by application of a meshed skin graft at the stump after it has been covered with granulations. After the skin is well healed, revision of the amputation can be carried out.

Open flap amputations

The technique of this type of amputation is somewhat similar to the circular amputation except that skin flaps of sufficient length are fashioned to provide wound coverage at the time of secondary closure. It is helpful to place half a dozen No. 1 sutures in the opposing parts of the skin flaps, but not to tie them. The dressing of the wound with nonadherent gauze and fluffed gauze as well as a stockinette for traction purposes is the same as in the circular open amputation.

After the wound has become covered with healthy granulations and there is no sign of infection, the previously fashioned skin flaps can be laid over the wound and the previously inserted sutures can be tied to keep the skin flaps in place. This procedure may eliminate the need for a second anesthesia for a secondary closure.

Toe amputations[2]

The amputation wound in toe amputations must be covered with a plantar skin flap. After removal of the normal tendon insertions, there is a tendency for the remaining parts of the toe to develop extension contractures, which may have to be treated with tenotomies. In vascular insufficiency, pressure necroses appear rapidly once the patient starts to wear closed shoes. Disarticulation in or amputation close to the metatarsophalangeal joint is, therefore, desirable in patients with vascular insufficiency. An exception is the first toe with its well-balanced proximal phalanx, which allows disarticulation in the interphalangeal joint.

Technique. The interphalangeal joint is opened through a dorsal incision and a plantar flap of sufficient length is outlined. The bone is dissected out of the plantar flap. The flexor tendon is pulled into the wound and transected; the digital nerves are cut above the level of amputation, and digital veins and arteries are ligated separately. If disarticulation is desired, the joint cartilage can be left in place as a barrier against infection. When diaphyseal amputation is required, the bone is exposed subperiosteally. Transection should be carried out with a microsaw since bone cutters lead to splintering of the bone. A drain is placed into the amputation wound and the plantar skin flap is attached to the dorsal skin by a few skin sutures. The drain should be removed within 24 to 48 hours.

Transmetatarsal amputation

Where a transmetatarsal amputation is possible in a well-vascularized and sensate foot, an excellent weight-bearing surface can be obtained. Coverage of the amputation site by plantar skin is required.

Technique. On the dorsum of the foot, the skin is at the level of the transection of the bones. The incision is carried through the tendons down to the bone. The blood vessels are ligated as they are encountered, and the transected nerves are trimmed back beyond the incision site. The metatarsal bones are transected with either a Gigli saw or an oscillating saw so they are of equal lengths. The edges of the cut surfaces are bevelled well. The distal ends of the metatarsals are avulsed out of the wound and the plantar flap is fashioned at or beyond the metatarsal heads. The common digital nerves and arteries are identified, the vessels are ligated, and the nerves are trimmed back as far as possible. The flexor tendons are resected after having been pulled into the wound, and the plantar skin flap is brought over the distal ends of the metatarsals. Drains are inserted into the wound and the skin is closed in layers.

Metatarsal ray resections[4,5,23]

In patients with plantar ulcerations and localized osteomyelitis large parts of the foot can sometimes be preserved by metatarsal ray resections. Following healing, the

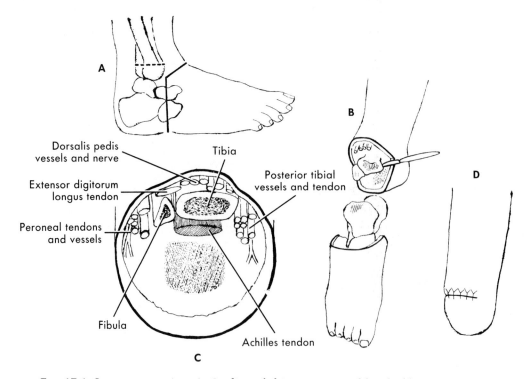

Dorsalis pedis vessels and nerve

Extensor digitorum longus tendon

Peroneal tendons and vessels

Tibia

Posterior tibial vessels and tendon

Fibula

Achilles tendon

FIG. 17-1. Syme amputation. **A,** Outline of skin incision and level of bone transection. **B,** Talus has been removed from ankle mortise and the calcaneus subperiosteally dissected from heel pad. **C,** Operative site prior to closure. **D,** Heel pad has been drawn over end of the stump.

patient will require a molded foot orthosis. Altered weight-bearing characteristics make amputation of the first or the first two rays unsuccessful because this leads to renewed breakdown over the remaining metatarsals.

Syme amputations

With the preservation of the skin pad covering the heel, proprioceptive feedback on weight-bearing is greatly improved. The surface of the tibia and fibula after the malleoli have been removed is large enough to allow end bearing.

In the one-stage Syme amputation (Fig. 17-1), the anterior part of the ankle joint is approached through an incision across the ankle joint, reaching from the tip of the medial malleolus to the area of the lateral malleolus. The ends of the anterior incision are then connected with an incision through the coronal plane of the plantar aspect of the foot. The extensor tendons of the foot are approached through the anterior incision, and the flexor digitorum longus and the anterior tibial tendon are tagged. The other extensor tendons are cut short. The dorsalis pedis artery is ligated, and the superficial branch of the peroneal nerve is dissected free and cut well above the level of the amputation. The ankle joint is then entered from anteriorly. The lateral collateral ligaments of the ankle and the deltoid ligament on the medial side are incised from the inside of the joint outwardly. Care has to be taken not to injure the posterior tibial artery since it provides the circulation for the heel pad. By a sharp plantar flexion of the foot, the posterior part of the ankle capsule can be opened; the tuber calcanei comes into view, and is stripped from all surrounding soft tissues subperiosteally. The Achilles tendon has to be separated from the tuber calcanei. All damage to the soft tissue at the sole of the heel is to be avoided. After talus and calcaneus have been shelled out of the pad, the amputated part of the foot is removed. The medial and lateral malleolus are sawed off, together with the subchondral bone at the distal end of the tibia, with a reciprocating saw. The cut is perpendicular to the line of weight bearing. The posterior tibial nerve, sural nerve, and saphenous nerve are transected well away from the amputation incision; the posterior tibial artery is ligated as are the veins on the dorsum of the stump. If a tourniquet has been used, it has to be released at this point to obtain meticulous hemostasis. A drain is introduced into the amputation wound, the anterior tibial and extensor digitorum longus tendons are sutured into the sole pad, and the skin is sutured with interrupted nonabsorbable sutures. A postoperative rigid dressing concludes the procedure.

Wagner[27] found that a two-stage Syme amputation has a better chance of success in diabetic patients. In this procedure the malleoli and the articular surface are left intact; the skin incision by necessity has to be slightly more distal. The second stage of the procedure is performed 6 weeks later after secure skin healing has been obtained. In the second procedure the malleoli are removed through two incisions on the medial and lateral sides of the amputation. At the same time, the flair of the tibia and fibula can be removed. Ambulation in a rigid postoperative dressing with a heel rocker can be resumed as soon as the patient is reasonably comfortable.

Below-knee amputations

Below-knee amputations are done most frequently of all the lower extremity amputations. In comparison with above-knee amputations, there is a saving in energy expenditure by the active use of the anatomical knee joint and the considerably smaller weight of the prosthesis. The procedure itself most often utilizes a long posterior flap.

Technique (Fig. 17-2). With the patient in a supine position, the diseased lower extremity is prepared and draped. A pneumatic tourniquet should be in place to be inflated when necessary. The level of transection of the bone should be determined by the greatest bulge of the calf musculature, that is, 12 to 16 cm below the tibial plateau. This area is marked anteriorly on the skin and a line is drawn from here posteriorly to the midmedial line. This outlines the anterior soft tissue flap. The posterior flap is considerably longer, reaching to the musculotendinous junction of the triceps surae. The anterior flap is incised down to bone. The fibula is exposed and transected 2 cm above the intended level of the transection of the tibia. The tibia is then transected and the anterior crest of the tibia is exposed in such a fashion that a 45-degree wedge can be cut to bevel the anterior part of the end of the tibial stump. After incision of the skin of the posterior flap, the posterior compartment muscles are then transected in such a way that they are beveled distally. Alternately, the bevel can be avoided and the soleus excised after the diseased part of the leg has been ablated. The anterior and posterior neurovascular bundles are then exposed and ligated and the nerves cut back well above the level of amputation. The sural nerve and saphenous nerve are excised in a similar fashion. If there is necrosis of the anterior compartment muscles, these can be excised without jeopardizing primary healing as long as there is adequate bleeding from the skin. Bleeding points have to be cauterized after the tourniquet has been deflated.

The wound is irrigated and the fascial layers are approximated with interrupted sutures after a suction drain has been introduced into the wound. The skin edges are approximated with absorbable subcutaneous sutures, and the skin itself is closed with interrupted, nonabsorbable sutures or Steri-Strips. A rigid dressing is applied.

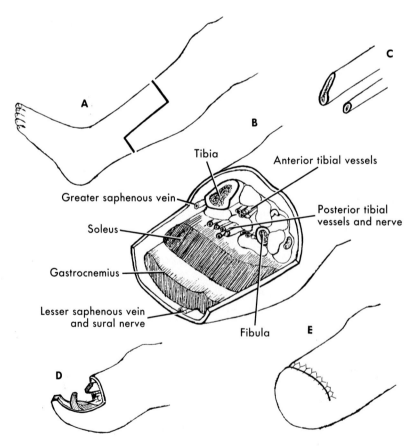

FIG. 17-2. Below-knee amputation. **A,** Outline of skin incision. **B,** Operative site following ablation of lower part of leg. **C,** Beveling of anterior part of tibia. **D,** Posterior soft tissue flap is approximated to anterior one. **E,** Skin closure.

Knee disarticulations

In those cases where below-knee amputation is impractical because of an insurmountable flexion contracture of the knee or an infection extending into the area of the below-knee amputation, an attempt at knee disarticulation should be made. Knee disarticulation provides a broad surface at the end of the stump, which is adequate for weight bearing. At the same time, this broad surface renders the stump end bulbous so that the patient may require special considerations in socket fitting.

A consideration in knee disarticulation is the fact that the long anterior flap for coverage of the stump end frequently becomes necrotic in patients with vascular insufficiency. It is, therefore, desirable to use either a long posterior flap or medial and lateral flaps of equal length (Fig. 17-3). The patellar tendon is sutured to the cruciate ligaments as are the tendons of the hamstring muscles. The patella is retained.

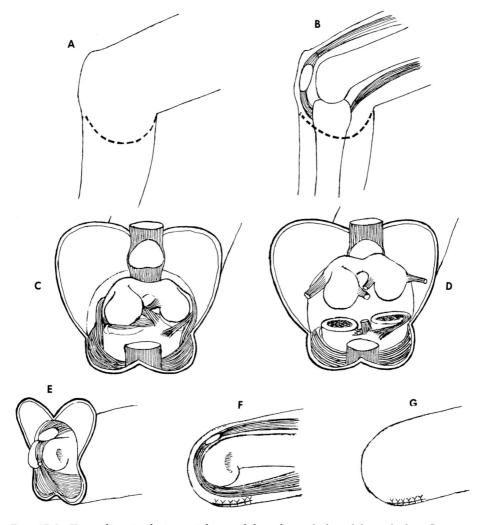

FIG. 17-3. Knee disarticulation with equal length medial and lateral skin flaps. A, Outline of skin incision. B, Insertions of subpatellar tendon as well as hamstrings have to be preserved. C, Knee joint has been opened and patellar ligament transected. D, Collateral and cruciate ligaments have been transected. E, Patellar ligament as well as hamstring tendons have been sutured to each other and to remnants of cruciate ligaments. F and G, Status following soft tissue closure.

Above-knee amputations

When disarticulation cannot be carried out, the area above the knee is the next level of amputation. Here, more than at any other level of amputation, the fixation of antagonistic muscles to each other is important to keep the femoral stump in the center of the soft tissue mantle. The more length that can be preserved, the easier it is for the patient to power the prosthesis. Thus, a stump of 5 cm or less as measured from the perineum cannot be considered for prosthetic fitting. Indeed, short femoral stumps present more of a nuisance than a help since with the severance of the insertions of the gluteus maximus and the hip

adductors, the hip quickly assumes a flexion and abduction contracture of extreme degrees, which creates a bothersome prominence.

Technique (Fig. 17-4). After skin preparation and draping, as well as the application of a pneumatic tourniquet, anterior and posterior skin flaps of equal length are fashioned to be slightly longer than one half the diameter of the extremity to be amputated. It may be advisable to make the anterior skin flap longer than the posterior one since the posterior skin retracts more after amputation. The muscles are beveled in such a way that a fish-mouth appearance is obtained. The bone is transected. The

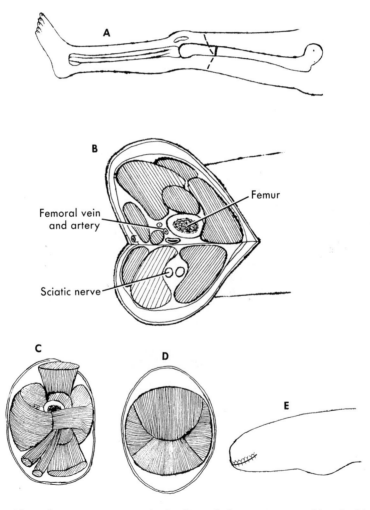

FIG. 17-4. Above-knee amputation. **A,** Outline of skin incision and level of bony transection. **B,** Operative site following ablation of leg. **C** and **D,** Myoplasty of medial and lateral **(C)** and anterior and posterior **(D)** structures. **E,** Skin closure.

major vessels need to be tied and the nerves cut back well above the level of the amputation. It is important to tie the sciatic nerve to avoid bleeding from the sciatic concomitant artery.

The fascial coverings of the opposing muscle groups are brought together after a drain has been introduced into the amputation wound. Subcutaneous tissue is closed with interrupted absorbable sutures, and the skin is closed with interrupted non-absorbable sutures. A postoperative rigid dressing is applied.

Hip disarticulation (Fig. 17-5)

The skin incision for this procedure is a racquet-type of incision starting at the anterior superior iliac spine and following the inguinal ligament to the perineum. It follows the inferior gluteal fold, turns upward, and connects with the beginning of the incision at the anterior superior iliac spine. The femoral vessels are exposed through the anterior part of the incision and are ligated and divided. The origin of the adductor muscles is divided at the inferior pubic ramus. Externally rotating the hip brings the lesser trochanter into view and the iliopsoas can be detached from it and from the adjacent part of the hip capsule. More laterally, the tensor faciae latae and the sartorius muscle are separated from the anterior superior iliac spine.

The patient is rolled further on the side, and the insertion of the gluteus maximus into the femur can be exposed and severed.

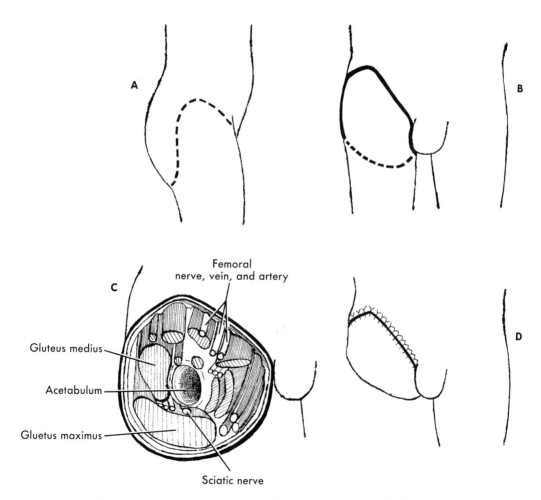

FIG. 17-5. Hip disarticulation. **A** and **B**, Outline of skin incision. **C**, Operative site after removal of limb. **D**, Skin closure.

The lesser trochanter comes into view and the abductors can be removed from it. Before severing the external rotators, it is advisable to find the obturator artery and ligate it before severing it since it tends to retract into the lesser pelvis and is difficult to ligate thereafter. After transection of the hamstrings at the ischium, the sciatic nerve and the gluteal vessels are ligated and separated as they emerge from the sciatic notch. The hip joint is then entered through the capsule, the round ligament is transected, and the amputation is completed.

Two drains should be introduced into the amputation wound, one into the area of the acetabulum and the other one under the muscle flaps. The abductors are sutured to the transverse acetabular ligament, and

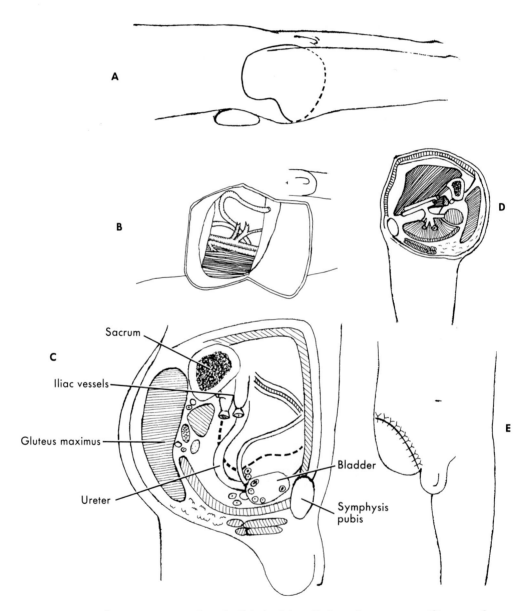

FIG. 17-6. Hind quarter amputation. **A,** Skin incision. **B,** Anterior exposure. Iliac vessels and spermatic cord are in view. Peritoneum is in upper edge of wound. **C,** Operative site after ablation of right hemipelvis. **D,** View of specimen. **E,** Skin closure.

the gluteus maximus is brought forward with the posterior skin flap and sutured to the anterior flap.

Hind quarter amputations (Fig. 17-6)

In the rare instances where this most mutilating of all amputations becomes necessary in an older person, it is done for primary malignant disease or overwhelming infection. The patient is placed on the sound side. An indwelling catheter, which has been inserted before the procedure, is taped to the sound thigh. In the male the scrotum is also taped to the sound thigh. The anus is closed with a single purse string suture, which has to be removed at the end of the procedure. The diseased extremity is draped free.

The skin incision starts over the anterior part of the iliac crest and moves forward across the anterior iliac spine and along the inguinal ligament to the adductor tubercle. Through the anterior part of the incision, the external iliac artery is exposed and clamped. The spermatic cord is identified and swept medially. The symphysis pubis is then isolated and transected. The urethra has to be protected during this procedure. The incision is then extended along the inferior pubic ramus into the perineum. The muscles on the floor of the pelvis are separated from the pubic ramus. The skin incision is continued along the inferior gluteal fold, swinging superiorly and anteriorly at its lateral end to meet the beginning of the incision at the iliac crest. By raising a large posterior skin flap, the abdominal muscles can be identified at the iliac crest and detached from it. The inside of the hemipelvis is now clearly visible. The external iliac vessels and femoral nerve are followed proximally, ligated separately, and transected. Transection of the femoral as well as obturator nerve is easier after the psoas muscle has been transected. The sacral plexus and the gluteal vessel have to be transected after ligation to expose the sacroiliac joint. The obturator vessels are ligated and the hemipelvis is disarticulated at the sacroiliac joint.

The previously raised posterior skin flap

is brought forward, the subcutaneous tissue is sutured to the stumps of the abdominal muscles, and the skin edges are brought together by interrupted sutures. It is important to introduce two to three drains in the wound cavity. The wound is dressed with a well-padded dressing that allows removal of the drains without disturbing it. The dressing should be kept in place for the better part of 1 week.

RESTORATION OF INDEPENDENCE
Postoperative care

The postoperative care begins ideally at the end of the surgical procedure while the patient is still in the operating room. At that time, a postoperative rigid dressing is applied to the stump. The rigid dressing provides an unyielding but form-fitting coverage for the remnant of the extremity, which decreases the postoperative edema and in many cases supplies the socket for a pylon that ultimately will allow early ambulation.[7,12]

Even in those cases where the application of an immediate postoperative rigid dressing is not feasible, a delayed rigid dressing should be considered within the first 3 weeks following the amputation. Such a dressing aids in the shrinkage and maturation of the stump. The immediate postoperative rigid dressing is maintained for the first 2 weeks. Thereafter it is removed, the wound is inspected, and a new rigid dressing is applied. If ambulation has not been started, it is well to start it at this point if the stump and wound appear to be doing well.

In those cases where more frequent changes in the rigid dressing are anticipated, a semi-rigid dressing can be applied.[11] This consists of the application of an Unna paste wrap, which has to be applied without any folds or creases over the postoperative dressing. It, too, is unyielding and serves to decrease the postoperative edema. It does not, however, allow the use of a pylon for early ambulation, and it requires the fabrication of a temporary socket if early ambulation is contemplated. Thus, the ease of application and economy of the semi-rigid dressing is offset by the cost of the fabrication of the temporary prosthesis.

In the case of an open amputation, the stockinette traction is also applied in the operating room. It must be kept in mind that in the postoperative period wound secretions from the open amputation accumulate at the lowest point under the stump and can lead to maceration of the skin unless the dependent area of the stump is kept meticulously dry. In open amputations in particular but also in primarily closed amputations, the possibility of postoperative bleeding must be kept in mind. If this hemorrhage comes from one of the larger vessels, it can prove disastrous. Therefore, a tourniquet should be kept at the bedside of the amputee, and the staff should be trained in the application of the tourniquet.

Drains should be removed during the first 24 to 48 hours. Suction drains can easily be led out over the brim of the rigid dressing. Penrose drains, too, can be secured with a long nylon suture, which can then be kept out of the rigid dressing. Thus, the Penrose drain, too, can be removed without needing to open the rigid dressing.

The amputation wound should not be the only cause for concern in the immediate postoperative period. The condition of the other leg and indeed the entire body of the patient should also be considered. First and foremost in the mind of the staff should be the prevention of decubitus ulcerations. Frequent turning and the use of eggshell mattresses are part of the preventive routine. Frequent rousing of the patient and breathing exercises are necessary to prevent hypostatic pneumonia.

Rehabilitation within the first 24 hours should include encouraging the patient to move from the bed to the chair.[16] If at all possible, the patient should start standing on the remaining leg and help in the transfer. Strengthening exercises for the upper extremities can be initiated as soon as the patient is sufficiently awake. During this period of time, frequent reassurances to the patient are advisable because of the sometimes rather marked phantom pain. The rigid dressing seems to decrease this pain.

It is, nevertheless, startling and often frightening to the point where the patient is unsure whether or not the amputation really has taken place. Unipedal ambulation between parallel bars and later on with a walkerette is the next step in the rehabilitation process.[19,26] Where it is feasible to attach a pylon to the rigid dressing, the patient may begin to touch the ground with the prosthetic foot. In patients who have undergone amputations for vascular insufficiency, it prudent to await the first change of the rigid dressing 2 weeks following the operation before ambulation is initiated. Once the wound is found to be healing well, the patient should start weight bearing to tolerance.

A particular advantage to the physical and psychologic rehabilitation of the patient seems to be the involvement of the patient in the fitting and manufacturing of the prosthesis whenever possible. This makes the patient feel that he is a member of the team and he will more readily volunteer information about discomfort in the prosthesis and about his worries and fears while he is wearing it. The aim is to make the patient an independent ambulator who ideally is functioning at home and in the community with minimal help from others.

MORTALITY

Postoperative mortality following amputations remains rather high. Intraoperative deaths are common; the long-term survival is poor.[6,9] In a study by Anderson and Ostberg[1] in 1972, only 57.5% of the elderly amputees survived the first year following surgery, a figure considerably lower than that for curative surgery of cancer. The figures vary, however, in large series, and range from 5% (Burgess, Ramano, Zettl, and Schrock)[4] to 13% (Couch, David, Tilney, and Crane).[6] The number of deaths following below-knee amputations is considerably lower than that after above-knee amputations or knee disarticulations.[13]

Of interest are the long-term effects of lower extremity amputation on the musculoskeletal system, in particular the axial skeleton. This problem has been discussed with particular intensity in the German literature.[3,15,17,28,29] A lateral deviation of the lumbar spine to the side of an above-knee amputation appears to be very common. It is considered to be the result of shortness of the prosthesis. However, in most cases, this lateral deviation is reversible. Degenerative changes on the concavity of the lateral deviation are also common. In spite of these findings and in spite of the common complaint of low back pain in amputees, back problems are rarely the cause for disabilities. Only where several factors coincide, such as flexion contractures of the remaining joints, poor prosthetic replacement, overweightedness, and constitutional factors, can back pain become a disabling factor in lower extremity amputees after many years of prosthesis wearing.

CONSIDERATIONS IN PROSTHETIC FITTING

There are three special considerations for the prosthesis of the elderly person: (1) weight of the prosthesis, (2) ease of application and removal of the prosthesis, and (3) safety in the use of the prosthesis. Unfortunately, all three determinants conspire against successful prosthesis wearing in the geriatric amputee.

The weight of the prosthesis is a cause for worry in diaphyseal amputations, in particular in short diaphyseal amputations. The dead weight of the prosthesis, even in a long and seemingly well-muscled stump, may present a problem for the older person. The inertia of this dead weight on a short stump may be more than the patient can control with the reduced muscle mass. Endoskeletal as well as exoskeletal prostheses, however, require enough structural stability and therefore mass to sustain the weight of the amputee.

The donning of the prosthesis, particularly one with a suction socket, may be too energy consuming for the patient whose cardiovascular system functions at a limited capacity. The alternative suspension systems may defeat the purpose by adding weight to the prosthesis, which again taxes the patient's cardiovascular output. Yet waist belts and silesean bandages are often necessary for above-knee prostheses for geriatric amputees, and a thigh lacer is sometimes unavoidable for a below-knee prosthesis when the knee has been saved by creating a short below-knee stump.

However, the suspension devices add to the feeling of security when the elderly patient walks with a strange device that replaces his own leg. Another component increasing the feeling of security for the amputee is a single-axis foot rather than a SACH foot. With the single-axis foot, there is less of a chance for the prosthesis to twist on the stump on heel strike. It does, however, add to the weight of the prosthesis. Raising the medial and lateral wall of the below-knee prosthesis sometimes adds to the feeling of stability in the knee. In the above-knee prosthesis, the knee axis must be well behind the center of gravity to allow full and stable extension of the knee at or slightly before heel strike. Sometimes a locking mechanism for the knee becomes necessary to allow the patient to stand for long periods of time; indeed, some amputees prefer walking with a locked knee, especially those who are household ambulators only. The release for the knee, however, should be located in such a way that the patient can reach it with ease. A silesean bandage may help in the suspension of the prosthesis, although it does not control rotation of the prosthesis.

References

1. Andersen, B., and Ostberg, J.: Long-term prognosis in geriatric surgery: 2-17 year follow-up of 7,922 patients, J. Am. Geriatr. Soc. **20:**255-258, 1972.
2. Baker, W.H., and Barnes, R.W.: Minor forefoot amputation in patients with low ankle pressure, Am. J. Surg. **133:**331-332, 1977.
3. Breitenfelder, J., and Wilcke, K.H.: Spätschäden am Stützapparat bei Beinamputierten, Mschr. Unfallheilk **77:**567-569, 1974.
4. Burgess, M., Romano, L., Zettl, H., and Schrock, D., Jr.: Amputations of the leg for peripheral vascular insufficiency, J. Bone Joint Surg. **53A:**874-890, 1971.
5. Condon, E., and Jordan, H., Jr.: Below-knee amputation for arterial insufficiency, Surg. Gynecol. Obstet. **130:**642-648, 1970.
6. Couch, P., David, J., Tilney, N.L., and Crane, C.: Natural history of the leg amputee, Am. J. Surg. **133:**469-473, 1977.

7. Devas, M.B.: Early walking of geriatric amputees, Br. Med. J. **1**:394 396, 1971.

8. Devas, M.B.: Geriatric orthopedics, Br. Med. J. **3**:190-192, 1974.

9. Ebskov, B., and Josephsen, P.: Incidence of reamputation and death after gangrene of the lower extremity, Prosthet. Orthotics Int. **4**:77-80, 1980.

10. Friedmann, L.W.: The indications for and modern management of conventional amputation, Talk given at the meeting of the American College of Angiology, New York, June 26, 1970.

11. Ghiulamila, R.I.: Semirigid dressing for postoperative fitting of below-knee prothesis, Arch. Phys. Med. Rehabil. **53**:186-190, 1972.

12. Golbranson, F.L., Asbelle, C., and Strand, D.: Immediate postsurgical fitting and early ambulation—a new concept in amputee rehabilitation, Clin. Orthop. **56**:119-131, 1968.

13. Hall, R., and Shucksmith, H.S.: The above-knee amputation for ischaemia, Br. J. Surg. **58**:656-659, 1971.

14. Harris, P.L., et al.: The fate of elderly amputees, Br. J. Surg. **61**:665-668, 1974.

15. Holland, C., and Wolck, H.: Oberschenkelamputation und Wirbelsäulenstatik, Arch. Orthop. Unfallchir. **62**:352-328, 1967.

16. Katrak, P.H., and Baggott, J.B.: Rehabilitation of elderly lower extremity amputees, Med. J. Aust. **1**:651-653, 1980.

17. Kruse, H., Baumann, W., and Groh, H.: Stützkräfte beim Beinamputierten, Mschr. Unfallheilk **74**:176-186, 1971.

18. MacBride, A., Rogers, J., Whylie, B., and Freeman, J.J.: Psychosocial factors in the rehabilitation of elderly amputees, Psychosomatics **21**:258-262, 1980.

19. Magato, R.S., and Rosenberg, L.: Evaluation of a training leg for above-knee amputees, A. J. Phys. Med. **46**:1219-1255, 1967.

20. Malone, J.M., et al.: The gold standard for amputation level selection: zenon-133 clearance, J. Surg. Res. **30**:449-455, 1981.

21. Miller, B.: Advanced occlusive arterial disease (gangrene) in the aged, and decision-making for amputation, J. Am. Geriatr. Soc. **23**:321-328, 1974.

22. Reyes, R.L., Leahey, E.B., and Leahey, E.B., Jr.: Elderly patients with lower extremity amputations: three-year study in a rehabilitation setting, Arch. Phys. Med. Rehabil. **58**:116-123, 1977.

23. Robinson, K.P.: Long posterior flap amputation in geriatric patients with ischaemic disease, Ann. R. Coll. Surg. Engl. **58**:440-451, 1976.

24. Scheibe, G.: Rheographische Bewertung der arteriellen Amputations-stumpf-Durchbluntung, Arch. Orthop. Unfallchir. **75**:264-272, 1973.

25. Smith, R.J.: Amputations in geriatric patients, J. Natl. Med. Assoc. **66**:108-110, 1974.

26. Traugh, H., Cocoran, J., and Reyes, L.: Energy expenditure of ambulation in patients with above-knee amputations, Arch. Phys. Med. Rehabil. **56**:67-71, 1975.

27. Wagner, F.W.: Amputations of the foot and ankle, Clin. Orthop. **122**:62-69, 1977.

28. Wilcke, K.H.: Die einseitige Beinamputation und ihre Chirurgisch-Orthopädischen Folgen, Mschr. Unfallheilk **74**:236-248, 1971.

29. Wilcke, K.H.: Anerkennung von Beinamputationsfolgen am Stützapparat, Mschr. Unfallheilk **77**:132-142, 1974.

chapter 18
STROKE: THE CHALLENGE

Brendan Clifford
Robert L. Waters
Christopher Jordan

Until recently, strokes have been of only peripheral interest to the medical community at large and to orthopaedic surgeons in particular. Strokes bore that intangible aspect of being a central neurologic insult in which the interrelationships of different neurologic dysfunctions (motor, perceptual, linguistic, gnostic) were incompletely understood and their relationships to overall patient function were unclear. Working with stroke patients imparted an uneasiness akin to laboring in a morass. Without a firm grasp of the underlying foundations of the disorder, it was impossible to initiate a decisive treatment program. From the point of view of the orthopaedic surgeon other neurologic syndromes were more easily understood and treated on both a physiologic and therapeutic basis. The isolated motor paralysis of the poliomyelitis patient or the discrete motor and sensory paralysis following peripheral nerve injury are examples of diseases in which involvement is restricted to a limited number of organ systems or anatomic regions. It is more difficult to treat stroke patients whose syndrome extends to nearly all organ systems and aspects of human function. Fortunately, recent advances in stroke rehabilitation have demonstrated the benefits that can accrue from a well-organized therapeutic program and the unique contribution that can be made by the orthopaedic surgeon.

The population of stroke patients has shifted towards the later decades, and there are approximately one quarter of a million stroke *survivors* per year in the United States alone. The overall incidence rate is 1 per 1000 annually. In contrast, the average yearly total number of spinal cord injuries is less than 10,000. In the past the typical stroke patient had painful contractures, was bedridden, and did not walk. Today, with the benefits of rehabilitation, 75% are able to ambulate at some level (Table 18-1).

This chapter will present an overview of the neurologic functional challenge that the cerebrovascular accident patient presents to the medical community. It will give a phylogenetic mode of understanding the complex neurologic mechanisms responsible for limb dysfunction and will review current concepts of treatment in stroke rehabilitation.

The dead neuron

The underlying problem in the patient with a cerebrovascular accident is the ischemic cortical neuron. Cerebral function is exquisitely dependent on abundant and continuous supplies of oxygen and glucose. The need for adequate cerebral blood flow to deliver these substrates is the "Achilles heel" of the central nervous system.[1]

The neuron, whether sensory or motor, can be deprived of its blood supply by different types of cerebrovascular accidents. Cerebral thromboemboli are the most common cause, accounting for more than two thirds of all strokes. Intracranial and subarachnoid hemorrhage are the next two

TABLE 18-1
Prognosis following CVAs

	Percentage of total number of CVAs (%)	Survival rate after			Functional prognosis of survivors (%)
		30 days (%)	5 years (%)	10 years (%)	
All CVAs		62			29 normal 33 able to work 3 total care
Thrombosis	71	90	43	22	27 normal 34 able to work 2 total care
Emboli	8	75	30	15	27 normal 34 able to work 2 total care
Hemorrhage, overall	16				49 normal 14 able to work 49 total care
Intracerebral bleeding		22	7	0	
Subarachnoid bleeding		55	37	30	

Modified from Matsumoto, N., Whisnant, J.P., Kurland, L.T., et al.: Natural history of stroke in Rochester, Minnesota, 1955 to 1969, Stroke **4:**20-29, 1973.

TABLE 18-2
Surgical morbidity in the stroke population

Patients	Number
Total	388
Receiving general anesthesia	370
Receiving spinal anesthesia	2
Receiving regional anesthesia	16
Deaths postoperatively	0
Intraoperative and postoperative medical complications	6.4% of patients

Modified from Garland, D.E., et al.: Clin. Orthop. **145:**189-192, 1979.

TABLE 18-3
Postoperative medical complications

Type of complication	Number
Total number of patients	388
Arrhythmia	6
Sepsis	5
Thrombophlebitis	5
Hypertension, labile	3
Pulmonary embolus	1
Respiratory failure	1
Upper gastrointestinal hemorrhage	1
Cholecystitis	1
Seizures	3
Pneumonia	2
Urinary tract infection	2
Epistaxis	1
Hyperthermia	1
Tachycardia	1
Acute urinary retention	1

Modified from Garland, D.E., et al.: Clin. Orthop. **145:**189-192, 1979.

most common etiologies. Predisposing risk factors include hypertension, birth control pills, hyperlipidemia, diabetes mellitus, smoking, and heart disease. There is no clear sex predilection.[1]

Survival and function vary, of course, with the location and extent of the vascular insult. Furthermore, it is of note that the rehabilitation outcome of patients with "bleeds" is poorer than for those with intracerebral thrombi. Cerebral thromboembolism, then, the most common cause of stroke, also carries the best functional prognosis. In turn, about 50% of the survivors have some neurologic residua, hemiplegia being the most common. These survivors are, as a whole, surprisingly good risks for elective surgical procedures (Tables 18-2 to 18-3).

The region of cerebral cortex supplied by the middle cerebral artery is most commonly affected. This gives rise to a clinical picture of contralateral hemiplegia, hemianesthesia, and homonymous hemianopsia. Depending on the hemisphere and extent of involvement, partial to global motor or sensory aphasia may be present (Figs. 18-1 and 18-2).

In contrast, the less common picture of anterior cerebral artery impairment gives rise to paralysis of the opposite lower limb and, to a lesser extent, of the upper limb. Patients with bilateral cortical involvement have mental impairment and frontal release signs and are often not rehabilitation candidates, since they are unable to remember and learn.[4]

Patterns of motor impairment

After a period of flaccid paralysis, there is an increase in tone in the adductors and flexors of the upper and lower limbs.[15] Hyperactive tendon reflexes ensue and this may be associated with clonus. If muscle tone does not appear within 6 weeks, the prognosis for motor recovery is grave.

Voluntary movement usually first returns at the shoulder. Recovery of voluntary movement then proceeds distally toward the fingers. In most patients the lower limb follows the same proximal-to-distal pattern of motor recovery.

Two types of voluntary motion may be present. Pattern movement is the first to recover and consists of mass flexor or mass extensor movements of the limb. Selective motor recovery (the ability to control individual muscles and joint movements precisely) depends on the extent of the cerebral cortical damage.

The patient's dependence on primitive limb synergies decreases as selective control recovers. The extent to which motor impairment restricts function differs between upper and lower extremities. The hemiplegic patient with even mild motor impairments and spasticity may prefer to perform activities with the opposite normal limb rather than fumbling with a hand that lacks motor control. On the other hand, gross limb synergies in the lower extremity may be quite adequate for walking.

Manual muscle stretch is the common clinical test of spasticity. Two types of responses occur, depending on the rate of stretch. If the muscle is quickly extended, velocity-sensitive components of the muscle spindle may be activated, giving rise to a phasic motor discharge and even clonus. If the muscle is slowly stretched below the threshold of velocity sensitivity, the spindle may still trigger a so-called tonic discharge in response to a change in the length of the muscle spindle, giving rise to clasp-knife resistance. This concept is important in determining range of motion. A joint should be slowly extended (or flexed) to minimize the phasic response and to obtain maximal range. Since tonic discharge may be continuous and remain even after the muscle is slowly extended in some patients, spasticity can be truly differentiated from myostatic contracture only by examining the patient under anesthesia or following peripheral nerve blocks (Figs. 18-3 to 18-4).[5]

Vestibular responses are increased following stroke, and spasticity is more dependent on body posture. It has been demonstrated that response of the triceps surae to quick stretch increased in the sitting or standing position versus the supine position. Polysynaptic spinal cord reflexes neurologically link muscles that are normally

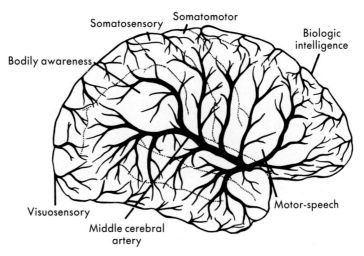

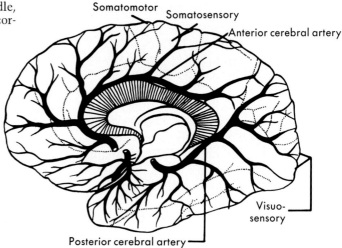

FIG.18-1. Territories of anterior, middle, and posterior cerebral arteries and corresponding centers of cortex.

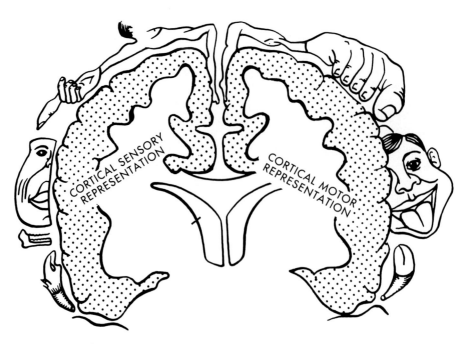

FIG. 18-2. Area of motor and sensory representation of hand as compared to foot. Notice their relationship to vascular supply shown in Fig. 18-1. (From Garland, D.E., and Waters, R.L.: Orthop. Clin. North Am. **9**:291-304, 1978.)

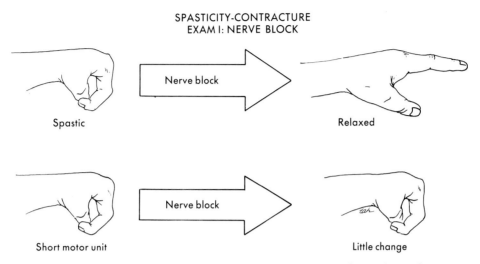

FIG. 18-3. Differentiation between spasticity and shortening of muscle tendon motor units is facilitated by a median nerve block, which releases hypertonicity without affecting motor unit length.

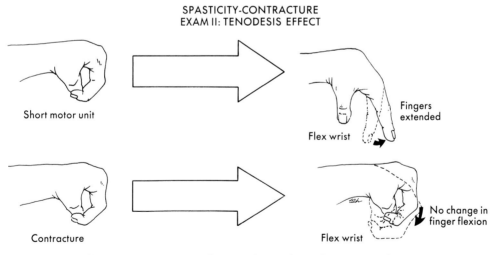

FIG. 18-4. Differentiation between shortened muscle tendon units and joint contracture is made by flexing proximal joints and noting resultant position of distal joints. Joint contracture is not affected by changing position of proximal joints. Shortened motor units allow distal joints to be extended as proximal joints are flexed. (From Braun, R.M., Mooney, V., and Nickel, V.L.: J. Bone Joint Surg. **52A:**970, 1970.)

synergistic and inhibit muscles that are normally antagonistic. Loss of cortical control following a stroke increases the dependency of spasticity (stretch response) on limb position. The extent of primitive reflexes generally varies inversely with the quality of selective control, which in turn is dependent on the extent of cortical loss.[7]

Because of the complex interrelationships of voluntary control and involuntary spinal reflexes, it is easy to understand why the single most important test of lower extremity function is the observation of the limb during intended use to ascertain the activity of the muscles. Dynamic electromyography provides the surgeon with more precise information on specific muscle actions. Assessment of the patient may include lidocaine nerve blocks to denervate muscles temporarily, enabling differentiation of spasticity from contractures.

Sensation/perception

The final process in sensory perception occurs in the cerebral cortex, where basic sensory information is integrated into complex sensory phenomena. The basic modalities of touch, temperature, and pain are often intact, but the higher discriminative aspects of sensation, such as shape, size, texture, point localization, and proprioception, which determine ultimate limb function, are often impaired or absent. Marked sensory loss precludes routine functional use of the hemiplegic hand. The importance of sensation to hand function is discussed in the section on the upper extremity (Fig. 18-5).

Prognostic rehabilitation determinants

It is the responsibility of the rehabilitation team to predict accurately who is a rehabilitation candidate and who is not.[6]

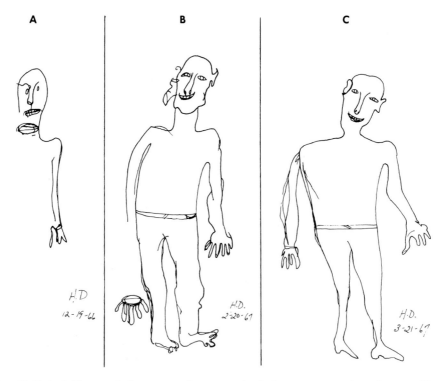

FIG. 18-5. A, Self-portrait demonstrating severe body image sensory impairment. Drawing was made on admission to Rancho Los Amigos Hospital about 2 months after acute onset of hemiplegia. Patient demonstrated marked sensory losses in all areas including sharp-dull sensation, position sense, and object identification. Note progress, **B,** after 2 months, and recovery, **C,** after 3 months of therapy.

The ability to perform accurate prognostications based on experience is one of the most important functions of a rehabilitation center. Inappropriate attempts to improve function waste time and revenue and demoralize the rehabilitation team. Poor prognostic indicators must be clearly recognized before embarking on a rigorous treatment program. However, a rehabilitation trial may be necessary in borderline patients whose rehabilitation potential is unclear.

Certain neurologic factors are now known to be particularly ominous with regard to rehabilitation potential. They include bilateral involvement with persisting frontal release signs (indicating the inability to retain information) and lack of bowel or bladder control past 1 month. Realistically, bowel and bladder incontinence often precludes satisfactory home management of a stroke patient. On a social level, family support is the key criterion determining the final disposition. Family involvement overlies all neural, psychologic, and social aspects of recovery and its presence or absence ultimately may determine the patient's domiciliary disposition.

THE LOWER EXTREMITY
Introduction

The process of bipedal evolution entailed neurologic and structural adaptation to holding the center of gravity aloft and balancing it precariously in the alternate manner on one foot in the single stance phase.[10] In developing the ability to walk with a bipedal gait, heel contact became essential (plantigrade gait) to increase the sagittal base of support in compensation for the loss of forelimb contact. In humans the hip and knee extensors fire before the heel strike to decelerate the swing limb and extend the knee preparatory to floor contact. Activity of the ankle plantar flexors is delayed until after floor contact to enable the heel to contact first. In contrast, quadrupeds fire the hip and knee and ankle plantar flexors before floor contact and are therefore toe (digitigrade) walkers. Human beings are the only bipeds who have heel-first contact, maintain heel and toe contact in midstance, and allow the knee to glide into full extension in stance. Forward motion in stance is carefully controlled by smooth dorsiflexion at the ankle, which is controlled by the triceps surae.

INHIBITORS OF REHABILITATION POTENTIAL

Severe inhibitors
    Severely impaired cognition and learning ability
    Decreased activity tolerance because of severe medical problems
Relative inhibitors
    Bilateral cerebral damage
    Obesity
    Contralateral extremity problems
    Body neglect
    Impaired balance
    Marked sensory impairment
    Prolonged flaccidity
    Placement in a nursing home

From Jordan, C., and Waters, R.L.: Orthopedic rehabilitation, St. Louis, 1980, The C.V. Mosby Co.

The fact that bipedal locomotion occurred simultaneously with the development of the newly evolved motor cortex with a relatively precarious blood supply accounts for a reversion to a more primitive quadripedal locomotor pattern following a cerebrovascular insult. After cerebral infarct the hemiplegic patient reverts to a mass extensor pattern, firing all extensors before heel strike, which explains why excessive plantar flexion and equinus are the most common gait disorders.[18]

The inadequate knee flexion often seen in the initial swing of the stroke patient also has underlying phylogenetic causes and inherent consequences. In quadrupeds there is no identifiable neurologic linkage between hip and knee flexors. Quadrupeds bear themselves in sustained knee flexion and have as a necessary consequence a requirement for a strong knee extension to maintain stability of the knee throughout stance. Minimal additional knee flexion occurs during swing and the knee extensors are also active to prevent excessive passive knee flexion secondary to forward thigh flexion. In contrast, humans lock the knee in full extension by simple joint compression and quadriceps activity is present only during initial stance and midstance. As a consequence of passively locking the knee in extension and decreasing the demand on the quadriceps, we pay the ambulatory price of requiring 65 degrees of knee flexion in swing to prevent toe drag. Quadrupeds have increased quadriceps activity during stance to maintain the flexed knee and increased quadriceps activity in the initial swing to prevent knee flexion. Dynamic electromyographic studies reveal that following a stroke, many hemiplegics revert to the more primitive quadripedal pattern of quadriceps activity, causing restricted knee flexion and a stiff-legged gait.[19]

In the quadriped the extensor activity at all joints persists throughout the weight-bearing period since the stance does not provide passive stabilization at the hip, knee, and ankle. In humans the upright posture and relatively extended position of the hip and knee enable passive stabilization and early termination of hip and knee extensor muscle firing. The reversion to a more primitive response after a stroke results in prolonged extensor activity at all joints, which further restricts the free passive knee flexion in swing that is needed to clear the ground and advance the limb.

Lower limb (functional requirements)

In order to walk independently, the hemiplegic patient requires the following:

Adequate balance to stand independently

Hip flexion to advance the limb

Intact strength in the uninvolved side

Based on these criteria and acceptable cognition, the orthopaedic surgeon can restore ambulation in most cases by prescribing appropriate orthotic aids and assistive devices.

Orthotic supplementation of gait

Support with an ankle-foot orthosis (AFO) is indicated for:

1. Inadequate calf strength. Some patients with inadequate triceps surae strength allow their ankles to collapse into dorsiflexion during stance, causing both knee and ankle instability. Most patients with calf weakness learn to hyperextend the knee after floor contact, thus passively locking the knee during limb loading. Gait can be aided by a rigid AFO, which stabilizes the ankle in neutral position.

2. Spastic calf. Again, a rigid AFO is needed. This time the rigid orthosis prevents ankle dorsiflexion and stretch on the triceps surae muscle spindles, eliminating the hyperactive stretch response as a mechanism for excessive muscle tone. This enables the foot to be positioned in neutral. Surgery may be required when spasticity is severe and the foot cannot be appropriately positioned.

3. Foot drop. Inadequate ankle dorsiflexion may be an isolated cause of gait dysfunction and should be treated with an AFO. A flexible orthosis (polypropylene) will allow ankle motion during stance and provides adequate dorsiflexion support in swing.

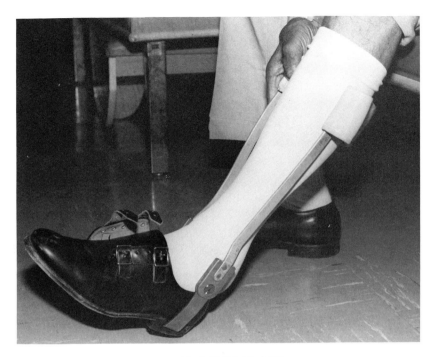

FIG. 18-6. BiCAAL AFO.

4. Varus. A mild varus deformity can be controlled by an AFO, but surgery is often needed for a severe deformity.
5. Decreased proprioception. Lack of proprioception in the lower limb can cause ataxic knee wobble during the stance phase. It can be corrected by the sensory input provided by a rigid orthosis. The AFO serves as a transducer that transmits pressure from the toe to the shank, thus giving sensory information to the anterior tibia.

The AFO supplies proprioceptive feedback and also is indicated most commonly to block excessive plantar flexion caused by excessive triceps surae spasticity. By preventing passive ankle dorsiflexion stretch on the triceps surae and its spindles, the AFO may be helpful in reducing excessive muscle tone (Fig. 18-6).

When inadequate dorsiflexion (foot drop) is the only gait problem, a lightweight flexible polypropylene (1/16-inch) orthosis with posterior trimlines is sufficient to provide toe pick-up during swing. Its flexibility enables ankle motion during stance (Fig. 18-7).

Mild varus during the swing phase is another problem manageable with a flexible polypropylene AFO. If varus is more severe, the rigid Bi-CAAL or rigid polypropylene orthosis is indicated, although these devices are commonly inadequate and surgery becomes necessary.

In contrast to the AFO, knee-ankle-foot orthoses (KAFOs) are rarely, if ever, indicated in the stroke population. They are difficult to don and to maintain. Their only function is that of a training aid when the quadriceps is weak. Stroke patients who have the ability to walk nearly always develop sufficient strength to extend the knee without the need for a KAFO.

The quad cane, a four-legged support structural base, is an important gait assist. It is the only effective means of substituting for the lack of hip abduction and extensor forces, since there is no passive orthosis that can directly affect hip function (Fig. 18-8).

During the initial phase of management patients may manifest various combinations of foot drop, knee and hip instability, and have fluctuating levels of propioceptive

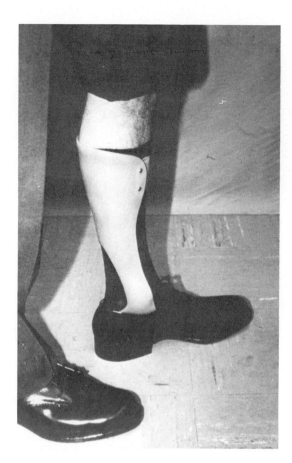

FIG. 18-7. Plastic posterior orthosis. It can be hidden completely in a man's sock or by his trousers and is not very conspicuous on a woman. Patient is free to wear almost any shoes desired, only constraint being use of shoes with same heel height. Plastic orthoses are contraindicated before patient's clinical picture has stabilized since none are adjustable. (From Waters, R.L., and Montgomery, J.: Clin. Orthop. **102:**133, 1974.)

FIG. 18-8. Quad cane. A variety of base modifications are available.

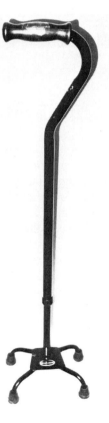

impairment. The Bi-CAAL is an optimum orthosis for this period since it can be used to correct all gait disorders requiring orthotic treatment and since it can be adjusted. Motor recovery occurs rapidly during the first 3 to 6 months. Polypropylene orthoses, which are not adjustable, are used following the period of neurologic recovery. For the same reasons definitive surgical procedures should not be contemplated until at least 6 months have elapsed.

A recent innovation is therapeutic electrical stimulation (TES). Applied through cutaneous electrodes, TES helps by maintaining the strength of flaccid muscles and preventing atrophy while also decreasing antagonist spasticity. TES also functions through a less well understood method of sensorimotor reeducation called carryover, which may hasten the return of volitional control.

The clinical uses of functional electrical stimulation (FES) are well documented. FES connotes an electrical stimulation used to supplement paretic muscles and improve function. Known therapeutic effects include muscle strengthening, inhibition of antagonist spasticity, correction of contractures, facilitation of voluntary motor control. FES can be visualized as an orthotic substitution in such syndromes as simple foot drop. The weight and bulk of these systems have led to poor patient tolerance. However, recent innovations in microcircuitry will most likely lead to their widespread use in the near future.

Surgical management of the lower extremity

Except for the correction of contractures still occasionally seen in neglected stroke patients, definitive procedures should be withheld for at least 6 months to allow a functional plateau to be reached. After this time surgery may safely be performed to improve usage in a functional limb. In a nonfunctional limb surgery may be performed to relieve pain or to correct contractures caused by spasticity. Most spastic contractural deformities in a nonfunctional limb are the result of an ineffective program of nonoperative care. To prevent these problems from developing, a program should include daily passive range-of-motion exercises, splinting, and limb positioning.[3]

The success rate of surgical procedures in the stroke patient can be enhanced by remembering that not only is simple paresis or paralysis present, but also the quality of existing muscle control is impaired. Some of the basic reflex mechanisms that should be checked before considering surgery include (1) slow stretch response, (2) fast stretch response, (3) volitional synergistic control, (4) selective cortical control, and (5) the influence of posture on stretch responses and volitional movement. Finally, as Perry[11] has pointed out, the single most important test of upper and lower extremity function is observation of the extremity during intended use to determine which muscles are overactive or underactive.

Unlike children in whom secondary bone and joint deformities develop as a result of the effect of muscle imbalances on growing bones, adults have strokes after skeletal maturation and there are no significant bone and joint changes. Consequently, in stroke patients bone and joint surgery is not required to correct limb deformities that may be corrected by soft tissue procedures.

The hip. Scissoring because of overactive adduction is the most common problem at the hip. It may be corrected by surgery or by serial obturator nerve blocks. Care should be taken not to release the adductor and not to perform anterior obturator neurectomies in patients whose adductor muscles are the sole means of limb advancement. Typically, such patients walk with a sideways gait, while patients who have a scissoring gait but who also have functioning hip flexors are able to walk directly forwards.

Fortunately, adductor spasticity, compared to other spastic syndromes, does not commonly interfere with hygiene in most stroke patients since such spasticity is usually unilateral, permitting personal skin care. However, if ranging and proning programs fail, flexion deformities may be dealt with by means of a surgical release incorporating an anterior approach.[17]

The knee. Inadequate knee flexion because of inappropriate quadriceps activity in late stance and early swing prevents knee flexion in some patients. To compensate, the patient must hike the pelvis or circumduct the leg to clear the foot during swing.

Electromyographic studies have shown that the abnormal activity is often restricted to the rectus femoris and vastus intermedius muscles (Fig. 18-9). If these isolated portions of the quadriceps are tenotomized, knee flexion will result and the so-called stiff-legged gait will be corrected.[19] If spasticity in the other quadriceps heads is noted, however, release of the rectus and vastus intermedius is not sufficient to restore knee flexion. Release of all four heads is not indicated since some extensor function must be preserved to stabilize the knee in stance.

The limited rectus and intermedius release is performed through an anterior midline incision from 4 cm above the patella going proximally, with subsequent isolation and resection of 2 cm of the muscle and tendon (Fig. 18-10).[19] Postoperative ambulation with a soft dressing is allowed as soon as tolerated.

Knee contractures in the ambulatory population increase the demand on the quadriceps and hip extensors, especially when the contracture exceeds 15 degrees. Hamstring or tendon release will enable full knee extension. Dynamic electromyograms enable precise identification of the muscles responsible for the deformity.

In nonambulatory individuals all hamstrings are released when knee flexion contractures cause a hygiene problem or interfere with limb positioning. Usually, in nonambulators knee flexion contractures are associated with hip flexion and adduction

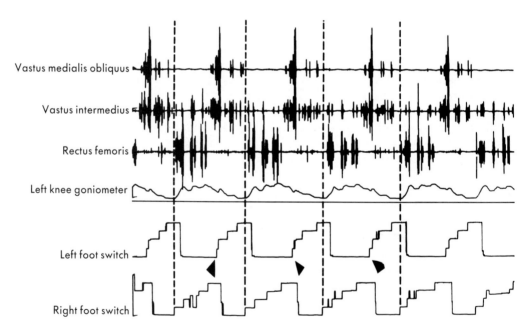

FIG. 18-9. Preoperative electromyogram of gait of left hemiplegic. Knee flexion corresponds to upward-deflection goniometer tracing. Foot-switch tracing indicates pattern of foot-floor contact in stance phase. Upward deflection arrow (↑) indicates beginning of swing phase and downward-deflection arrow (↓) indicates time of floor contact and end of swing phase. Each vertical broken line indicates contralateral heel-strike and beginning preswing phase. Note clonic motion at knee in response to clonus, shown in electromyogram of rectus femoris. Stance-phase activity in vastus medialis obliquus ends before beginning of terminal stance. Activity in vastus intermedius persists during terminal stance phase and swing phase. (From Waters, R.L., et al.: J. Bone Joint Surg. **61A:**927, 1979.)

contractures. Such surgical releases are needed less often now with the advent of better nursing care[17]

Surgical correction of equinus is indicated when the foot cannot be maintained in the neutral position with the heel in firm contact with the sole of the shoe despite a well-fitted orthosis. Often pistoning resulting from excessive spasticity is not manifested until after 50 to 60 steps, so the examination should include observing the patient walk a hallway, and not merely observing him in the examination room (Fig. 18-11).

Despite the wide variety of methods designed to weaken the triceps surae, none has proven to be more effective in adult patients than Achilles tendon lengthening (TAL). Closed percutaneous TAL is a simple and safe procedure. Triple hemisection tenotomy is performed via three stab incisions, with the most distal cut based medially to alleviate varus pull of the soleus (Fig. 18-12). Tenotomies are performed while slight tension is placed on the Achilles tendon so that it bowstrings posteriorly from the neurovascular structures. Following tenotomy, the foot is dorsiflexed to the neutral position with the knee extended and then a short leg cast is applied in 5 degrees of plantar flexion. Care should be taken to prevent further lengthening, which may lead to permanent plantar flexion weakness that can be more disabling than the original deformity.

The postoperative regimen consists of a short-legged cast for 6 weeks, followed by a Bi-CAAL, AFO for an additional 4½ months, supplemented by a posterior shell night splint. At the end of this period, orthotic-free ambulation may be possible in some patients with intact proprioception.

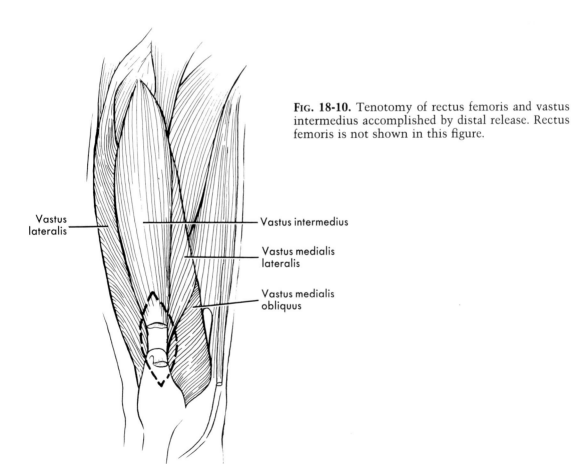

FIG. 18-10. Tenotomy of rectus femoris and vastus intermedius accomplished by distal release. Rectus femoris is not shown in this figure.

Vastus lateralis

Vastus intermedius

Vastus medialis lateralis

Vastus medialis obliquus

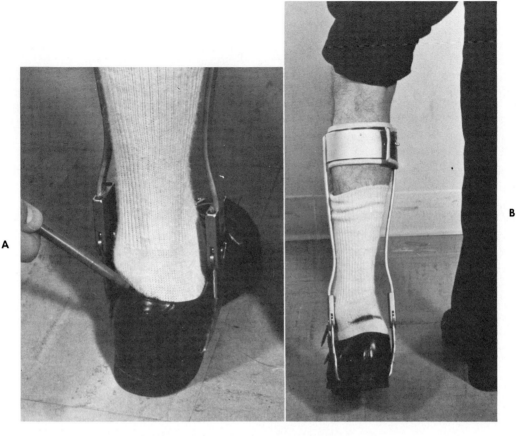

FIG. 18-11. A, Mark is placed on patient's sock while patient is standing with heel in firm contact with sole of shoe. B, Heel pistons out of shoe when patient walks. (From Waters, R.L., Perry, J., and Garland, D.E.: Clin. Orthop. 131:57, 1978.)

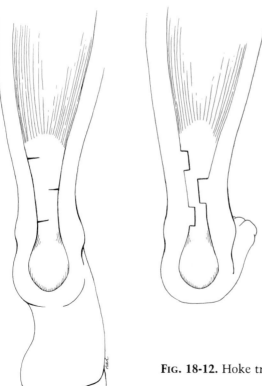

FIG. 18-12. Hoke triple hemisection tenotomy.

A posterior tibial lidocaine block is a valuable tool here. It demonstrates preoperatively the ankle range of motion that can be obtained through surgical intervention. For instance, if after a lidocaine block the patient is able to dorsiflex the ankle to neutral, then the potential exists for the patient to be a brace-free ambulator postoperatively. However, most patients who lack sufficient active dorsiflexion during this test will require permanent orthotic support to correct foot drop after Achille's tendon lengthening.

If there is toe flexion during gait, the extrinsic long toe flexors are divided prophylactically at the time of the TAL, because increased ankle dorsiflexion increases the tension on the extrinsic long toe flexors and may cause painful excessive toe flexion. The long toe flexors are released in the arch of the foot by an incision over the interval between the first metatarsal and abductor hallucis longus muscle. The interval between the second and third layers of muscles is developed and a 1-inch segment of the toe flexor is removed (Fig. 18-13). Surgeons who prefer the open TAL procedure commonly perform release or lengthening of the toe flexors through the incision above the malleolus.

Varus. Surgical correction of varus is indicated when varus is not corrected by a well-fitted orthosis or to enable the patient to walk without an orthosis when varus is the only significant problem.

The anterior tibialis, posterior tibialis, flexor hallucis longus, flexor digitorum longus, and soleus are responsible for varus. Electromyographic studies (Fig. 18-14) in most stroke patients show that the posterior tibialis is inactive or minimally active. When the soleus and extrinsic toe flexors significantly contribute to varus, the patient will have evidence of equinus and/or excessive toe flexion. When the tendons of these muscles are lengthened or released to correct equinus or toe flexion, their contribution to varus is abated. The anterior tibialis is the key muscle responsible for varus and in most patients this is easily confirmed by visual examination or palpation while the patient walks.

Split anterior tibialis transfer (SPLATT) converts a deforming force to a corrective force.[9,13] Approximately two thirds of the tendon is transferred to the third cuneiform and cuboid. The lateral two thirds of the tendon is detached, stripped proximally, and delivered through the second incision, or the shank, over the musculotendinous

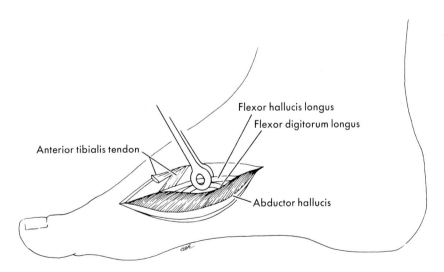

FIG. 18-13. Flexor hallucis longus and flexor digitorum longus are released in interval between first and third layer of plantar muscles. Abductor hallucis is reflected plantarward. Same incision is used to detach lateral part of tibialis anterior for SPLATT procedure.

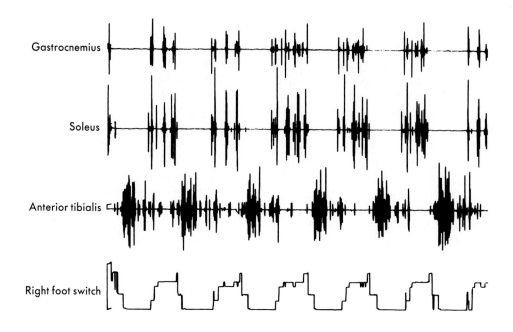

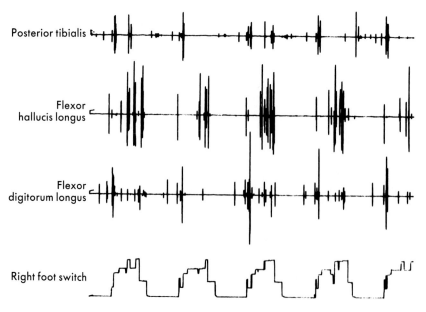

Fig. 18-14. Normal dynamic electromyogram of major muscles responsible for equinus and varus. Lowest tracing is foot switch, which records swing phase (baseline), heel strike (first level), metatarsal head contact (second level), and first toe contact at roll-off (highest level). Gastrocnemius and soleus are firing inappropriately in late swing, anterior tibialis firing continuously, posterior tibialis with little activity, and toe flexors firing inappropriately in late swing and early stance.

junction of the anterior tibialis. The detached portion of the tendon is then reinserted through drill holes in the third cuneiform and cuboid bones and the tendon is sutured to itself. Special care is taken to pass the tendon on top of the extensor retinaculum to avoid the formation of adhesions between the tendon and surrounding tissues, which may occur when the tendon is passed beneath this structure. Postoperative care is the same as for the TAL (Fig. 18-15).

Equinovarus. Treatment of equinovarus consists of the TAL and SPLATT procedures. At surgery the anterior tibialis is secured under sufficient tension to hold the foot in neutral. After healing, many patients are able to walk without an orthosis. However, there is a gradual tendency for the anterior tibialis to stretch in patients with a weakly contracting anterior tibialis. The extrinsic toe flexors, which are often inappropriately active in the swing phase, can be transferred anteriorly to augment dorsiflexion force in younger stroke patients. Activity of the long toe flexors in the swing phase of any gait may be surmised by visual inspection of the toe while walking; however, this is best determined by electromyography (Fig. 18-16).[12]

Planovalgus. Patients with preexisting pes planus may develop an increase of deformity and pain following stroke. Planovalgus occurs for several reasons. First, the calcaneous is in the valgus position and the Achilles tendon (particularly those fibers from the gastrocnemius) tends to exert a valgus pull on the heel. If the triceps surae is spastic, this will result in further valgus deformity. Second, gait electromyography

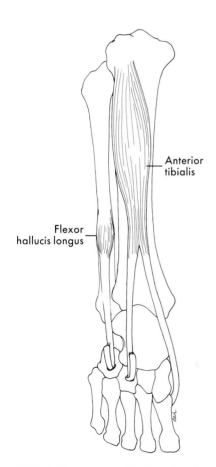

FIG. 18-15. Split anterior tibial tendon transfer.

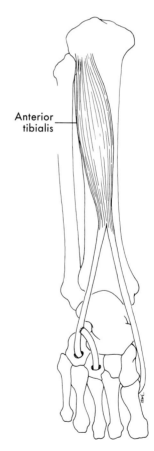

FIG. 18-16. SPLATT reinforced with flexor hallucis longus transfer.

on patients with painful planovalgus reveals that the peroneal muscles are usually overactive and this is associated with minimal or no activity in the posterior tibialis muscles.

Surgical treatment of planovalgus is Achilles tendon lengthening using the same technique described for correction of equinus deformity with the following exception. The most distal cut is based laterally to alleviate valgus pull of the triceps surae. If the peroneal tendons are active during the stance phase, both tendons are lengthened. This procedure will be sufficient to relieve pain in most all patients. It is rarely necessary to perform triple arthrodesis or other bony procedures for planovalgus in adult patients.

Toe flexion deformity. Electromyographic studies reveal that both long and short flexors are generally active and responsible for toe flexion deformities. Treatment consists of dividing the long and short flexors via transverse incisions over the volar aspect of each toe. For the great toe, release of the flexor hallucis longus only is performed. For an associated hallux valgus deformity, adductor release is performed. For an associated significant bunion deformity, a Keller procedure is recommended along with flexor hallucis longus release.

THE UPPER EXTREMITY

The unique selective control of the hand owes its dexterity to the large "newly" developed motor area of the cerebral cortex. The motor and sensory area for the upper limb receives its vascular supply from the vulnerable middle cerebral artery, which accounts for the relatively poor prognosis for upper extremity function after a cerebrovascular accident. From a phylogenetic point of view, we are all paying the price of the biologic recentness of the conversion of our upper extremities from locomotor appendages.

McCullough[6] noted that two thirds of stroke patients will recover partial use of the limb sufficient to assist the normal extremity while one third will develop a permanently functionless limb. The problem

is not only the loss of motor function but also the loss of sensation. The normal upper extremity relies on the brain's rapid ability to interpret large numbers of afferent impulses. Bunnell called sensation the "soul of the hand." This becomes obvious when a patient loses the ability to assimilate basic sensory input as a result of the infarction of the parietal area of the cerebral cortex and is therefore unable to perceive two-point discrimination, stereognosis, and proprioception. In such a patient, motion will be intact and tasks with the affected hand can be performed utilizing the eyes as visual feedback augmentors. However, such a patient will rarely utilize the limb spontaneously for habitual activities.

Other ancillary syndromes also have a detrimental effect on successful limb rehabilitation. Homonymous hemianopsia on the paralyzed side limits visual feedback until the patient has learned to compensate by turning the head or eyes. Also, nondominant (generally right) hemispheric infarcts may subtly affect higher integrative function, destroying special relationships and detrimentally influencing upper limb function. These higher perceptual defects can be studied by observing the patient's ability to organize a task in a sequential manner.[8]

Because of the complexity of impaired sensorimotor and integrative functions, rehabilitation of the upper limb entails training the patient first to function one-handed, pending evidence of adequate neurologic recovery of the affected side.

Early treatment

With the knowledge that the bulk of spontaneous neurologic recovery will appear within the first 6 weeks to 3 months, the rehabilitation team must prevent the development of ultimately disabling contractures. In the paralyzed limb, return of voluntary motion first appears as flexion of the shoulders, followed in sequence by flexion of the elbow, wrist, and fingers, and then forearm supination. At this early stage, any movement of the affected extremity results in simultaneous flexion of all joints. The presence of flexor spasticity in the absence of extensor movement will lead to the rapid onset of contractures if the joints are not passively extended on a daily basis.

Once established, contractures lead to the vicious cycle of pain and increased spasticity, with ensuing increased loss of motion. Contractures must be prevented by limb positioning, range-of-motion exercises, and splinting at this early stage. As the shoulder will tend to assume the position of adduction and internal rotation, it must be positioned in abduction, while the wrist should be supported in neutral. The shoulder, forearm, wrist, finger, and thumb joints will require manual stretching.

Range-of-motion exercises should be permitted only in the painfree arc to avoid an exacerbation of spasticity. Suspension slings may be used to reduce shoulder subluxation and to provide total arm support for the patient in a wheelchair, while shoulder abduction can be aided by reciprocal pulley systems when the patient is in and out of bed. These devices should be discontinued when sufficient tone for antigravity support is noted in the deltoid and proximal musculature. Note that for an ambulatory patient a "hemi-sling" serves the same purpose.

Extensor motion at the shoulder and elbow usually occurs by the time flexor synergy extends to the wrist and fingers. At this stage, the initial flaccid paralysis of the limb, which was followed by spasticity, evolves into a well-defined pattern of synergistic volitional control. There is a delay of several seconds between the command to execute a movement and the time when muscle contraction or relaxation occurs.[16]

The ability to flex the shoulder, elbow, wrist, and fingers selectively without invoking total flexor synergy returns first at the shoulder and elbow. As selective extension develops, there is a concomitant amelioration of flexor spasticity and an improvement in precision and speed.

Next, simultaneous flexion and extension of all fingers occurs, followed by the ability to flex and extend each finger selectively and independently with the index and middle fingers preceding the others.

This marks a critical stage. Most hemiplegics will not routinely use the extremity unless recovery reaches this point. Selective finger or thumb extension must be present without simultaneous elbow mass extensor patterning.

The longer the initial period of flaccid paralysis and delay in motor recovery, the poorer the prognosis, and if flaccidity persists beyond a few weeks, there is little chance for functional recovery. At least partial selective volitional control of the shoulder, elbow, and hand are prerequisites for useful upper extremity function. When recovery is arrested at a level where some selective extension of the fingers or thumb is present but incomplete because of mild flexor spasticity, the surgeon can improve function by lengthening the flexors to increase active extension.

Sensory perception

As alluded to previously, sensory integration is the key to upper limb function, and although perceptual defects may resolve in the early weeks after a cerebrovascular insult, their presence past 3 to 4 months is ominous. Furthermore, if documentation by trained clinical personnel reveals a neurologic plateau for 6 weeks or longer, the outlook for further useful function is grim.

Assessment of the stroke requires detailed sensory evaluation by an occupational therapist. However, if a patient's two-point discrimination and proprioception are intact, it is likely that other more complex functions will also be present and intact and that limb awareness will be sufficient to enable automatic or habitual use of the hand.

During this initial recovery phase of expectant waiting, the sound side must not be neglected. Upper limb impairment necessitates that the patient function in activities of daily living with one limb while ranging and strengthening exercises to the affected limb are carried out.

At this point, if spasticity of the wrist and finger flexors is severe, full-time splinting may be needed. Active strengthening of muscles with some voluntary control will help overcome the tendency to spastic contractures and prevent atrophy until further neurologic recovery occurs, enabling the patient to use the limb.

Management of the upper extremity

The shoulder. The shoulder is the joint most likely to develop symptoms of pain from contractures. Other causes of shoulder pain, such as subdeltoid bursitis, bicipital tendonitis, and acromioclavicular arthritis, should not be forgotten. Management of these other syndromes should be conventionally treated by appropriate local steroid injections, nonsteroidal antiinflammatory medications, and range-of-motion exercises. Chronic painful subluxation is rarely encountered in patients who have received appropriate early treatment.

Surgical release of the spastic, contracted shoulder is indicated to improve hygiene or relieve pain. There are several different mechanisms resulting in shoulder pain in the stroke patient, including inferior glenohumeral subluxation, shoulder-hand syndrome, central pain, aggravation of preexisting degenerative conditions about the shoulder, and spasticity. When abduction is less than 45 degrees, it can be assumed that the spastic deformity is superficially contributing to the pain (in the absence of central pain syndrome) and that pain can be alleviated by tendinous release. Electromyographic studies have indicated that the pectoralis major, subscapularis, teres major, and latissimus dorsi contribute to spastic adduction and internal rotation in stroke patients. All four muscles are gen-

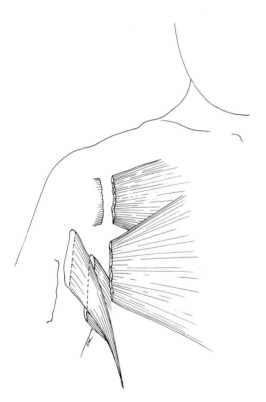

FIG. 18-17. Surgical release of spastic adducted shoulder. Division of pectoralis major and tenectomy of subscapularis should be accompanied by release of latissimus dorsi or teres major tendons whenever these muscles are found to be contributors.

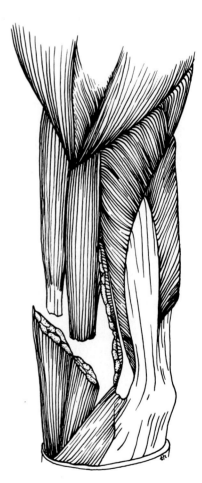

FIG. 18-18. Elbow flexion contractures corrected by releasing origin of brachioradialis, performing myotomy of brachialis, and releasing biceps tendon. (From Waters, R.L.: Clin Orthop. **131**:30, 1978.)

erally released by an incision over the deltopectoral groove and a simultaneous musculocutaneous neurectomy can be carried out at that time if indicated (Fig. 18-17).

The elbow. Dysfunctional and unaesthetic elbow flexion may be present in patients with nonfunctional upper extremities. The operative procedure depends upon the amount of contractural deformity. Lidocaine block of the musculocutaneous nerve helps differentiate between dynamic and fixed contractural deformities. If there is less than 90 degrees of fixed contractural deformity following the block, musculocutaneous neurectomy is performed. Residual contracture is corrected following surgery by serial or dropout casts. When the fixed deformity is greater than 90 degrees, biceps tendon lengthening, brachioradialis

release, and brachialis myotomy are performed. This surgery uses an anterolateral incision over the distal humerus (Fig. 18-18). Residual contracture is corrected with postoperative casting.

Flexion deformities of the wrist and fingers. The sublimis-to-profundus transfer is an excellent means of obtaining the necessary amount of tendon lengthening to correct combined wrist and finger flexion deformities (Fig. 18-19). A volar forearm incision is made, the sublimis tendons are divided distally, the profundus tendon is divided proximally, and they are sewn to each other totally. Via the same incision, the wrist flexion tendons may be lengthened by Z-plasty and the flexor pollicis longus may also be lengthened if the thumb is flexed in the palm.[2]

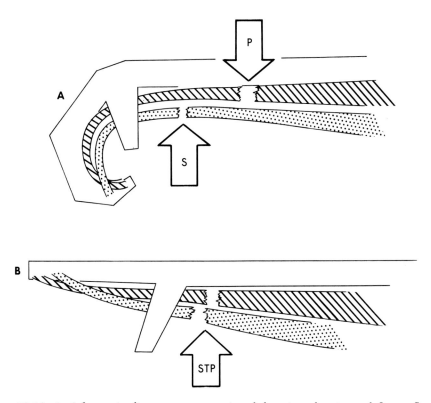

FIG. 18-19. A, Schematic diagram representing deformity of wrist and finger flexion. Profundus mechanism is transected in proximal forearm. Superficialis is transected at its musculotendinous junction in distal part of forearm. Palmaris longus is transected. Wrist flexors and flexor pollicis longus are lengthened. **B,** Schematic diagram illustrating extension of wrist and fingers to corrected position. An anastomosis is made between distal profundus tendons and musculotendinous junction of superficialis. Superficialis tendons retract into palm as fingers extend. (From Braun, R.M., Mooney, V., and Nickel, V.L.: J. Bone Joint Surg. **56A:**466, 1974.)

Intrinsic spasticity is often masked by extrinsic finger and thumb flexion. Following surgery for the extrinsic flexors alone, the patient may develop an intrinsic-plus posture of the fingers. Neurectomy of the motor branch is carried out if there is presumptive evidence of intrinsic spasticity. The thumb should be checked for adductor spasticity in the first dorsal interosseous muscle and adductor brevis muscle. When adductor spasticity in the thumb is seen, intrinsic spasticity is probably present in the finger intrinsics as well. A neurectomy of the motor branch of the ulnar nerve is carried out. This releases the adductor spasticity of the thumb and results in a more pleasing cosmetic appearance of the fingers following extrinsic tendon lengthening. Most patients require postoperative splinting in an orthosis to prevent recurrence of the deformity if they lack the extensor tone to maintain the wrist in the neutral position following flexor release. Tenodesis of the wrist extensor tendons can also be performed to hold the wrist in the neutral position.

Transfer of wrist flexor tendons to the extensors is not recommended in adult patients with acquired spasticity. The level of spasticity is variable throughout the day and is dependent upon many factors such as limb posture and the level of patient activity. It is not possible to place the transferred tendon under the proper amount of tension that will enable its muscle to exert the exact amount of tension suitable to hold the wrist in neutral and prevent either overcorrection or undercorrection.

Functional hand. Functional use of the hand depends upon adequate cognition, motivation, intact sensory and perceptual awareness, relative absence of restrictive spasticity, the ability to place the hand, and some selective extension of the fingers or thumb. As a general rule, if proprioception is intact and two-point discrimination is less than 1 cm, the patient with sufficient cognitive perceptual skills will utilize the hand if adequate motor function is present. In stroke patients there is generally a reciprocal relationship between the quality of extensor control and antagonistic spasticity. Presence of selective extension ensures that antagonistic spasticity is not too severe, that flexor control is adequate for grasp or pinch, and that the patient can extend the fingers or the thumb while maintaining the correct position for hand placement without the arm extending in a mass extensor synergy. Patients with an opposite uninvolved hand prefer to perform tasks one-handed rather than attempting tasks awkwardly with a hand with more than a slight degree of spasticity and impairment of motor control.

Automatic habitual use is the most important preoperative requirement for hand function. Patients who have automatic use of the hand will benefit from surgical procedures that will improve motor function. Patients who do not have some habitual use are rarely candidates for surgical procedures.

Finger extension loss. When some selective extension is present but incomplete, surgical lengthening is carried out. Because overlengthening results in loss of flexion or grip strength, the amount of lengthening performed is approximately one half of the amount necessary to extend the fingers from their preoperative position of maximal extension to the neutral position.

When more than two fingers are involved, fractional lengthening is used. Transverse cuts in the tendon are made just proximal to the most distal insertion of muscle or tendon. The fingers are extended to obtain the desired amount of tendon lengthening and then they are splinted in this position postoperatively for 3 weeks. A postoperative therapy program is essential to train the patient to utilize the increased extension range and to restore flexor strength and range of motion.

Wrist extension loss with adequate finger extension. Manual palpation often reveals that the flexor carpi radialis, palmaris longus, and/or flexor carpi ulnaris restrict wrist extension. During attempted finger extension, abnormal firing patterns can be detected by electromyography. Lidocaine blocks of the ulnar and median nerves can determine the relative importance of the different wrist flexors. The wrist flexor tendons are lengthened the full amount of tendon lengthening necessary to extend the wrist from the point of maximum preoperative wrist extension to the neutral position.

The thumb. Surgery is most commonly indicated to improve thumb extension so that the patient can perform lateral pinch between the thumb and the side of the index finger. Spasticity is commonly present either in the adductor pollicis and the first dorsal interosseous or in the flexor pollicis longus muscles. When spasticity is present, primarily in the adductor pollicis and the first dorsal interosseous, the thumb metacarpal is positioned close to the second metacarpal and it may not be possible for the patient to extend from this position voluntarily even in the presence of some volitional thumb extension. A lidocaine block of the motor branch to the ulnar nerve at the wrist will temporarily paralyze the adductor pollicis and first dorsal interosseous muscles and enable thumb extension. If improved extension occurs, then release of the adductor and the first dorsal interosseous is performed.

Spasticity in the flexor pollicis longus often restricts thumb extension and may be present alone or in association with spasticity in the above-mentioned intrinsic muscles. Spasticity in the flexor pollicis longus is manifested by excessive flexion at the thumb interphalangeal joint on attempted extension. Preoperative block of the median nerve at the elbow is performed, temporarily paralyzing the flexor pollicis longus, to demonstrate improved thumb extension. If positive results are obtained, the lengthening of the flexor pollicis longus is performed. The interphalangeal joint of the thumb is fused simultaneously.

SUMMATION

Rehabilitation begins at the inception of the stroke. Recognition of the characteristic patterns of motor and sensory involvement and the evolution of neurologic dys-

function serves to take the mystery out of an otherwise baffling syndrome. A multidisciplinary approach to stroke rehabilitation continues to be the key to maximizing ultimate patient function.

References
 1. Block, R., and Bayer, N.: Prognosis in stroke, Clin. Orthop. **131:**10, 1978.
 2. Braun, R.M., Mooney, V., and Nickel, V.L.: Flexor-origin release for the pronation-flexion deformity of the forearm and hand in the stroke patient, J. Bone Joint Surg. **52A:**907, 1970.
 3. Frazier, J.: An electromyographic analysis of the ankle and foot in the hemiplegic patient, Orthopedic Seminars, Rancho Los Amigos Hospital, Downey, Calif., 1978.
 4. Garland, D.E., and Waters, R.L.: Orthopedic evaluation in hemiplegic stroke, Orthop. Clin. North Am. **9:**291, 1978.
 5. Jordan, C., and Waters, R.L.: Stroke. In Nickel, V., editor: Orthopedic rehabilitation, St. Louis, 1981, The C.V. Mosby Co.
 6. McCollough, N.C., III: Orthopaedic evaluation and treatment of the stroke patient. In American Academy of Orthopaedic Surgeons: Instructional Course Lectures, vol. 24, St. Louis, 1975, The C.V. Mosby Co.
 7. McCollough, N.C., III: Orthopedic management in adult hemiplegia, Clin. Orthop. **131:**38, 1978.
 8. Moberg, E.: Criticism and study of methods for examining sensitivity in the hand, Neurology **12:**8, 1962.
 9. Mooney, V., Perry, J., and Nickel, V.: Surgical and non-surgical orthopedic care of stroke, J. Bone Joint Surg. **49A:**989, 1967.
10. Napier, J.: The antiquity of human walking, Sci. Am. p. 56, 1967.
11. Perry, J.: Lower extremity management in stroke examination: a neurologic basis for treatment. In American Academy of Orthopaedic Surgeons: Instructional Course Lectures, vol. 24, St. Louis, 1975, The C.V. Mosby Co.
12. Perry, J., Waters, R.L., and Perrin, T.: Electromyographic analysis of equinovarus following stroke, Clin. Orthop. **131:**47, 1978.
13. Roper, B.A., Williams, A., and King, J.B.: Surgical treatment of equinovarus deformity in adults with spasticity, J. Bone Joint Surg. **60B:**533, 1978.
14. Tower, D.B.: Effects of ischemia or tissue hypoxia on the neuron. In Goldstein, M., et al. editors: Advances in neurology, vol. 25, New York, 1979, Raven Press.
15. Twitchell, T.E.: The restoration of motor function following hemiplegia in man, Brain **74:**448, 1951.
16. Waters, R.L.: Upper extremity surgery in stroke patients, Clin. Orthop. **131:**30, 1978.
17. Waters, R.L., and Montgomery, J.: Lower extremity management of hemiparesis, Clin. Orthop. **102:**133, 1974.
18. Waters, R.L., Perry, J., and Garland, D.E.: Surgical correction of gait abnormalities following stroke, Clin. Orthop. **131:**54, 1978.
19. Waters, R.L., et al.: Stiff-legged gait in hemiplegia surgical correction, J. Bone Joint Surg. **61A:**927, 1979.

part IV

NURSING CARE AND REHABILITATION OF THE ELDERLY

chapter 19

NURSING CONSIDERATIONS IN THE GERIATRIC ORTHOPAEDIC PATIENT

Eileen Triolo

The nursing management of the geriatric orthopaedic patient presents a unique challenge to the professional nurse. In order to plan, deliver, and evaluate quality care, the nurse must have an extensive knowledge base. The geriatric patient will have age-related physiologic changes and health problems that differ from those of the younger patient. The elderly patient may have multiple medical problems, nursing needs, and psychologic and socioeconomic problems requiring nursing intervention. All of the nurse's resources, varied knowledge base, and skills are used to provide quality care to the older patient. The nurse attempts to understand the total person and to meet the multidimensional needs of the elderly patient through the nursing process.

THE NURSING PROCESS

The nursing process is a problem-solving approach to nursing management and includes four basic elements: assessment, planning, intervention, and evaluation. The assessment phase of the nursing process may be divided further into three steps: the interview or data collection, the analysis of data, and the identification of needs. Following the assessment phase, the nurse develops a nursing care plan to meet the needs identified, carries out that plan of care in the intervention phase, and then evaluates the effectiveness of the care delivered. It is in the evaluation phase of the nursing process that the nurse asks questions such as: Have the established goals been met? Is the intervention effective? Has the problem been resolved? The nurse may find that the answer is not always in the affirmative and will then have to reassess, alter the plan of care, and change selected nursing interventions. The nursing process is thus cyclic, ongoing, and dynamic in nature.

The nursing process permits individualization in the delivery of nursing care. Specific goal setting and planning that is individualized communicates to the older person the nurse's interest in and awareness of him as a unique individual.

Before beginning the assessment phase of the nursing process, the nurse caring for the elderly patient should have a knowledge base that includes an awareness of the theories of aging, the biologic and psychosocial changes that occur with age, and the communication skills that enhance the health assessment.

Assessment interview

The nursing assessment usually begins with the patient interview. The nurse should start with a brief, friendly social interaction and then proceed to more goal-directed communication. Goals should be developed mutually and pursued by both the nurse and patient. The nurse should establish the appropriate climate, facilitate accuracy in communication, validate information received, and evaluate the results.

A major obstacle to overcome in communicating with the elderly person is focusing on the age of the patient. Frequently, nurses bring to interactions with an elderly patient their stereotypes and perceptions of how they believe an elderly person should think, act, or feel. Nurses may see themselves and their own aging process projected in the patient. This will put a nonverbal dimension into nurses' communication style and content, which may have a negative effect on the therapeutic relationship. If nurses are aware of their own feelings and attitudes toward the aging process, they can then appreciate the uniqueness of this life experience for each individual older adult.

The nurse must be alert to nonverbal communication as well as to verbal statements. It is often the nonverbal part of the interaction that expresses further meanings, feelings, or emotions attached to ideas. Many times, people communicate messages that show inconsistency between the verbal statements and the nonverbal body language that accompanies these statements. Nurses should be aware of their own body language as well as of the patient's during the interview. The nurse can help promote wellness in the older patient by maintaining the person's self-esteem and dignity. Touching can be reassuring and help communicate acceptance. The nurse should attempt to communicate acceptance and respect for the feelings and values of the older patient.

In the elderly reminiscence can be a valuable therapeutic tool and communication outlet. Reminiscence and reviewing one's life occurs as part of the process of understanding events. It helps the elderly person to maintain self-esteem and reinforces a sense of identity. This reviewing of the past provides an outlet for coping with the stresses of today. The information revealed can provide a link between past and present that enables the nurse to understand the patient's current behavior or response to illness.

Data collection and assessing needs. The nurse-patient relationship begins during assessment, and the data obtained provides information about the patient's level of functioning and life satisfaction. The nursing history and assessment should focus on the meaning of illness to the person as well as on the pathology. Although the form used will vary from institution to institution, the information collected will be similar in content.

The health history usually begins with identifying data such as name, address, sex, and age. A concise statement should be made as to the patient's reason for seeking medical care or hospitalization. The patient's perception of the problem and his health status is important in learning the meaning of illness to this person. The nurse should ask the patient to describe the problem or illness that brought him to the health agency. It is also important to ask about the patient's past medical history and illnesses. The information obtained should include previous hospitalizations, previous surgery, medical conditions, and psychiatric and obstetric history if applicable. The patient should be asked about routine or periodic examinations, the last Pap smear, and any recent exposure to known cases of illness or communicable diseases. The patient should be questioned carefully about allergies including information on the causative substances and the reaction they produced. Measurement of vital signs should include blood pressure, pulse, respirations, temperature, height, and weight.

The nursing history should also include information about personal habits such as the use of tobacco, alcohol, and medications. The nurse should determine what the patient knows about medications, including the purpose and common side effects, and the present schedule and dosage for each medication taken. Over-the-counter drugs are often not considered medications by patients, and the nurse must inquire specifically about such items as laxatives, aspirin, or vitamins.

It is important to determine what the elderly person is able to do and how that individual feels about what he can do. In general, most older persons are realistic about their health status, but elderly persons will at times overestimate their health and ignore symptoms or attribute them to the aging process. They will frequently assume that symptoms are age related and not worth mentioning.

The orthopaedic nurse will be particularly interested in functional capacity and in assessing the person's ability to carry out activities of daily living. Posture and gait can usually be assessed immediately upon meeting the patient. The assessment should include a determination of range of motion in all joints and of muscle strength.

The nurse should be particularly alert to any abnormal movements including the presence of tremors, spasticity, and/or rigidity. Peripheral sensation should also be assessed. The nurse should question the patient about the use of assistive devices for mobility and about any prescribed exercise programs.

Many orthopaedic disorders cause pain and this area of concern to both patient and nurse should be assessed. Pain is a subjective experience and the nurse must question the person thoroughly but tactfully. The nurse should include questions about the quality, intensity, and location of pain and about measures used to alleviate pain and their perceived effectiveness. Many nurses use a PQRST approach to assessing pain. This involves the obtaining of information about what promotes or palliates the pain, the quality of the pain, the region of pain and whether it radiates, any signs and symptoms that accompany the pain, and the temporal aspects of the pain, such as when the pain occurs or how long it lasts.

The patient's skin condition should be assessed and information obtained about previous skin conditions, current skin problems, general skin care needs, and any areas of ulceration, discoloration, redness, or scar tissue.

In the elderly the nurse should also assess for the presence of sensory deficits. The elderly patient may have impaired hearing, vision, speech, taste, or touch.

The nursing assessment of functional ability in activities of daily living should be thorough and specific. The nurse might begin collecting data about activity patterns by asking how the patient spends an average day. It should be determined whether the patient perceives present behavior and activities to be altered from the previous level of functioning. The degree to which the elderly individual is able to carry out such activities of daily living as hygiene, walking, eating, and dressing should be ascertained. The nurse should use questions for each area of activity. For example, when evaluating the ability to perform personal hygiene independently, one might ask about the ability to bathe, shave, comb and wash hair, or brush teeth. A patient who can feed himself may still not be independent in meeting nutritional needs. The patient should be asked if he can shop for groceries, prepare meals, feed himself, cut the food, or use ordinary utensils. Dressing can be very difficult for patients with limited mobility, pain, or limited range of motion, and the nurse should ask: Is the patient able to get into a bra, underclothes, shirt, dress, trousers, shoes, and socks? Can the patient fasten buttons, snaps, or zippers? Is the patient capable of applying the brace, sling, or corset?

It is important to include data on activity patterns during the night and to obtain a sleep history. Older people tend to have sleep disturbances. The elderly person often sleeps less at night, has difficulty staying asleep, and naps during the day. Physical disorders or medications may interfere with the sleep cycle. Older persons experiencing chronic pain may report multiple arousals during the night. The patient should be asked about methods used at home to facilitate sleep and their effectiveness.

Nutritional status and fluid intake should be evaluated. Those patients on prescribed special diets should be assessed by a dietician during their hospital stay. The elderly are susceptible to food faddism, particularly diets that promise to improve health and cure disease. Older adults may not have an adequate total fluid intake, and diuretics may tend to further deplete fluid reserves. The patient should be questioned about the amount of salt used and about any problems with weight gain, poor appetite, constipation, or excessive flatulence.

Psychosocial aspects of the nursing assessment. The nursing assessment should include information about the patient's present life-style. A description of the home environment, family life, affiliations, and occupation should be obtained. The patient should be asked about religious preference and special interests or hobbies. It is important to determine the number and types of social contacts as well as the following information: Does the client live alone? Is there a friend or relative nearby to provide assistance? What is the home environment like? Are there stairs to climb or potential safety hazards? Can the nurse assist the patient with home care arrangements? How has the present health problem affected the person's life-style?

The nurse should remember that every stage of life presents its own special conflicts and needs. The interpersonal experiences of the elderly may assist or hinder resolution of the conflicts of old age. The major task during this stage includes attempts to accept and integrate past life experiences with the present situation. The elderly person needs to adjust to physical changes, loss of loved ones, and social role changes. Illness and hospitalization may intensify difficulties in conflict resolution and result in depression, withdrawal, loss of self-esteem, bitterness, or anger. Nursing approaches to the elderly should maximize the person's sense of worth and self-esteem.

Planning, intervention, and evaluation

The nursing care plan is the documentation of the application of the nursing process. When the assessment has been completed, the nurse will organize the data collected, identify problems or concerns, and begin to plan care. The written care plan reflects the fact that the nursing process has been used as a basic framework in the delivery of care. The nurse formulating a care plan will begin with a set of identified needs, establish priorities among needs, formulate goals or objectives, select nursing interventions, and choose appropriate evaluation methods.

Selecting priority needs. The professional nurse frequently uses Maslow's hierarchy of needs as a basis for priority selection. All people have certain basic needs that must be met in order to maintain homeostasis. According to Maslow, there is a hierarchy among needs, moving from lower physiologic needs to the highest psychologic need of self-actualization. Lower ranking needs must be partly or wholly satisfied before higher needs emerge and exert their influence. This hierarchy of needs can be viewed as a series of steps with physiologic needs emerging first, followed by needs related to safety and security, then love and belonging, self-esteem, and finally self-actualization or self-fulfillment of one's potential.

Physiologic needs are of utmost importance and they will emerge first and will dominate the conscious mind if unmet. Once basic physiologic needs are satisfied, the concern for safety and security emerges. The need for love and belonging will be of concern after physiologic and safety needs have been met. The need to preserve self-esteem emerges when lower order needs have been satisfied. Finally the need for self-actualization becomes apparent.

The nurse can apply this hierarchy of needs to setting priorities among the patient's health care needs. Physiologic needs would be given high priority and must be met first. Safety and security needs would have the next priority, and then would come the need for love and acceptance, the need to preserve self-esteem, and finally the need for self-actualization.

Formulating goals. After ranking problems according to priority, the nurse should establish the goals and write an objective for each problem or concern identified. The nurse first determines the outcome or change desired in the patient. The desired outcome may be in the area of knowledge, skills, or attitudes. The goal may be that the patient acquire knowledge about a health problem, perform a particular activity, or alter his attitude about a prescribed therapy.

Whenever possible, long-term and short-term goals should be established. Goals or objectives should be patient centered, mutually set, realistic, and measurable. Goals should be compatible with the overall therapeutic regimen. Goals that are specific, observable, and measurable will facilitate later evaluation of the nursing care.

Intervention and evaluation of the plan of care. Once specific goals have been formulated, the nurse will select a nursing approach and nursing interventions that will help the patient achieve the goals. The nursing approach and actions to be carried out are documented in the care plan. These nursing actions or interventions are designed to meet stated objectives. They should be specific to the individual's needs and communicate what to do and how to do it. The nursing actions if followed by all who care for the patient will provide continuity in nursing care. It is during the intervention phase of the nursing process that the nurse carries out selected actions and implements the plan of care.

Evaluating the patient's response to nursing interventions is essential to the nursing process. The selection of evaluation methods is part of the care planning process and should reflect desired outcomes or goals. The evaluation is based on criteria derived from these goals and objectives of care. In order to evaluate whether a nursing intervention has been successful, the nurse needs clearly stated, measurable objectives of care.

It is in this evaluation phase of the nursing process that the nurse compares present nursing management with the ideal and attempts to determine the extent to which goals have been achieved. This is the final step in the nursing process, but it can be the indicator of a need to reassess, select new nursing interventions, and alter the plan of care.

NURSING CARE OF THE ELDERLY PATIENT UNDERGOING ORTHOPAEDIC SURGERY

Older persons tolerate elective surgery surprisingly well despite the psychologic and physical stresses imposed by surgery. With aging there is a loss of physiologic reserve and the homeostatic mechanisms are less efficient. The ability to return to normal when external stress occurs is less than in younger persons.

The dangers of surgery for the elderly patient are increased in the presence of multiple medical problems. The severity of coexisting disease, along with the nature and duration of the procedure, will affect surgical risk. Lower reserve capacity in renal and cardiopulmonary systems increases surgical risk. The older person requires more time for the body to recover and return to normal after illness. Alterations in the immune mechanism may lower resistance to infection and prolonged healing time can result from diabetes, atherosclerosis, or nutritional deficiency. In the elderly patient the hazards of urinary retention, oversedation, overhydration, and immobility must be avoided. The nurse must keep in mind this decrease in physiologic reserve when planning and providing preoperative or postoperative care to the elderly patient.

Preoperative nursing care

The nurse should attempt to prevent unnecessary demands on adaptive capacity. The patient's ability to maintain homeostasis in the presence of continued strain is lessened with age. Long-range goals include the prevention of complications, regaining the preoperative level of functioning, or improving functional capacity. In order to restore the patient to independent functioning the nurse must obtain the patient's active cooperation.

The nurse will discover more optimistic outlooks in patients who realize that the proposed surgery is less hazardous than the disease it is designed to remedy. The nurse can do much to alleviate anxiety by providing adequate preoperative teaching and preparation.

Preoperative preparation should include an explanation of the plan of care. The patient should be told what to expect before surgery, including skin preparation, preoperative medications, intravenous therapy, and whether the patient will be in the recovery room after surgery or in a post-surgical intensive care area. The anticipated presence of dressings, drainage tubes, special positioning, and exercises should be explained and demonstrated if possible.

The nurse should teach deep breathing and coughing techniques to prevent pulmonary complications. If respiratory treatments, such as intermittant positive pressure breathing (IPPB), will be used, the patient will need an explanation of their purpose and instruction in their use. This should be started before surgery so that detailed instructions need not be imposed immediately postoperatively.

The elderly patient may require repeated explanations, clarifications, and reassurances. The nurse should provide clear, simple explanations in a soothing voice.

When multiple diseases affecting vital systems exist, thorough preoperative medical evaluation may be necessary. Ideally, deficiencies are corrected before surgical intervention, but this is not always possible. The cardiovascular, renal, and respiratory systems along with the nutritional status are evaluated. The anesthesia plan and surgical procedure are discussed with the patient by the appropriate health team members. Abnormal laboratory values, symptoms of infection, and abnormal vital signs should be brought to the physician's attention preoperatively.

Postoperative nursing care

Postoperative care of the elderly is similar to that given other patients, and nurses should apply their knowledge of basic postoperative management when dealing with this group of patients. It is necessary to provide additional support, however, to body systems with impaired function. It is important to focus care on the prevention of complications since older patients' decreased reserve capacity makes them more vulnerable to system failures.

Cardiovascular concerns. Cardiovascular disease is a common problem among elderly patients. The heart, brain, and kidneys are very sensitive to a reduction in perfusion and oxygenation. Postoperatively, blood pressure, pulse, respiratory rate, temperature, and urinary output must be monitored carefully. Deviations from normal should be reported promptly. The older person does not tolerate hypotension and reduced blood volume, so blood pressure must be maintained near normal values. The urinary output should be measured and recorded, as it is an indicator of adequate perfusion and blood volume. When shock is treated with fluid replacement, the central venous pressure should be measured frequently to prevent circulatory overload.

The neurovascular status of the extremities should be assessed frequently. Peripheral pulses, color, temperature, movement, sensation, and circulation to all limbs are evaluated. For example, the patient is instructed to avoid positions that encourage venous stasis. For example, the patient should avoid crossing his legs while sitting. Also, the head and foot of the bed should not be elevated simultaneously because this position promotes stasis in the pelvic veins.

The nurse should attempt to prevent venous complications, such as thrombophlebitis, in patients requiring bed rest. Preventive measures include frequent position changes, elastic stockings, leg exercises, avoidance of pressure on the calves of the legs, and adequate hydration. Anticoagulation therapy may be used to prevent vascular clotting. Activity promotes good circulation; therefore, active exercises and early ambulation are desirable.

Respiratory concerns. The older patient is at particular risk for pulmonary complications because of age-related changes in the lungs and chest. The lungs in the elderly have lost some of their elastic recoil, lung compliance is reduced, and there may be a progressive decline in vital capacity. Decreased lung expansion, weakness, and a drug-depressed cough reflex will contribute to complications such as atelectasis and pneumonia.

The nurse must observe the nature and quality of respirations as well as the respiratory rate and should note any dyspnea, rapid shallow respirations, coughing, or sputum production. It is important to ensure adequate hydration and promote aeration with frequent turning, coughing, and deep breathing exercises. Early ambulation will help prevent pulmonary complications.

Fluid and electrolyte balance. Intake and output should be accurately measured and recorded. Intravenous fluids and transfusions must be administered at a slow rate; the older person's circulatory system and heart will not tolerate overloading, and excessive fluid or too rapid infusion rates may result in pulmonary edema. Symptoms of this serious complication include shortness of breath, wheezing, cough, frothy sputum, sensation of pressure in the chest, elevated pulse, and rapid respiratory rate. Monitoring of central venous pressure will also indicate circulatory overload.

If an indwelling urinary catheter is ordered, the nurse must be certain that strict asepsis is maintained in its insertion and care. A closed drainage system must always be used and adequate fluid intake encouraged.

Gastrointestinal and nutritional concerns. Gastrointestinal distention and ileus may follow major surgery and general anesthesia, extensive trauma, and intraabdominal procedures. Lack of muscle tone of the large bowel, fecal impaction, and the use of narcotics that reduce peristalsis may cause ileus.

In the elderly sluggish peristalsis in the colon may result in imcomplete evacuation, retention of fecal matter, and impaction. Reduced activity and having to use a bedpan will also promote constipation. A laxative that supplies bulk or lubrication may be necessary. To help prevent or alleviate constipation the nurse should encourage adequate fluids, fruit juices, and a diet with adequate bulk.

The nurse should not give fluids or food by mouth until the gastrointestinal tract is functioning normally. Normal function is indicated by the presence of bowel sounds, absence of distention, and the passage of flatus or feces from the rectum.

When first beginning oral fluids, the nurse should restrict the amount to approximately 30 ml per hour. Fluids should be discontinued if the patient vomits or the abdomen becomes distended. Adequate nutrition is important for wound healing and prevention of infection. The diet is increased as the patient tolerates it, and the selection of a well-balanced diet is encouraged.

Wound and skin care. The nurse should routinely observe dressings postoperatively for bleeding or drainage. Frequently after major orthopaedic surgery a wound drain and suction apparatus is used. The use of wound suction decreases the likelihood of wound hematoma. The drainage tube from the wound is usually attached to a low-suction device. The nurse must carefully observe wound drainage and measure and record its amount. Fluid that is excessive in amount or bright red must be reported promptly. The wound suction is ordinarily discontinued 48 hours after surgery.

The nurse should maintain strict aseptic technique when changing dressings to prevent wound infection. Encouraging adequate fluid intake and nutrition will promote wound healing and decrease the possibility of infection. In elderly patients the temperature-regulating mechanisms are less reliable as indicators of infection. Since an elderly patient may show little change in body temperature in response to an infection, the nurse must therefore be alert to subtle increases in respiratory rate or pulse rate.

Skin care is very important, and the nurse is responsible for preventing decubitus ulcers. Decubiti may be caused by any of the following: immobility; diminished circulation; irritation or abrasions; poor nutritional status; pressure on bony prominences; incontinence; reduced sensation to pressure or pain; debilitation; rough, moist bed linen; and shearing forces. The goal is to maintain skin integrity and preventive measures must be implemented. Bony prominences should be inspected and massaged regularly. Daily skin care, cleanliness, frequent position changes, and adequate nutrition are essential. The use of sheepskin or an alternating air pressure mattress may be helpful. The affected limb should be inspected for signs of pressure and circulatory status should be monitored conscientiously. Ambulation should be initiated as soon as possible after surgery.

Pain management. The nurse should make every effort to treat pain promptly. Patients should be made aware of the fact that medication is available to relieve pain and that they will receive more relief from analgesics if the pain has not become too severe. Intense pain that is unrelieved may cause weakness, pallor, sweating, nausea, and vomiting.

The elderly patient should receive enough medication to relieve pain but not so much that it depresses respirations. Pain relief with analgesics should promote activity and facilitate rest. The side effects of narcotics can be dangerous, and any signs of respiratory depression or the presence of stupor should be reported immediately.

Exercise and ambulation. Early ambulation is most instrumental in the prevention of complications. Ambulation should be started as soon as the patient's condition permits. The nurse should remember that the elderly patient with preexisting pulmonary or cardiac problems must be watched carefully. Ambulation and periods out of bed should be gradually increased to avoid overexertion. Vital signs should be monitored and used as a guide to the elderly person's response to exercise and activity. Those patients for whom bed rest is prescribed are particularly at risk for the development of complications. Activity in bed should be encouraged including turning, position changes, flexing and extending the arms and legs, and deep breathing and coughing. Sitting positions that promote venous stasis must be avoided. The over-

head trapeze is helpful for the patient in raising up and strengthening the upper extremities. Muscle strength and joint function must be maintained. Range-of-motion exercises to all joints should be part of the care plan.

The nurse must be aware of what surgical procedure was performed and what activity is allowed. Information as to the exact position of the extremity, the amount of weight bearing permitted, and turning and transferring techniques should be clearly written in the nursing care plan.

Summary

The elderly patient undergoing orthopaedic surgery requires knowledgeable, skillful nursing management. The nurse must have a firm knowledge base in orthopaedic care as well as in geriatric nursing concepts. The elderly frequently have multiple problems that require nursing interventions. The nurse who provides individualized care to this rapidly growing patient population will discover a most rewarding professional experience.

References

1. Brunner, L.S., and Suddarth, D.S.: Textbook of medical-surgical nursing, ed. 4, Philadelphia, 1980, J.B. Lippincott Co.
2. Burnside, I.M., editor: Nursing and the aged, ed. 2, New York, 1981, McGraw-Hill Book Co.
3. Combs, K.K.: Preventive health care in the elderly, Am. J. Nurs. **78:**1340-1341, 1978.
4. Forbes, E.J., and Fitzsimons, V.M.: The older adult: a process for wellness, St. Louis, 1981, The C.V. Mosby Co.
5. Hilt, N.E., and Cogburn, S.B.: Manual of orthopedics, St. Louis, 1980, The C.V. Mosby Co.
6. Mezey, M., Rauckhorst, L., and Stokes, S.: Health assessment of the older individual, New York, 1980, Springer Publishing Co.
7. Mischel, W., and Mischel, N.: Essentials of psychology, New York, 1977, Random House.
8. Murray, R., Huelskoetter, M.M., and O'Driscoll, D.: The nursing process in later maturity, Englewood Cliffs, N.J., 1980, Prentice-Hall, Inc.

chapter 20
REHABILITATION

SECTION I
Concepts of Rehabilitation
Vernon L. Nickel
Erin McGurk-Burleson

In classical rehabilitation a variety of allied health professionals are needed to achieve the best results, that is, the least amount of permanent physical disability with maximum independence and at the least cost both of money and of social disability. These specialists are the rehabilitation nurse, physical therapist, occupational therapist, speech therapist, social worker, clinical psychologist, and vocational counselor.

In modern rehabilitation centers it has been shown that subspecialization by disease categories, such as spinal cord injury, brain injury, stroke, and amputation, leads to optimal results. Examples of highly successful categorical programs are spinal cord injury, hand rehabilitation, and sports medicine.

The classical orthopaedic problem in the geriatric patient, however, can usually be well served by the maximal intervention of the physical therapist, and therefore the role of the physical therapist will be highlighted in this chapter. It is also particularly fitting that the close association between the orthopaedic surgeon and the physical therapist be emphasized since the beginning and development of the field of physical therapy was in very large measure the result of direct collaboration with the early orthopaedic surgeons. Yet it must be emphasized that we clearly recognize that the utilization of other allied health professions may not only be most helpful to geriatric patients, but also that it is often absolutely essential.

ROLE OF THE PHYSICAL THERAPIST

Of all the health professionals who might engender an attitude of obtaining maximal function and preventing unnecessary complications, the physical therapist is best suited for such a role. It is an excellent idea to have a physical therapist consult with a physician regarding a patient who suffers from a disorder that results in physical deconditioning so that such a patient does not reach the stage when unnecessary complications such as significant contractural deformities, fractures as a result of falls, or pressure sores develop. Even a minor hip, knee, or ankle flexion deformity can very significantly reduce the ability of a person to perform functional activities of daily living such as ambulation, and in conditions where general paresis is present, such as after a stroke, this kind of deformity can effectively prevent ambulation. Prevention of complications must be aggressively addressed or if they have already occurred immediate action should be taken to correct them. With the intervention of physical therapy, maintenance of the geriatric person's maximal level of physical activity can be encouraged so that even with overlying medical problems deconditioning will be minimized.

MAINTENANCE OF ACTIVITY AND PREVENTION OF DECONDITIONING

As an individual becomes older, there is a natural wasting of muscle tissue. Therefore, it is important to institute a reasonable exercise program compatible with the person's maximal level of activity. This is particularly true in those who have suffered an additional physical disability. With the

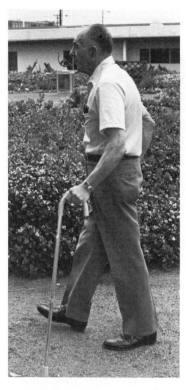

FIG. 20-1. Walking can be an excellent form of exercise.

proper instruction and supervision from a physical therapist, a program of physical exercise can be instituted and maintained. The exercises should be done at least once a day and for an adequate period of time. It has been well established that cardiopulmonary reserve is beneficially affected by such an exercise regimen. Associated with this are significant psychosocial benefits including the reduction of depression, an improved self-image, and a generally improved mental outlook.

If the person is able to walk, walking can be one of the best exercises for such a directed exercise program (Fig. 20-1). The optimal situation would be for the physical therapist to initiate the walking program while the individual is in the hospital and then to continue supervision into the patient's home situation through occasional reevaluations to see that the exercise program is maintained and upgraded appropriately.

If the person is nonambulatory, the exercise program should include a combination of exercises for stretching flexibility, coordination, and strengthening to be accomplished in the bed, on a mat, and/or sitting in a chair (Fig. 20-2). It is important

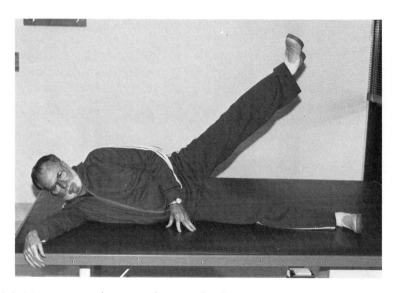

FIG. 20-2. Mat exercises for strengthening, flexibility, coordination, and stretching are an important component of all exercise programs, especially for nonambulatory individuals.

```
            EXERCISES TO OBTAIN NORMAL RANGE OF MOVEMENT IN JOINTS


Do the exercises marked by the instructor or therapist.  Repeat each exercise the number
of times indicated by the instructor.  At end of each exercise, return to original position.

Exercises

1.  Neck:
    a.  Bring head and neck forward touching chin on chest.
    b.  Bend head and neck backward as far as possible.
    c.  Tilt head and neck toward left shoulder; avoid raising shoulder toward head.
    d.  Tilt head toward right shoulder; avoid raising shoulder toward head.
    e.  Turn face to left side, then to right side, keeping neck, shoulders, and trunk
        straight.
    f.  Roll head in circular pattern, first in one direction, then in other.

2.  Shoulder:
    (Exercise may be done while sitting, standing, or lying down.)
    a.  With arm straight at side, raise it forward and upward overhead, keeping trunk
        straight.
    b.  With arm straight at side, raise it sideways and upward overhead, keeping trunk
        straight.
    c.  Put palm of hand on or near back of neck; then rotate arm downward and place
        hand in small of back.  Place hand on hip if lying down.

3.  Elbow:
    a.  Bend elbow until finger tips touch shoulder if possible; fully straighten arm.
    b.  With upper part of arm at side of body and elbow bent to a right angle, turn palm
        upward; turn palm downward.

4.  Wrist:
    Keep upper part of arm at side of body, bend elbow to a right angle, and hold hand
    out straight with thumb side of wrist up.
    a.  Move hand toward body as far as possible; move hand away from body.
    b.  Move hand upward as far as possible; move hand downward as far as possible.
    c.  Move wrist so that hand describes a cone-shaped pattern.
    d.  Turn palm upward; turn palm downward.

5.  Fingers and thumb:
    a.  Bend fingers making a fist; fully straighten fingers.
    b.  Keep fingers straight and spread them wide apart; bring fingers together.
    c.  Keep fingers straight and bend hand at knuckles.
    d.  Keep thumb bent and placed against palm; pull it across palm toward little finger.
    e.  With thumb straight and lying parallel to and on palmar side of index finger,
        raise it straight up from palm.  Pull down.
    f.  Touch tip of thumb to tip of little finger; open hand wide; repeat, touching each
        finger with thumb.

6.  Hip:
    a.  Lie on back with knee bent; bring knee toward body as far as possible.
    b.  Lie on back; move leg out to side as far as possible, keeping knee and hip straight
        and toes pointed straight upward.
    c.  Lie on back; roll leg inward as far as possible, then outward.
    d.  Lie on abdomen; raise leg straight upward as far as possible, keeping knee straight
        and pelvis and abdomen flat on table.
    e.  Sit with hip and knee bent and lower part of leg hanging over edge of chair or bed;
        move one foot inward in front of other leg, which will rotate thigh outward.
    f.  Sit with lower part of leg hanging over edge of chair or bed; move one foot outward,
        rotating thigh inward.
    g.  Sit with lower part of leg hanging over edge of chair or bed; raise knee and thigh
        upward toward chest.
```

FIG. 20-3. Sample exercise program for strengthening and stretching.

Continued.

EXERCISES TO OBTAIN NORMAL RANGE OF MOVEMENT IN JOINTS—cont'd

7. *Knee:*
   a. Sit on table; bend knee as far as possible, then straighten it.
   b. Lie on abdomen; bend knee as far as possible, then straighten it.

8. *Ankle and foot:*
   Sit on table with foot hanging free.
   a. Raise toes and foot upward as far as possible.
   b. Bend toes and foot downward as far as possible.
   c. With foot at right angle to leg, turn sole in toward other foot.
   d. With foot at right angle to leg, turn end of foot outward away from other foot.
   e. Turn end of foot in and up, keeping toes bent.
   f. Move ankle so that big toe describes a circle (circumduction).

9. *Trunk:*
   a. Stand with feet about 2 inches apart; bend forward, arms hanging down; attempt to touch toes but avoid bending knees.
   b. Stand with feet about 2 inches apart; bend backward, arms hanging down; avoid bending knees.
   c. From standing position, bend upper part of body to left.
   d. From standing position, bend upper part of body to right.
   e. Twist upper part of body to left without turning pelvis.
   f. Twist upper part of body to right without turning pelvis.

Fig. 20-3, cont'd. Sample exercise program for strengthening and stretching.

to utilize exercises aimed at all of the major joints and muscle groups to obtain an optimal overall conditioning effect rather than to emphasize solely one exercise aspect, such as strengthening at the expense of losing range of motion. This more stationary type of exercise regimen should also be incorporated into the ambulatory person's walking program in a shortened version in order to establish a well-rounded exercise routine. It can be utilized effectively as the warm-up for the ambulation exercise (Fig. 20-3).

PRONING

Another simple practice that has numerous beneficial results is proning; that is, when the individual lies on his stomach for a significant period of time. Proning is a valuable technique that aids greatly in the prevention of contractural deformities. For example, proning has the remarkably beneficial effect of preventing or even correcting the marked tendency of the elderly to develop hip and knee flexion and ankle plan-

tar flexion deformities. Proning is also an effective way to decrease focal skin pressure points. The most obvious advantage of proning is that the skin of the buttocks and sacrum is completely relieved of any pressure and thus it has the opportunity to dry thoroughly and be aerated.

The geriatric person typically does not prone as frequently as is recommended and often may not prone at all. However, with training even very elderly and quite ill patients can be taught to prone for appropriate periods of time in intervals throughout the day and night.

The appropriate position for proning is with the feet projecting over the edge of the mattress and the knees and hips straight (Fig. 20-4). Preferably, the thighs are also abducted slightly to decrease pressure on the medial part of the knees and to encourage abduction range. Care should be taken to check the skin over the anterior iliac crests, knees, and dorsal aspects of the feet for redness after proning. If there is a tendency for redness, pillows should be placed under bony prominences before proning to aid in relieving pressure (Fig. 20-5). Most patients feel quite comfortable proning for up to an hour several times a day. During proning, it is recommended that the patient elevate both arms over the head, which effectively aids in maintaining range of motion at the shoulder joints, which exhibit a tendency toward increased tightness as age progresses and activity lessens (Fig. 20-6).

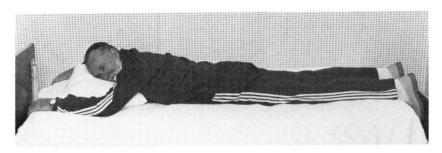

FIG. 20-4. Proning is a valuable technique to aid in maintaining normal range of motion.

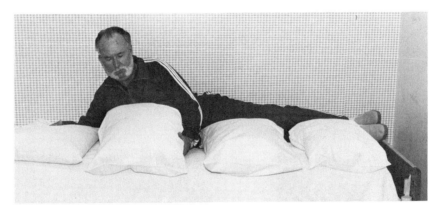

FIG. 20-5. If there is a tendency for redness, pillows should be placed under bony prominences before proning to help in relieving pressure.

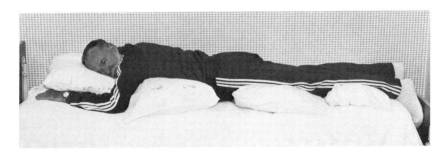

FIG. 20-6. It is beneficial to elevate both arms overhead during proning to aid in maintaining normal range of motion in shoulders.

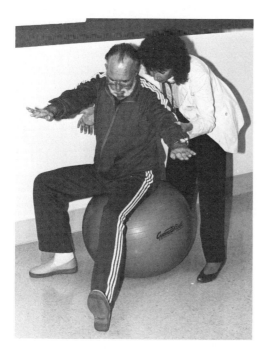

Fig. 20-7. Formal physical therapy treatments can be directed toward improving balance and coordination.

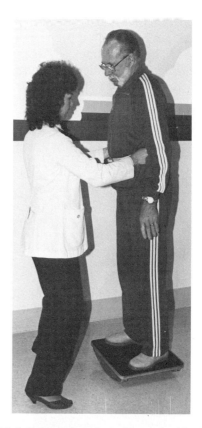

Fig. 20-8. Balance board can be a valuable device to aid in stimulating balance reactions.

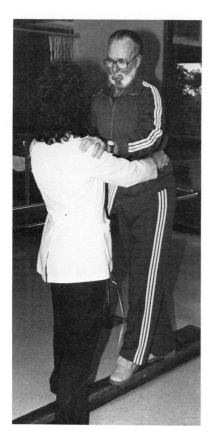

Fig. 20-9. Physical therapist can be instrumental in incorporating balance and coordination exercises into a daily exercise program.

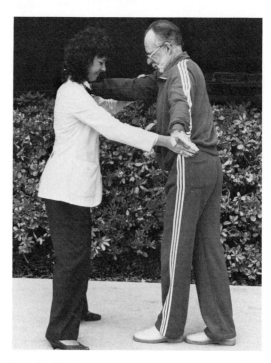

Fig. 20-10. Exercise program can progress from simple weight shifting in stance to practicing more difficult tandem and cross-stepping gait techniques.

BALANCE, COORDINATION, AND PROPRIOCEPTION

With advancing age balance becomes an important problem, and numerous falls and fractures occur when individuals are not able to balance appropriately. In addition, decreased coordination skills and reduced proprioception often complicate this balance problem. The physical therapist can be instrumental in incorporating balance and coordination exercises into a daily exercise program to stimulate improvement in these areas (Figs. 20-7 to 20-9). The exercise program can progress from simple weight shifting in stance to practicing more difficult tandem and cross-stepping gait techniques (Fig. 20-10). Completing repetitions of reciprocal limb movements and patterns of stepping through a floor ladder are examples of exercises utilized to improve coordination (Fig. 20-11).

The therapist can also teach the patient and the family safety techniques and make them aware of potential safety problems. For example, one preventative measure that can be recommended to the elderly when balance becomes a problem is discontinuing the use of throw rugs in the home (Fig. 20-12). A physical therapist can effectively evaluate the patient's home environment to determine hazards and can give recommendations for ensuring the patient's safety.

The physical therapist might also suggest that the individual sit up for a period of time before standing to prevent lightheadedness and possible fainting, which is a frequent complaint of geriatric individuals. Use of a bedside commode when getting up during the night may be recommended to the patient. Fainting episodes are common in the elderly population and except for the danger of patients' falling and injuring themselves, which is of course most serious, the problems, such as cardiovascular collapse associated with fainting episodes, are generally overrated.

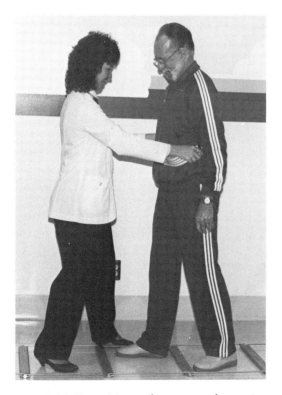

FIG. 20-11. Repetitions of patterns of stepping through a floor ladder are useful for improving coordination skills.

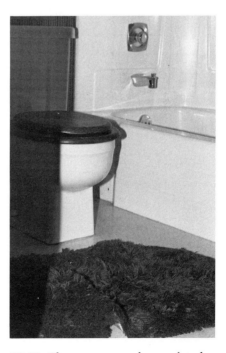

FIG. 20-12. Throw rugs can be a safety hazard, especially for people with balance and gait problems and visual impairments.

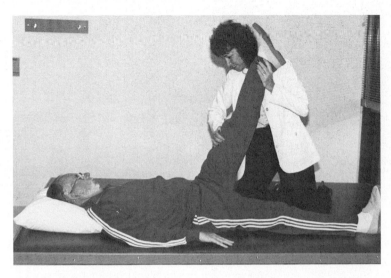

Fig. 20-13. Physical therapist can teach family members or attendants how to perform range-of-motion exercises with patient to aid in prevention of joint deformities and contractures.

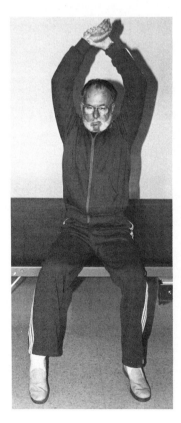

Fig. 20-14. Patient with hemiplegia can perform range-of-motion exercises with involved extremity by using uninvolved arm.

Contractural Deformities

Contractural deformities are unfortunately all too common in the geriatric population and they are frequently present in the chronically disabled. Yet, it is a fact that except in instances of severe spasticity such contractures can usually easily be prevented.

To prevent such contractural deformities, it is essential that a range-of-motion program be instituted and carried out, preferably at least once a day. It is a clinical fact that almost any joint that is taken through a full range of motion once a day will not develop a contractural deformity. In those unusual instances where a single range of motion is not adequate more frequent ranging should be instituted. Here, again, a physical therapist may be a key person in teaching the patient, family, and attendants about the devastating effects of contractural deformities and the method of preventing them (Fig. 20-13).

For those individuals who require another person to do their daily care activities, such as bathing, it is an excellent procedure to teach such helpers to incorporate a full range of motion of all the major joints into the bathing routine. It has been established that a properly instructed person can accomplish the range-of-motion exercises by adding less than 3 minutes additional time to the daily dressing or bathing procedures. Patients who are physically able to do their own range-of-motion exercises should be taught the importance and precise mechanism of doing so. For example, a patient with hemiplegia could range the involved arm with the opposite arm and could also learn specific range-of-motion exercises to do with the paretic lower extremity (Fig. 20-14).

Patients with arthritis, both degenerative and rheumatoid, need to be very aggressively educated about the importance of performing range-of-motion exercises, since the tendency for losing range in the involved joints is inevitable.

A very common practice in caring for an elderly person is to put pillows under the person's knees when the person is supine. This is actually quite harmful because the position leads to flexion deformities of the hips, knees, and ankles. Obviously, discontinuation of this practice, in addition to the proning and range-of-motion exercises described previously, is beneficial in reducing problems, with contractural deformities.

PRESSURE SORES

Pressure sores, as the name implies, are caused by pressure. The use of the word "decubitus" is often a misnomer and has euphemistic overtones that fail to emphasize the fact that pressure sores are caused by pressure. In actual fact, a pressure sore is an area of tissue necrosis that has resulted from the loss of blood supply secondary to pressures that exceed capillary blood flow, which has been calibrated at approximately 40 mm Hg. Studies of such pressures have demonstrated that these pressure curves are sharply aggravated over bony prominences and, in actuality, pressure sores almost always occur in such places. The skin is most vulnerable to the development of pressure sores when it is damp, particularly when it is macerated,

when it is locally hot, and, of course, when there is an actual decrease in local circulation, such as in a patient with diabetes or peripheral vascular disease. Local shear forces increase pressure areas very significantly and make the development of necrosis more likely.

Pressure sores can be classified according to their four stages: The first is a slight reddening, the second is early blistering, the third is superficial skin necrosis, and the fourth is major ulceration. The early erythema that results from pressure to tissue should be a clear warning that aggressive measures need to be taken immediately to prevent further damage. The development of pressure sores is commonly blamed on a lack of adequate time to undertake appropriate measures to prevent them; yet, in actual fact, such ulcerations have occurred, the personnel time used to treat them far exceeds the time that would have been involved in their prevention.

The monetary costs of caring for such pressure sores are truly enormous, and often major surgical procedures have to be undertaken. Once a pressure sore has occurred, and even if it has healed, the tissues in the area will always be more vulnerable to ulcer recurrence. Again, it must be emphasized that those elderly individuals suffering from diabetes, peripheral vascular disease, or other causes of peripheral vascular insufficiency such as paralysis of a part of the body, decreased circulation, and poor nutrition are more vulnerable and less responsive to treatment, and therefore it is all the more urgent to practice rigorous preventative measures. If a patient requires the use of an orthosis or even a prosthesis, the same rigorous measures to prevent skin breakdown must be instituted since such patients are particularly vulnerable to skin breakdowns.

There are several things that can be done to promote good skin integrity. Regular exercise can help to increase circulation and to maintain good cardiovascular reserve. Careful skin checks around bony prominences, under braces and prosthetic devices, and in other potentially problematic

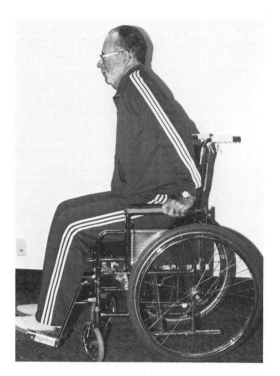

FIG. 20-15. Press-ups on arms of wheelchair will help relieve pressure on ischial tuberosities and sacrum and aid in prevention of pressure sores.

areas and subsequent relief of the cause of the pressure will help prevent pressure sores. If patients sit for long periods of time, especially if they are nonambulatory and wheelchair-bound, they should change their position frequently to shift the pressure and provide weight relief. Press-ups on the arms of the chair every 15 minutes will help to relieve the weight on the ischial tuberosities and sacrum, and frequent proning will provide intermittent pressure relief (Fig. 20-15).

It is also advisable to use a sufficiently dense foam or suitable air seat cushion to help in the reduction of pressure on the ischiums and greater trochanters. The cushion should be cut out around the bony areas, if necessary, to reduce the pressure to less than 40 mm Hg (Fig. 20-16). A physical therapist can be of value in suggesting the appropriate cushion, cutting it out, and measuring the subsequent pressure produced when the patient is in the sitting position.

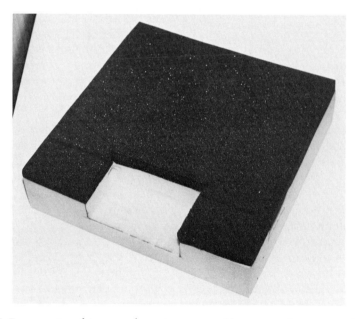

FIG. 20-16. Foam seat cushions can be cut out around bony prominences, such as ischial tuberosities, to reduce sitting pressures.

HOME EVALUATION

The physical therapist can be helpful in the evaluation of the elderly person's home, its degree of safety, and the patient's level of performance in the home situation. The areas to evaluate are the entrance to the dwelling, the stairs and other architectural barriers, the width of doorways and halls if the person is in a wheelchair, the ease of movement in significant areas as a result of the arrangement of furniture, and safety hazards in the bathroom (Fig. 20-17). Also important is the accessibility of clothes, kitchen utensils, food, telephones, light switches, faucets, and stove dials (Fig. 20-18). The height of tables, toilets, and bathtubs and the number and placements of emergency exits should be evaluated.

There are numerous home modifications that can be suggested for patients with specific medical disorders. For instance, a patient who has had a stroke should have his bed arranged so that he can get out on his most functional side. Other valuable modifications are the utilization of grab bars in

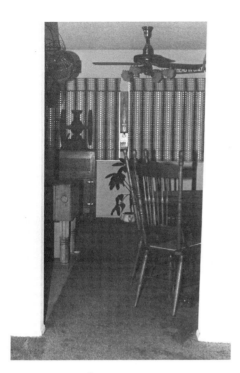

FIG. 20-17. Poor furniture arrangement or narrow doorways can have a detrimental effect on mobility of persons with gait difficulties or of those in wheelchairs.

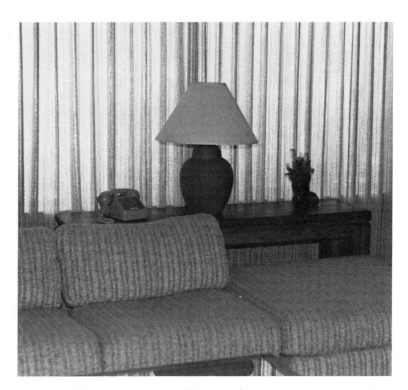

FIG. 20-18. Accessibility of telephone, light switches, faucets, and stove dials are important safety concerns, especially for a person in a wheelchair.

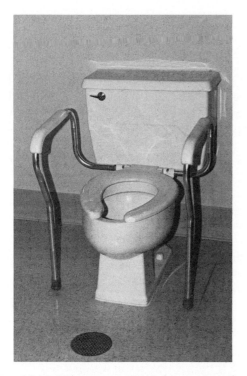

FIG. 20-19. Safety arms or raised seats on toilets can be valuable adaptation for a person with problems in balance or rising to stance.

strategic areas so that the patient can move securely from one area to another with a safety handhold. There are a number of adaptive devices for the bathroom including safety rails near the commodes, raised toilet seats, and adaptive bathing equipment especially designed for the patient's particular disability (Figs. 20-19 and 20-20). One of the most common unfortunate accidents with elderly patients occurs when the individual has difficulty in controlling hot water or moving out of the way of a running hot water tap and is therefore burned. There are special adaptions for faucets, and the physical therapist can also help to prevent such accidents by teaching the patient safety techniques. Teaching patients a pattern of where the furniture is located is quite helpful so that individuals with decreased mental and physical abilities, as well as those with visual and hearing deficits, develop habit patterns that result in more normal functioning.

In the aggressive attempt to maintain disabled individuals in a home situation, numerous community resources can be utilized. For example, the Meals-on-Wheels program will help the patient to maintain adequate nutrition. The patient may be able

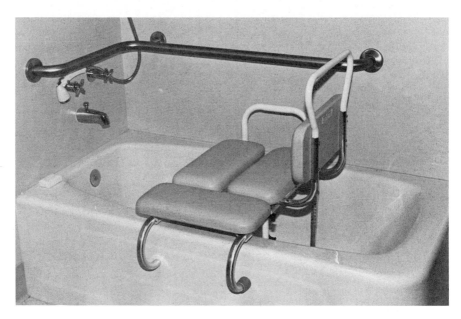

FIG. 20-20. Many adaptive devices are available to ensure safety and increase independence in bathing.

to take advantage of special adaptations such as books for the blind and visually impaired. The community often has support groups, such as stroke clubs or arthritis associations, that can be helpful in offering suggestions and support.

ADAPTIVE EQUIPMENT

The physical therapist is uniquely qualified to evaluate and recommend professional adaptive equipment, to aid in the procurement of these devices, and to institute a training program in their use. For example, the use of the appropriate type of crutches and instruction in crutch walking, with the authorization of a physician, allows the appropriate amount of graduated weight bearing that is needed in the treatment of the patient with a fractured hip. A quad cane will greatly aid the hemiplegic patient in ambulation. The physical therapist, working with the orthopaedist in ordering appropriate orthoses, such as an ankle-foot orthosis for drop-foot associated with hemiplegia, can help the patient to achieve more independent ambulation. The role of the physical therapist in training patients in the use of prosthetic devices has long been established.

Wheelchairs if they are to be used more than temporarily should be specifically fitted to the patient and have the appropriate adaptations needed by patients with that particular disability (Fig. 20-21). These adaptations include an appropriate cushion to prevent skin pressure. The appropriate seat measurements, height from the floor, type of arm and foot rests, and method of propulsion (one-handed wheelchair or electric chair) must be carefully determined according to the person's level of function. Often, wheelchair mobility is markedly reduced when appropriate equipment has not been provided.

References

1. Lister, M.J.: The physical therapist. In Nickel, V.L., editor: Orthopedic rehabilitation, New York, 1982, Churchill Livingston.
2. Nickel, V.L.: Orthopedic rehabilitation, New York, 1982, Churchill Livingston.

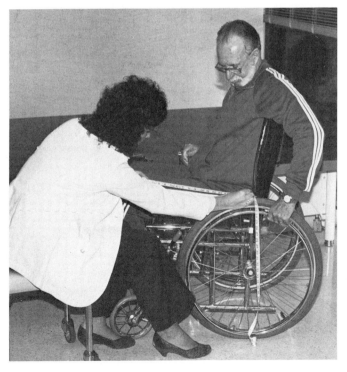

FIG. 20-21. Wheelchairs with appropriate adaptations should be specifically fitted to a patient to maximize independence and mobility.

SECTION II
Exercise and the Geriatric Patient
Cynthia D. Sculco

During the last decade, increasing emphasis has been placed on the importance of exercise, and adults of all ages have become involved in recreational and conditioning forms of exercise. Rather than becoming an exclusive domain of the young, exercise should be practiced by all age groups and the older adult, a person over 60 years of age, should definitely be included. For the older adult exercise is particularly important since it can provide the continued musculoskeletal function necessary for independent existence. It is not uncommon for an inactive elderly person to fall and fracture a hip and despite an uneventful recovery from a surgical stabilization not achieve the prior level of independent function. The cardiovascular conditioning provided by an exercise regimen has also been well documented.

How do we learn the importance of exercise as an essential ingredient in a healthful way of life? Research has supported the notion that activity habits learned at a young age are responsible for the orientation that one has toward activity in adulthood. Children exercise just for the joy or the sensation of movement. Exercise is incorporated as a part of their play and for them it also becomes a time for socialization. The principles children learn and use early in their lives are most applicable to the older adult. The practice of exercise just for the joy of being in touch with the body needs to be reemphasized in the older adult and it should also provide a time for socialization.

Through midlife, exercise methods are often quite competitive and in many instances involve significant body contact. These competitive sports are also self selecting and limited in total years of useful participation. Additionally, the principles of exercise as a means of maintaining one's body in a healthful state and as a method of developing cardiovascular reserve and endurance are often not emphasized. The importance of *winning* in competitive long

distance swimming, bike riding, track, and tennis is stressed but not the physiologic benefits. Young people should be encouraged to develop an exercise program that they can actively participate in for the remainder of their life and it should become a routine part of one's daily activities just like brushing one's teeth. The person who continues to exercise throughout adult life usually has selected an activity that can be continued and truly understands the importance of exercise as an essential component to a healthy existence.

PHYSIOLOGICAL CHANGES WITH AGE

It has been demonstrated that working capacity does decrease with age; however, with exercise a well-trained 65-year-old can have a greater physical work capacity than an untrained 35-year-old. One's physical capacity does not have to be determined by chronologic age, and most of the loss of physical capacity that the older adult experiences is a result of disuse rather than the age of the individual. Chronologic age should not be used as the yardstick of one's potential to achieve physical fitness.

Maximum heart rate lessens with age and cardiac output decreases about 1% per year. Muscular endurance will decrease with aging but less dramatically than the cardiovascular parameters. Respiratory rate and efficiency also decrease markedly. It should also be noted that 3% to 5% of active body tissue is lost per decade. It is reassuring, however, that the studies done by de Vries[7] show that older adults who are involved in an exercise program demonstrate marked improvement in aerobic capacity, muscular fitness, and flexibility. It appears that the problem of aging is more closely associated with loss of functional capacity than structural tissue alterations.

PHYSICAL FITNESS AND ITS RELATIONSHIP TO THE AGING PROCESS

The importance of exercise in retarding the aging process has been known for many years. Hans Kraus[11] noted that the physically inactive individual shows signs of aging earlier in life, exists physiologically at a lower level of potential, and is less well equipped to meet the daily stresses of life. The diseases that can result from lack of activity include myocardial infarctions,[12] hypertension, obesity,[9] musculoskeletal pain, headache,[2] and nervous tension.[13] Disorders from disuse or hypokinetic problems do result from lack of exercise. The more time an older person spends sitting in the chair, the more difficult it will become to get out of that chair, and therefore the more time he will spend in a chair.

Aesclepeades (124-56 BC) is called the father of geriatrics because of his interest in studying and treating chronic disease in the elderly.[10] He noted that nature can do harm as well as good and recommended that his patients be prudent in their diet, bathe regularly, and take massage and exercise. He stressed the importance of exercise for all older adults including both the sick and the well. He recommended what he called transportation therapy, whereby an ill person would be carried in a transportation device for the benefit of the swinging and vibration of the movement. Cicero also recommended walking and composed many of his speeches while walking and dictating to his secretaries.

Walking can be one of the best conditioning exercises for the older adult. A brisk walk for at least 30 minutes can have a conditioning effect. Cooper[4] in his well-known books on aerobics has outlined an extensive program based on walking. de Vries,[8] an authority on the physiology of exercise, noted that the older person is definitely trainable and the percentage of improvement is similar to that of the young.

Along with the physiologic benefits of exercise are important psychologic benefits. In a double-blind study, exercise had a greater tranquilizing effect than meprobamate. It was noted that a 15-minute walk at a moderate rate would raise the heart rate to 100 per minute and provided a tranquilizing effect for up to 1 hour.[6] Additional studies consistently report that patients feel better about themselves with exercise and note a lesser degree of depression, a common element in the aging process.

NURSES AND EXERCISE

Most older adults are not informed regarding the benefits that exercise can have on their lives. Nurses have an opportunity to put into practice some of the preventive health practices so important to their geriatric patients. During the assessment phase the nurse can easily incorporate an evaluation of activity. This will provide valuable information regarding the patient's functional capabilities and abilities to carry out activities of daily living. It is also important to ascertain whether patients have altered their life-style in any way because they are physically unable to do a particular activity, for example, the elderly woman who is becoming socially isolated because she is unable to walk the two blocks necessary to visit her closest friend. Another question to ask is whether the older adult engages in any form of regular exercise, such as swimming, brisk walking, tennis, bicycle riding, or jogging.

It is also important to inquire how the patients spend their day. From the response the nurse will be able to determine whether the individual is basically sedentary, moderately active, or very active. *Sedentary activities* would include reading, playing cards, or watching television. *Light activities* would include activities such as preparing meals, dusting, walking slowly, or activities that require some movement of the upper extremities. Making beds, light carpentry work and gardening would be classified as *moderate activity*. *Vigorous activity* would involve scrubbing floors and walking briskly, and finally playing singles tennis, jogging, and riding a bicycle would be considered *strenuous activities*.

Before older adults begin an exercise program they should have a complete physical examination, which should include a stress test. Physical fitness has been defined as the general capacity of an individual to adapt and respond favorably to physical effort.[1] Obviously a person's degree of physical fitness depends on the individual's state of health, personal constitution, and present and previous activity. The importance of the individual's activity history as well as medical history becomes obvious.

A person who works from early morning until bedtime is less in need of an extensive exercise program than the person who is basically sedentary. The nurse is in the ideal position to do case finding in this area.

The nurse also needs to know what facilities are available for exercise. One of the best resources available is the YMCA/YWCA or the YMHA/YWHA since many of these centers have special programs for the older adult. Senior citizens' clubs and church groups may also have exercise programs for the older adult. Dancing, which is very popular with senior citizen groups, provides good exercise as well as excellent socialization opportunities. If there are no programs available, the nurse should consider the possibility of beginning a group in the community. A local physician or a physical education person or both would be excellent team members in this endeavor. It is important to note that many simple exercises can be done alone or with a friend.

PRINCIPLES OF AN EXERCISE PROGRAM FOR AN OLDER ADULT

A basic exercise program usually consists of three parts: a warm up period, an aerobic period, and a cooling down period. The purpose of the warmup exercises is to put joints through their full range of motion and stretch the muscles. All muscles should be stretched slowly. It is better to stretch slowly and hold that position than to stretch while bouncing, which can result in tearing of tendon and ligament. The warm up period provides an increase in body temperature, more oxygen being delivered to the tissues, and a dilatation of the blood vessels with an overall increase in the metabolic rate. The warmup period should last about 10 minutes and should prepare the body for the more strenuous aerobic portion. The nurse should also remind patients never to hold their breath while performing exercises because this can result in the Valsalva-type response and cause increased strain on the cardiovascular system. The patient should also be reminded to exhale while performing any type of flexion exercise.

A person who has adequately warmed up is ready to begin the aerobic portion of the exercise regimen. Aerobic activities include jogging, swimming, bicycling, and walking. One of the most beneficial activities for the older adult is walking, which appears to be once again becoming a popular form of exercise. People like Edward Payson Weston who was one of the most famous pedestrians of the 1920s and lived to be 90 years of age truly have a message for the American people. At the age of 74 Weston was invited to dedicate a new athletic building in Minneapolis and decided to walk the 1,500 miles from New York, which he did in 60 days. He truly believed that walking was the best way to stay in condition and with this type of regular exercise a man could actually improve with age.

If the older adult has received medical clearance to begin an exercise program, there is no reason why this person should not begin a walking program immediately. It is important to remind patients that they should maintain good posture and pull in the stomach and buttocks when they walk. This is especially important if they have had a back problem. Walking for 30 to 60 minutes with a heart rate of 100 to 120 is enough to improve cardiovascular and respiratory function. A walking program for the older adult could be started in the house or apartment. This becomes an important consideration for those who are recovering from an illness or have been sedentary for a long time and may be fearful of leaving their home. The patient can select a route, which could be in the home, and walk that route as many times as possible without fatigue. Keeping a record of the number of times this is done will document gains and setbacks. This activity should be repeated three or four times each day; patients should rest if they experience fatigue. Walking to music can also be an incentive and make the exercise more enjoyable.

Activities such as walking, swimming, bicycling, and jogging are all excellent ways of increasing cardiorespiratory endurance. If the older adult has not been active in the past, walking and swimming are the best activities and will put less stress on joints. As the older adult begins this segment of the program, he or she can learn about monitoring heart rates. For a conditioning effect the heart rate should be maintained between 70% and 85% of one's maximum heart rate for at least 15 minutes three times per week. The maximal heart rate is that rate beyond which the heart cannot increase and when it is at its peak ability to provide maximum oxygenation of the blood. The maximal heart rate is approximately 220 minus the patient's age. In the beginning the person should engage in activities that increase the maximum heart rate to only 60%. If the older adult follows this type of regimen, peak physical condition can be reached within 3 to 6 months. Although a stress test can determine more exactly what the target heart rate should be for an individual, it is important to remember that these tests are usually performed in an air conditioned environment and therefore must be readjusted downward for very warm or very cold weather. Older adults especially must learn to listen to their bodies and should always be reminded not to push themselves beyond the point of fatigue.

To determine whether the aerobic portion of the exercise period has been adequate, the individual needs to be taught to count radial pulse for 10 seconds and then multiply that number by six. The heart rate is taken for this shorter period because once the exercise is stopped the heart rate will drop very rapidly. It is not advisable to teach patients to take a carotid pulse because they can stimulate the carotid body resulting in bradycardia or may push too hard on the carotid artery and reduce the blood flow to the brain.

The third segment of all exercise programs should be a cooldown period to return the body to the nonexercising state and allow the cardiac rate to return to normal. The heart rate should be below 120 for 5 minutes after stopping the exercise and 100 after 10 minutes. The cooldown period should be at least 5 to 10 minutes and possibly longer at the onset of exercise programs. During this period the blood that has been drawn into the muscles is allowed to return to the central circulation. If one stops exercising suddenly, the blood may pool in the extremities and the individual may feel faint. Slow walking is an excellent way to cool down after the aerobic segment of the exercise.

Patients should be informed that if at any time they feel dizzy, nauseated, have palpations or a pain in their chest, they should stop exercising and if these symptoms persist they should consult their physician. It should also be pointed out that symptoms from exercising can occur from 2 to 24 hours after the exercise period. Examples of delayed symptoms are prolonged fatigue up to 24 hours, or insomnia that was not present before starting the program. These symptoms will disappear with rest and reduction of the exercise regimen. Patients should also be reminded to wear proper shoes and loose fitting clothing when exercising. Because asymptomatic atherosclerosis increases in frequency and degree with age, the possibility of cerebral ischemia during strenuous exercise is a potential problem. If the basic principles of exercising are adhered to, elderly people should find increased enjoyment in their life as they increase their cardiovascular reserve and improve the flexibility and strength of their muscles.

In assisting older adults in becoming interested in exercise one must take into consideration their personal reaction to aging. When trying to individualize reasons to motivate patients toward fitness, one should know some background information about the person such as the type of life-style he leads, his interests, habits, and present physical condition; what his stated expectations are, and his personal goals if he changes his life-style toward one of increased activity. This information can be included very easily in an assessment.

Selected Techniques to Share with Elderly Clients

The older adult who may be recovering from an illness can still participate in a limited exercise program. Many of these simple exercises can be taught to the older patient before discharge from the hospital or on a followup home visit by the public health nurse. Many simple warmup exercises can be done while sitting in a chair. It is of course understood that the patient is not recovering from a condition in which these exercises would be contraindicated.

The following are some examples of simple exercises that can be done while sitting in a chair. The older adult can sit in a straightback chair, bring the knee up to the chest or as far as possible holding under the knee with both hands and then slowly stretching the leg out as straight as it will go. This activity should be repeated five times. Another exercise is to raise the left arm and left leg. This exercise can be repeated 10 times and then done with the right arm and leg. All upper extremity joints should be put through a complete range of motion and as much range as possible should be achieved with the lower extremity.

Elderly patients must also be better informed about how to use their bodies properly. They must be conscious of their posture and the importance of using correct body mechanics. As people get older they tend to be less active and as a result they experience increased weakness of the muscles that support the back and shoulders. This may lead to poor body posture and an increase in thoracic kyphosis. Change in posture can further effect poor expansion of the lungs, which can reduce respiratory function and influence the level of wellness. Also, as the older person becomes less active the weakness of the back and hip muscles increases, which in turn leads to increased difficulty in standing up or sitting down. It is this lack of understanding of proper body mechanics that results in an increased tendency of the older adult to fall while trying to sit in a chair or get into and out of a car.

A good support chair with arms and preferably a high seat should be used. The elderly individual should feel the back of the chair with the calves, be certain she is centered in the middle of the chair, bend the knees and the body at the same time, sticking the chin out and gradually lower himself into the chair with both hands holding the armrest. It is important for the patient to realize that getting up is more difficult than sitting down. The person should always be forward in the chair with his feet securely under him. It is important to bend the body forward and push with the hands when getting out of the chair. Elderly persons who practice this technique, should eventually be able to do it without using the hands. These same principles apply when trying to get into a car. It is important for the elderly person to have his backside as close to the car seat as possible with the feet firmly on the ground and then slowly lower himself into the car as he bends forward.

As adults become older they experience an increase in problems related to the back because of the reduction of strength in the muscles of the lower back and abdomen, an increased incidence of lumbosacral osteoarthritis, and osteoporosis. Many geriatric patients have back problems resulting from weakness in the muscles of the back and therefore need information specific to this area. It is also important to remind all older patients to bend the knees slightly when trying to do most standing exercises such as touching toes or knees, since this will take direct strain off the lower back region.

Specific exercises that the older adult can do increase the muscle strength and tone in the lumbosacral area. Strengthening these groups of muscles will also help to improve the patient's posture. Three simple effective exercises for the low back are the pelvic tilt, single and double knee raise, and the bent knee situp. This exercise program should be done every day for maximum benefit and twice a day for the first 3 months. If the patient experiences any discomfort while exercising, he should be advised to discontinue that particular exercise for several days.

The pelvic tilt is a simple exercise done while lying on the floor with the knees bent. First, the patient should squeeze the buttocks together tightly as if trying to hold a coin between them. While holding the buttocks together, the patient should pull in the abdomen. The lower back should now be flat against the floor. This position should be held for a slow count of five. This exercise should be repeated three times with a gradual increase to 20 repetitions. The pelvic tilt will strengthen the gluteal and abdominal muscles.

The second exercise is the single knee raise. This will stretch the soft tissues of the lower back. The patient should lie on the floor with knees bent. The buttock should be squeezed and the abdomen tightened. One knee is then raised over the chest. With both hands over the knee, the knee is pulled slowly toward the axilla. This is held for a count of five and repeated three times in the begining, progressing to 20 times. The same exercise is repeated with the other knee. Once this exercise can be done with relative ease, the patient can begin to do the double knee raise. The only difference is to hold the position for a count of 10 rather than five.

The third basic exercise is the partial to full situp. The patient lies on the back with both knees bent. Once again the buttocks are squeezed and the abdomen tightened. Head and neck are slowly raised then shoulders, as the patient extends hands to the knees. The low and middle back should be kept on the floor. This position is held for a count of five. It should be repeated three times, advancing to 10. If 10 repetitions can be done easily, before long the patient can advance to a full situp, which means that the nose comes close to touching the knees. The patient may never reach this point but that is not important. The partial situp is sufficient to increase strength in the abdominal area. If patients follow these simple exercises, their posture as well as their low back pain should improve dramatically.

THE SECOND FORTY YEARS CAN BE THE BEST

The responsibility for assisting the older population in making the second 40 years as healthy as possible rests with the health professionals. This can be done by sharing with the elderly person specific information regarding the benefits of exercise. The patient should be provided specific information regarding the type of exercise best suited.

Increased activity has been correlated with increased self image. The lowering of one's self image with aging is one of the major obstacles to overcome with the older adult. It is important to emphasize to the older adult the benefits of exercise as well as its role in socialization and recreation. Older patients should be aware of the fact that according to de Vries[5] the decline of efficiency experienced by aging can be inhibited by 25 years or more provided there is a systematic and lasting application of sensible physical training. The older adult needs to be reminded that unlike a machine the human body *needs* activity. It is important to understand the principle that *energy initiates more energy* and inactivity will not sustain the human body but lead to an earlier deterioration.

References
1. AMA Committee on Exercise and Physical Fitness: Is your patient fit? JAMA **201**:131-132, 1967.
2. Appleton, L.: Study on fitness or performance of West Point cadets, New York, 1956, New York University Press.
3. Butler, R.: Why survive? Being old in America, New York, 1975, Harper & Row, p. 366.
4. Cooper, K.: The new aerobics, New York, 1970, Bantam.
5. de Vries, H.A.: Physiology of exercise for physical education and athletics, Dubuque, 1966, William C. Brown.
6. de Vries, H.A., and Adams, G.M.: Electromyographic comparison of single doses of exercise and meprobamate as to effects on muscular relaxation, Am. J. Phys. Med. **51**:130-141, 1972.
7. de Vries, H.A.: Vigor regained, Englewood Cliffs, 1974, Prentice Hall.
8. de Vries, H.A.: Physiology of physical conditioning for the elderly. In Harris, R., and Frankel, L., editors: Guide to Fitness After 50, New York, 1977, Plenum Press, p. 49.

9. Johnson, M.L., Burke, B.S., and Mayer, J.: The prevalence and incidence of obesity in a cross-section of elementary and secondary school children, Am. J. Clin. Nutrition **41**:231-238, 1956.

10. Kamenitz, H.: History of exercises for the elderly. In Harris, R., and Frankel, L., editors: Guide to fitness after 50, New York, 1977, Plenum Press, p. 16.

11. Kraus, H.: Preservation of physical fitness. In Harris, R., and Frankel, L., editors: Guide to fitness after 50, New York, 1977, Plenum Press, p. 35.

12. Morris, J.N., and Crawford, M.D.: Coronary heart disease and physical activity of work: evidence of a national necropsy survey, Br. Med. J. **2**:1485-1496, 1958.

13. Sainsbury, and Gehson, J.G., J. Neurol. Neurosurg. Psychiatry **17**:216, 1954.

chapter 21

LONG-TERM CARE CONSIDERATIONS IN THE GERIATRIC ORTHOPAEDIC PATIENT

M. Joanna Mellor

The term "long-term care for the aging" has undergone a metamorphosis in meaning over the last few years. Long-term care once referred to institutional care provided over a period of time within the nursing home milieu, and it was thus defined in contrast to the short-term health care provided within the acute care setting of a hospital. As the aging population continues to grow in absolute and relative numbers, it has become apparent that nursing home care is limited to a small proportion of the aging population. Only 5% of those over 65 years of age live in an institutional setting. However, 80% of all those over 65 years of age suffer from at least one chronic health condition, and it is estimated that one third or 8 million persons require one or more forms of service support.[2] It is clear that the vast majority of the aged in need of health care services on a long-term basis reside in the community. Long-term care, therefore, has broadened its meaning to include all those services, both formal and informal, that are targeted at the well-being of the older population.

Brody[2] defines long-term care as those services "provided on a sustained basis in order to maintain (older persons) at their maximum levels of health and well being." The goals of these services are to "close the gap between actual and potential functioning" and to "meet residual dependencies (of the older person) in such a way as to promote independence and well-being." Thus long-term care today encompasses institutional services of the hospital, rehabilitation or nursing home settings, and services available within the community, such as adult day care, home care, and visiting nurse services. Furthermore, long-term care includes both the services available through the formal system of health services and those services provided by the informal system—the wide array of support and help given by family, friends, and neighbors. The General Accounting Office estimates that 80% of all home care required by frail elderly persons is provided by this informal system.[16]

As the age cohort of those over 65 years continues to grow, there will be an accompanying growth in demand for long-term care services. Medical advances mean that the older patient is not necessarily entering the health care system as one step in the inevitable process of dying but may realistically expect to receive care that will help to sustain him as a functioning adult during an additional 15 to 20 years of life. The prime indicators of an individual's need for assistance over a long period of time are levels of mobility and activity, both factors that distinguish the geriatric orthopaedic patient group.

Studies have shown that, in general, frail elderly persons and their families prefer to have the older person continue to live at home within the community rather than to be institutionalized. Even when the older person requires a great deal of "hands on" care, families will often opt for care at home and be willing to undergo extreme changes in life-style in order to accomodate the older person.[12] A second more pragmatic reason for long-term care in the community is the cost. As health costs continue to spiral upward, there is interest in cost containment, whether the financial burden is carried by the patient, the insurance company, or the government through Medicare and Medicaid. A variety of studies throughout the country are currently assessing the difference in total cost between institutional and community-based care.

On both humanitarian and financial grounds it seems expedient to promote care in the community and toward this end to utilize the array of services, both medical and social, formal and informal, that exist. The viability of this type of care is dependent on functional and creative coordination of services tailored to the individual patient's needs. The most effective methods of implementing and managing this coordination of services and providing individualized case management are still being sought. At present long-term care suffers from fragmentation, an overreliance on medical care, lack of continuity, limited access to supportive services, and frequently inappropriate nursing home placement. There is often too much care as well as too little. The overarching concern is to coordinate services to provide the needed amount of help in the most effective and practical way possible.

The medical and health care professions come in contact with the geriatric patient at a pivotal point in the individual's life and they hold a special responsibility for indicating the optimum plan of care. No matter who becomes responsible for establishing and maintaining a plan of care—social

worker, insurance company, or family member—effectiveness of the plan is dependent upon interdisciplinary collaboration and communication during every phase of the patient's care. Collaboration between disciplines is necessary for a holistic assessment of patient needs at the outset. Once this occurs, coordination and linkage of services are then essential to sustain the frail elderly person over a long period of time.

Hospitalization may be only one phase in the extended care of a patient, or it may mark the point at which the geriatric patient first enters the health care system. This is especially true of the otherwise healthy older person who suffers a fracture. In these circumstances if hospitalization occurs, it is occurring at a crisis point and marks the beginning of the patient-doctor involvement.

Ideally, planning for the long-term care of the geriatric patient will take place during this initial hospital stay. In theory a plan will be established, support services will be located and contracted, and all will be prepared to move smoothly into place at the exact moment at which the patient is discharged from the hospital. In reality this rarely occurs. Hospital social workers and discharge planners are generally overworked and have insufficient time to tailor services to the patient's individualized needs. Medical personnel and those responsible for a discharge plan may not have shared relevant information, not by intent but through omission. Frequently patients are discharged from hospitals to nursing homes or to the community, and a plan of care is initiated in stages by the patient and his family in response to one crisis after another.

Agencies providing information and referral services to the aged are very familiar with the panic call from an adult daughter:

Mrs. A. calls the agency in alarm. She reports that her mother has suffered a hip fracture and is in the hospital. When she visited the hospital today, her mother told her that she will be sent home tomorrow. Mrs. A. has no idea what to do since her mother cannot walk unaided and lives in a fourth floor walk-up apartment. Mrs. A. herself works and lives some distance from her mother. The mother could stay with Mrs. A. for a while but there is no one to keep her company and, besides, the mother maintains that she can manage and wants to return to her own home.

The daughter is facing the fraility of her mother for the first time. She is unaware of any service that might be available, she does not know where to seek help, and both she and her mother are confused and angry. Under these circumstances, the daughter's first recourse in obtaining help can be to the hospital social services department. If the older person has not been hospitalized, there is even more likelihood that there will be no opportunity or effort made by representatives of the formal system to assess needs and coordinate the necessary care.

Failure to plan is the general rule even though all parties recognize the dysfunctional aspects of this failure. An older person with health care needs is vulnerable. The absence or inefficiency of needed support services creates a climate that is detrimental to increased functioning and well-being and this can exacerbate the initial medical problem. Failure to plan effectively may be the result of overburdened, overworked health and service personnel or a haziness about who is responsible for the planning, but more often it is caused by lack of knowledge by the relevant actors as to what information is needed to effect a total plan of care. Understanding the various facets necessary for planning may encourage increased collaboration between patient, family, and hospital/medical personnel. This chapter will suggest some of the factors that should be considered when establishing a long-term care plan in order to meet the needs of the individual older patient as efficiently and cost effectively as possible. Much of what will be detailed is not limited to the older orthopaedic patient but is applicable to all geriatric patients, whether they enter the long-term care arena through an initial hospitalization or through a visit to a community clinic or physician's office.

Needs Assessment and Planning

A plan for long-term care can only be formulated after a thorough assessment of the patient within his setting. Blumenfield[1] suggests that "in any assessment, we are dealing with the characteristics of the person/family, the illness, the environment, the social system, the needs of the person/family, and the resources available." All these factors combined will affect the ability of the patient to function and will indicate the service needs. In the hospital setting it will be the responsibility of the social worker and/or discharge planner to perform the assessment. The worker will need to interact with other members of the hospital treatment team in order to gather the pertinent information.

Coulton[6] has proposed a conceptual framework in which to view the patient's needs. She speaks of a "person-environment fit," by which she means the correspondence or congruence between the individual and his environment. Ill health will create a lack of fit, and a lack of fit in itself can result in ill health. It is therefore desirable to seek means by which, after the trauma of hospitalization a "fit" can be attained between the patient and his environment. With this concept in mind, assessment can be made of various factors, and the findings will point to the needed resources and services that combined will form the optimum long-term care plan. Brody[3] states, "The major task to be accomplished is to blend or mix medical and social care to create living arrangements and to provide individualized, unfragmented coherent packages of services in accordance with the social and medical needs of each older person."

Each set of needs is integrated with others and services can be planned to meet several needs simultaneously. The home care worker who shops and cooks for the older person in his home will be meeting physical survival needs and may also be meeting the need for companionship and emotional support. However, for purposes of assessment it is helpful to distinguish several discrete areas of need and the existing resources available to meet them.

Functional abilities and the environment

The functional abilities of the patient are critical in planning care. The level of functioning, rather than the nature of the ill health itself, determines care needs. As Brody and Brody[4] emphasize, the level of functioning

affects every aspect of life: self-esteem, status, capacity for work and role fulfillment, income, living arrangements and overall life-style. The older person's functional capacity also has a direct impact on the family: the nature of relationships, the number of contacts, living arrangements, finances and even the mental and physical health of family members.

Is the patient capable of caring for himself? Can he take care of his personal needs? Can he walk? Can he shop, cook, and maintain his home environment? In order to assess these abilities the functional capabilities of the patient need to be measured and the patient's home surroundings will also have to be evaluated. An older person suffering from arthritis that makes walking difficult who lives in an apartment building with elevator service on a busy street with shops will be far less vulnerable than a patient who lives in a home in the suburbs with three steps leading up to the front door. After assessing the abilities of the patient to meet basic survival needs within his or her specific living situation, the areas in which help will be required become clear.

If the patient is to live in the community and is unable to meet some or all of the survival needs, persons able to fulfill these needs must be identified. If the patient is married or living with others, many of these daily survival needs may already be met by others. Even if the patient lives alone, family members may be available to help. The belief that the caregiving role of the family has been taken over by institutions and formal service programs and that older people are generally isolated and abandoned has been modified by a number of researchers over the past two decades.[13,15] Older persons may live alone but strong family ties are maintained. As mentioned earlier, it is estimated that the informal system of family, friends, and neighbors provides 80% of all home care for the elderly.[16]

The danger of ignoring the role of family members is equally offset by the danger that once a family member is identified, it will be assumed that the necessary care is available. This may not be true. A son and daughter-in-law may visit the patient regularly during evening visiting hours but be unavailable during the day because of employment or other caregiving commitments. The patient may be married but the spouse may be in ill health and ill equipped to shoulder the caring responsibilities. No one can mandate how much care family members can or should provide, as every situation will be unique. To overload the family by expecting too much is as dysfunctional as ignoring the family members altogether. Ideally the family members should meet with the hospital discharge planner to clarify what service needs they can supply.

In general, family members tend to assume an enormous burden in caring for frail elderly relatives out of a sense of love, commitment, and familial duty. The professional worker must be alert to factors that may combine to make the caregiving role a dysfunctional burden and be ready to suggest alternatives. Are there other caregiving commitments? Will the health of the caregiver suffer? Can several family members be encouraged to share the caregiving tasks? What community services are available?

Once the amount of care available from the family is known, additional service gaps may be met through the formal support services. The long-term care plan can include linkages to home care services, home health visitors, or adult day centers, depending upon the specific needs. The existence of such services is frequently unknown to the patient and family, who may suddenly be faced with negotiating an unfamiliar world of formal services and selecting appropriate care. Sharing of information by the health team—physician, nurse, therapist, and social worker—with the patient can help to ensure that the most appropriate type and amount of service is sought. The social worker and/or discharge planner then has the particular responsibility of aiding the patient and the family in negotiating the various agency systems and fashioning the optimum plan of care.

Mr. O. is a 74-year-old man suffering from arthritis. Mr. O. lives alone and his married daughter comes every evening to cook and clean. Mr. O. is practically immobile until his daily warm bath, after which he can move around a little with the aid of a walker and can carry out a daily exercise routine. The physician has recommended home care, and 4 hours of home care are provided every afternoon, during which time Mr. O. is assisted in bathing. Mr. O. dislikes this dependency and insists that he can manage alone. The social worker helps Mr. O. and his daughter to request home care for 2 hours only but during the early morning hours. This provides the necessary help with bathing, which frees Mr. O. to function on his own for the remainder of the day.

Other service supports that can be utilized in planning a total care plan are the semiformal services. These include Meals-on-Wheels, friendly visiting services, escort aides, and shopping or transportation help. The availability of such services varies from one community to another, and the patient and the family may be unaware of what exists in their neighborhood. Once again, it becomes the responsibility of the social worker and/or discharge planner to be familiar with the existence of such services and to aid the patient in securing those that are needed.

Long-term care for the geriatric patient in the community is likely to include all these facets of help—informal, semiformal, and formal. The task is to recognize what services are needed and what services are available and to weave the two together creatively.

Medical health needs

The provision of long-term care is tied to a medical model approach, since it is often the medical needs of the geriatric patient that alone factor in the decision as to whether the patient enters a nursing home or a rehabilitation center or receives visiting nurse services and home health care in the community. In the attempt to emphasize the importance of assessing other areas of interest when planning long-term care, the medical needs must not be minimized. Health professionals must continue to take the leadership role in determining the amount and level of medical and nursing care needed. The point to be emphasized is that a choice between nursing home placement or home care in the community is not solely dependent upon the assessment of medical needs. Many levels of care can be provided in the home setting as well as in the nursing home.

The geriatric patient in the community will require ongoing medical attention that may necessitate visits to the doctor and/or the therapist. This generally entails some difficulty, especially if the patient is immobile. Frequent loss of work time is reported by family members who take time from their jobs to transport and escort a frail older relative to medical appointments. Until transportation becomes readily accessible to this population on an universal basis, such situations will continue to persist. The medical team can ease the problem by scheduling tests and clinic and office visits on the same day, thus avoiding the need for a family caregiver to lose several days of work each month.

The geriatric orthopaedic patient may be involved in a daily exercise routine or the use of equipment, such as canes, walkers, or braces. The proper use of such equipment and an understanding of the prescribed exercises and medication, including potential side effects, are necessary for the patient and the family. Clear explanations are required. The social worker often has a mediating role between the physician and the patient. The physician is an authority figure and the aura that surrounds him or her frequently prevents a patient from asking questions. A social worker is not accorded the same respect as the physician, but this is advantageous since it allows the patient to confide concerns. A frequently heard explanation is "I didn't want to bother the doctor, who is so busy." It becomes the task of the social worker to encourage the patient to ask the correct questions and to seek explanations.

Patients and their families are also often unclear about the appropriate level of physical activity allowed the patient. This is especially true if the older person has suffered a sudden loss of physical functioning through accident or surgery. After discharge from hospital, the patient may hesitate to resume activities or family members may contribute to a slow recovery by being willing to "do" for the patient and by being overeager to compensate for the patient's loss of capacity. It is generally home care workers or social workers who have the opportunity to view this interaction in the home setting, but they lack the physician's medical expertise and are thus not able to evaluate whether a geriatric patient is doing too much or too little. Once again, interdisciplinary collaboration is essential so that information can be shared and utilized for the overall benefit of the patient.

Psychosocial considerations

The psychosocial needs of the geriatric patient tend to be overlooked when planning for care, even though the vital role such needs play in the rehabilitation and overall functioning of the patient is well recognized.

For the orthopaedic patient, hospitalization may be the point of entry into the medical health system. Records are initiated and impressions are formed that may be used in any future deliberations concerning treatment. Since this is the case, it is particularly important that hospital personnel, including physicians, nurses, therapists, and social workers, recognize that hospitalization marks a sudden loss in the patient's physical and social functioning and that the patient's behavior is related to this crisis situation. Assessment of overall functioning must be sensitive to the patient's "change in fortune." Although the manner in which the patient handles the situation will reflect a past history of coping mechanisms, hospital personnel are first viewing the patient in the midst of a personal crisis situation. Family and friends are invaluable

at this juncture in identifying "normal" behavior of the patient, thereby aiding in a realistic appraisal.

The experience of hospitalization encourages dependency and depersonalization. Blumenfield[1] theorizes that this effect may be even greater on the geriatric patient, who in all likelihood has already suffered "losses and assaults on his self-esteem." Hospitalization is viewed as one aspect of declining health, which leads inevitably to death. Erik Erickson[8] contends that old age has the developmental task of maintaining a "sense of integrity rather than a sense of despair." This developmental task should be a factor in the care plan for the period after the hospitalization. Opportunities should be sought to allow the geriatric patient to maintain some autonomy and control over his environment. This can take the form of including the patient, if possible, as the principal actor in the planning process for his care.

The geriatric patient in the nursing home or in the community who is receiving home care services also suffers from loss of control. It is the need for autonomy, coupled with anger and fear over one's own frailty and lost capacities, that often results in "awkward" patients.

Mrs. C. is severely incapacitated and is confined to her home where she is cared for by her adult daughters and a home health aide. One daughter, employed full time, lives with Mrs. C. She wakes Mrs. C. in the morning and feeds her breakfast before leaving for work. The home health aide arrives soon after and helps Mrs. C. to bathe, dress, and get up for the day. The daughter experiences a great deal of anxiety because Mrs. C. does not seem to be able to keep any one home health aide for any length of time. Mrs. C. complains constantly and every few weeks fires the aide or the aide herself refuses to continue working, stating that Mrs. C. is demanding, rude, and irritable. This pattern has continued for a year. Friends of the family view Mrs. C. as a charming, if strong-willed, lady and concur in a belief that the home health care agency is poorly staffed.

In this situation, if the community plan of care is to be maintained, some attention must be paid to Mrs. C's self-destructive behavior. Understanding on the part of the aide and the daughter of the reasons for this difficult behavior will ease the tension, and ways can be sought to give Mrs. C. control in areas of her life over which she can exercise some authority. This may be as simple as enabling her to make up the weekly shopping list, to plan meals, or to determine if and when the television will be switched on.

In addition to this loss of autonomy, the geriatric patient may experience loss of socialization opportunities. Each individual will vary as to how much companionship is sought or needed. In some cases, nursing home placement might be desirable because it can provide companionship that may be lacking in the home environment. In other cases, socialization needs can be met through a friendly visiting service or participation in an adult day center.

Economic considerations

Having considered the physical, medical, and psychosocial aspects of care, a detailed plan of care can be tailored to the individual. The efficacy of this is generally heavily dependent upon financial resources and this area cannot be overlooked. It is especially critical when dealing with geriatric patients since members of this age group are facing increasing medical costs at a point in their lives when they are experiencing a decrease in income as a result of retirement or loss of employment. A recent study of why residents of one Veterans Administration domiciliary chose not to live in the community determined that "fear of lack of money" was the major factor.[9]

Federal programs covered under Medicaid provisions tend to favor institutionalization. Though some home health care is available through Medicaid, it requires a great deal more paperwork and recertification processes. After hospitalization it is frequently simpler to opt for nursing home placement. Economic considerations with a bias towards nursing homes will have to be removed if patients and their families are to have the freedom to choose the optimum plan of long-term care. A number of demonstration projects are currently being administered throughout the country to test the belief that community home care can be less costly than institutional care. If this hypothesis is proven, it is hoped that the findings will result in altered regulations that will encourage rather than mitigate against long-term care in the community setting.

Those aiding the patient and family in planning must explore the financial needs. Older persons and their families are often unaware of what services are available under Medicaid regulations. Perhaps the hardest hit financially are those whose annual income sets them just above the Medicaid eligibility levels but whose income is insufficient to meet the service costs. These persons are often those who have worked and saved all their adult lives in order to be self-sufficient. Now, in their nonproductive years they find that they are penalized for having saved a little against retirement and that they cannot afford to continue living independently. Health service personnel must be aware of the possibility of financial strain and the fear this engenders.

ASSESSMENT PROCESS

Information from these major areas will provide the guidelines for the most appropriate plan of care. Assessments of functional abilities, the physical environment, medical care needs, psychosocial functioning, and financial considerations are all vital in forming an overall picture. The hospital setting provides an opportunity for all relevant actors in the assessment process to share information. That this rarely occurs is due to time constraints and often a lack of clarity concerning who is responsible for coordinating the overall assessment and formulating a plan of care. When the medical personnel and social worker are in contact, this often occurs just before discharge of the patient, which allows little time to coordinate support services and contributes to the pressure surrounding discharge planning.

Ideally, initial assessment of the case should take place as soon as possible after hospitalization occurs. Pertinent information about the patient needs to be shared. Stewart claims,[14] "Assessment of the need for continued care postdischarge is subjective and somewhat random." However, although no general standardized form is yet in use, there are assessment indicator forms covering the major areas that have been highlighted here. It is the responsibility of the discharge coordinator (nurse or social worker) to coordinate information and fill out these assessment forms. In order to do this, the orthopaedist must necessarily be contacted for input on the functional ability and medical care needs of the patient. The sharing of this information may be accomplished informally but the hospital setting does allow for more structure and formal discussions and/or team meetings, including all relevant personnel, can be the means for gathering information and establishing care plans. If such meetings are not part of the organizational fabric of the hospital, the orthopaedic surgeon holds a responsibility to the patient for contacting the discharge coordinator and setting in motion the assessment procedure.

If the geriatric patient is not hospitalized but is in need of long-term care, the possibility that careful coordinated planning will take place is even more unlikely. The patient and family, often those persons with the least knowledge of available resources and possible solutions, become the major planners. Crisis planning is the result. In such instances the orthopaedic surgeon has an even greater responsibility to the patient. If the patient, the family, and the physician concur that home care is the preferred care plan, links must be formed with an appropriate home health care agency and contact must be established with the staff person responsible for an assessment interview in the home. This may be a visiting nurse, social worker, or case manager. Of necessity this process will be more informal and requires greater initiative on the part of the orthopaedist, often involving frequent telephone contacts. The effort and time spent in this procedure will be well repaid by the advantages accruing from a plan of care tailored to the individual's needs.

MAINTAINING THE LONG-TERM CARE PLAN

Involvement by the formal service sector in the long-term care plan does not end with discharge from hospital. Events and happenings in any facet of the patient's life will affect the overall plan of care. Reassessment must be a continual activity. Community support services combined to form the total care plan are multidimensional and varied, but this very characteristic permits a flexibility that can be sensitive to changing circumstances.

The necessity of ongoing case management of long-term geriatric patients is acknowledged, and debate is taking place as to where in the system this responsibility should lie. Case management is probably best handled by the patient and the family if they possess the necessary information and knowledge to deal effectively with the formal system. Educational programs targeted at the family caregivers can provide the needed information and skills.

Informal caregiving is critical to the success of any community long-term care program. Any breakdown in the informal care giving structure will result in the collapse of the care plan. Paralleling the growing understanding of the role of the family and neighbors in caring for the frail elderly, there is a recognition of the enormous stress that informal caregivers experience in providing this care.[12] Horowitz[10] states, "It is clear that caregiving takes an extensive emotional toll on the caregiving relative who is attempting to cope. . . . The emotional strains emerge as the most pervasive and appear to be the most difficult for the caregiver to deal with." In addition, the very act of providing care allows little opportunity for the caregiver's own needs to be met. The financial and physical strains of providing care may be considerable, but these tend to be overshadowed by the fact that neither time nor emotional space exists for the caregiver to retain a sense of self-identity. "No time for oneself" and "living another's life" are some of the phrases used to express the deeply felt curtailment of the ability to be an individual in command of one's own life.[18] Caregivers identify the greatest need for themselves as a need for some form of respite from their caring responsibilities to enable them to continue coping. Currently there are few respite programs in effect, but those that do exist may offer respite in the home or take the form of temporary institutionalization for the geriatric patient. Respite may be for a few hours, a week, or an occasional weekend to enable the caregiver to take a brief vacation. Without scientific control studies it is impossible to measure the real effect of such respite help, but caregivers frequently suggest, through such statements as "I don't know how I would have continued without you," that without this respite they would be unable to bear the burden of caregiving for any length of time. When the long-term care plan for the patient involves substantial caregiving by members of the patient's informal system, the effects on the caregivers must be acknowledged. The need for respite should be included in the overall plan of care. In effect, the caregivers, as well as the patient, must be viewed as the recipients of the long-term care services.

POLICY AND PLANNING ISSUES

The demand for long-term care is likely to increase dramatically in the next few decades as the aging population increases.

The preceding discussion concerning the development of individualized long-term care plans has presumed an ideal world in which all needed services are both accessible and available. In this best of all situations, the holistic assessment of a patient and the family results in the implementation of a care plan to meet all medical and social needs. Reality, not surprisingly, falls far short of this ideal.

Service programs identified as belonging to the arena of long-term care have been added incrementally to the existing service system, generally in response to a specific need. A national committee charged by the Federal Council on Aging to study the need for long-term care concluded:

Although many good things are accomplished by these programs, they never seriously address the central problems of long-term care. Every program and every funding resource relates to something else—a particular diagnosis, specific income, a special type of building assistance. Each of the programs is limited, restricted and focused primarily on some purpose other than the delivery of long-term care to the people who need it.[7]

This means that fragmentation, duplication, service gaps, and confusion reign. The federal programs that underlie the services have no provisions for assessing the older person's needs holistically. Each service program has its own eligibility requirements. To understand and fashion a comprehensive long-term care plan, the worker requires an understanding of the financial and administrative parameters of federal entitlements—Title XVIII (Medicare), Title XIX (Medicaid), and Title XX (Social Services) as well as knowledge of the regulations governing income maintenance, transportation, housing, and health programs.

The Medicaid program will shoulder the full cost of nursing home care if the patient is eligible, but even when the patient is impoverished, it will rarely finance the total array of services needed in the community setting. Thus nursing home institutionalization is favored even though there is a shortage of adequate nursing home beds and in spite of the fact that such care is not the preferred choice of most disabled elderly individuals.

Even if community-based services were to be publicly reimbursible, there is still an additional drawback to home health care, which is that the community-based services that now exist are insufficient. Before long-term care in the community can be a universal and viable alternative to institutionalization for functionally disabled patients, sweeping changes will have to be made in the emphasis and administration of health and social services. This necessity is recognized and efforts are being made on a national level, through the funding of long-term care demonstration projects, toward improved delivery and coordination of programs. Nevertheless, progress is slow.

The 1971 White House Conference on Aging recommended that long-term care be legislated and financed through a national health insurance plan. This would ensure availability and accessibility of services and establish the center of responsibility for the overall coordination of long-term care. Lowy[11] declares that "Rapid movement toward this objective is a sine qua non, if long-term care is to be a viable aspect of a coordinated, comprehensive and continuous system of health care." Over a decade after the conference the same problems still exist, while the older population and the demand for long-term care continue to grow.

Meanwhile the majority of long-term care services continue to be provided by the informal network of family and friends. No matter what public programs are initiated, the role of the informal caregiver will remain. A report of the Select Committee on Aging of the U.S. House of Representatives[17] stressed this role and spoke of the need to "empower available natural support systems (to enable them) to provide the bulk of such services at the local level." Education and skills training by the formal service sector and the provision of concrete services such as counseling, advocacy, and respite care are means that can be used to empower informal caregivers. The efficacy of providing family members with financial incentives or reimbursements for the care they provide is also being studied.[5] Findings indicate that family members provide care regardless of reimbursement and that while welcoming financial help they state a preference for service supports to fill service gaps that they are unable to provide for by themselves, either because they lack the skills or ability or because they have other commitments such as work or child care responsibilities.

Summary

The notion of long-term care and its accompanying issues characterizes the health care system of the older person more than any other age group. Although the social welfare needs of other age groups are part of the maintenance of their physical well being, it is the large number of chronically ill elderly patients with their burgeoning social and economic needs that highlights the necessity for a combined service approach. Medical health care and social service programs need to be interwoven for maximum effectiveness.

This stance invites little argument. Long-term care for the aged with its attendant philosophy of a holistic approach has become a fashionable concept. The continuing debate is concerned with the ways in which professional collaboration, coordination, and service delivery can be operationalized for the optimum results.

The task is herculean. The health care system is marked by inconsistencies and cumbersome regulations. However, an understanding of the various components involved in an older person's care needs can still lead to improved planning and implementation of a more appropriate long-term care plan. While policy planners, legislators, and program administrators move the system towards the functioning ideal, the practitioners—physicians, nurses, therapists, and social workers—at the cutting edge of service delivery can become more effective with an increased sensitivity to the factors that feature in the long-term care needs of each older patient.

References

1. Blumenfield, S.: The hospital center and aging: a challenge for the social worker. In Getzel, G. and Mellor, J., editors: Gerontological social work practice in long-term care, New York, 1983, Haworth Press.
2. Brody, E.: Long-term care of older people. A practical guide, New York, 1977, Human Sciences Press.
3. Brody, E.: Long-term care of the aged: promises and prospects, Health Social Work 4:25-59, Feb. 1979.
4. Brody, E., and Brody, S.: Proceedings of the Anglo-American conference on new patterns of medical and social supports for the aging. In Lewis, M.A., editor.: The aging: medical and social supports in the decade of the 80's, New York, 1980, Fordham University.
5. Community Council of Greater New York: Financial incentives for informal caregiving, Proceedings of a research utilization workshop, New York, Oct. 1981.

6. Coulton, C.: Person-environment fit, Social Work **26:**26-35, 1981.

7. Department of Health and Human Services: The need for long-term care, A chartbook of the Federal Council on the Aging. DHHS Publication No. (OHDS) 81-20704, Washington, D.C., 1981, U.S. Government Printing Office.

8. Erikson, E.: Childhood and society, New York, 1963, W.W. Norton Co., Inc.

9. Ewalt, P.L. and Honeyfield, R.M.: Needs of persons in long-term care, Social Work **26:**223-231, 1981.

10. Horowitz, A.: The role of families in providing long-term care to the frail and chronically ill elderly living in the community, Final report submitted to the Health Care Financing Administration, Department of Health and Human Services, May, 1982.

11. Lowy, L. and Helphand, M.: Matching community resources and patient needs. In Sherwood, S., editor: Long-term care. A handbook for researchers, planners and providers, Holliswood, N.Y., 1975, Spectrum Publications, Inc.

12. Mellor, J., and Getzel, G.: Stress and service needs of those who care for the aged. Paper presented at the thirty-third annual scientific meeting of the Gerontological Society of America, San Diego, Nov. 1980.

13. Shanas, E.: Family relationships of older people, Chicago, 1961, Health Information Foundation.

14. Stewart, J.E.: Home health care, St. Louis, 1979, The C.V. Mosby Co.

15. Sussman, M.B.: Relationships of adult children with their parents in the United States. In Shanas, E., and Streib, G., editors: Social structure and the family: generational relations, Englewood Cliffs, N.J., 1965, Prentice hall Inc.

16. U.S. General Accounting Office. Report to the Congress on the well-being of older people in Cleveland, Ohio, Washington, D.C., 1977, U.S. Government Printing Office.

17. U.S. House of Representatives: Future directions for aging policy, a human service model, Report of the subcommittee on human services of the U.S. House of Representatives Select Committee on Aging, May 1980.

18. Zimmer, A., and Mellor, J.: The role of the family in long-term home health care, Pride Institute J. Long Term Home Health Care **1**(2):20-25, Fall 1982.

Additional readings

Kane, R.L., and Kane, R.A.: Values and long-term care, Lexington, Mass., 1982, D.C. Heath Co.

Kauffman, A.: Social policy and long-term care of the aged, Social Work **25:**133-137, 1980.

Pegels, C.C.: Health care and the elderly, Rockville, Md., 1980, Aspen Systems Corp.

INDEX